CoL.

363.8013
MUR

D0510892

'THE NATION'S DIET'

The Social Science of Food Choice

edited by Anne Murcott

Longman
London and New York

Addison Wesley Longman Ltd
Edinburgh Gate
Harlow
Essex CM20 2JE
United Kingdom
and *Associated Companies throughout the world*

Published in the United States of America
by Addison Wesley Longman, New York

© Addison Wesley Longman Limited 1998

The right of Anne Murcott to be identified
as editor of this work has been asserted by
her in accordance with the copyright,
Designs and Patents Act 1988.

All rights reserved; no part of this publication may be
reproduced, stored in a retrieval system, or transmitted
in any form or by any means, electronic, mechanical,
photocopying, recording, or otherwise without either
the prior written permission of the Publishers or a
licence permitting restricted copying in the United
Kingdom issued by the Copyright Licensing Agency
Ltd, 90 Tottenham Court Road, London W1P 9HE.

First published 1998

ISBN 0 582 30285 4

British Library Cataloguing-in-Publication Data

A catalogue record for this book is available from the British Library

Library of Congress Cataloguing-in-Publication Data

The nation's diet: the social science of food choice/edited by Anne
    Murcott.
        p. cm
    Includes bibliographical references and index.
    ISBN 0-582-30285-4
    1. Diet–Social aspects–Great Britain. 2. Nutrition–Social
aspects– Great Britain. I. Murcott, Anne.
TX360.G7N37 1998
363.8'5'0941–dc21   98-11982
                                                                         CIP

Set by 57
Printed in Malaysia, PJB

Contents

List of figures

List of tables

The Editor

Anne Murcott, Director of the ESRC Research Programme 'The Nation's Diet, is MA in Social Anthropology and PhD in Sociology. She is the author of many articles in sociology on various aspects of health, and on diet and culture. She co-authored *The Sociology of Food: Eating, Diet and Culture* with Stephen Mennell and Anneke van Otterloo. From 1982 to 1987 she was the editor of *Sociology of Health & Illness* and from 1995 to 1997 a co-executive editor of *Appetite*. Having taught sociology, other social sciences and medical/health professional under- and postgraduates in the University of Wales (Cardiff) for more than 20 years, she now holds a research post as Professor of the Sociology of Health at South Bank University, London.

The contributors

Annie S. Anderson, School of Management and Consumer Studies, University of Dundee
Hannah Bradby, MRC Medical Sociology Unit, University of Glasgow
Robert G. Burgess, Centre for Educational Development, Appraisal & Research, University of Warwick
Michael Burton, CAFRE, School of Economic Studies, University of Manchester
Helen Bush, MRC Medical Sociology Unit, University of Glasgow
Pat Caplan, Institute of Commonwealth Studies, University of London
Mark Conner, Department of Psychology, University of Leeds
G. Jill Davies, Centre for Nutrition, South Bank University, London
Richard Dorsett, Policy Studies Institute, London
Alan Dowey, Department of Psychology, University of Wales, Bangor
John Eldridge, Department of Sociology, University of Glasgow
Ben Fine, Department of Economics, School of Oriental and African Studies, University of London
Andrew Flynn, Department of City and Regional Planning, University of Wales, Cardiff
Leslie Gofton, Department of Social Policy, University of Newcastle upon Tyne
Susan Gregory, Department of Sociology, University of Surrey
Malcolm Hamilton, Department of Sociology, University of Reading
Michelle Harrison, Department of City and Regional Planning, University of Wales, Cardiff
Michael Heasman, School of Oriental and African Studies, University of London
Spencer Henson, Department of Agricultural Economics & Management, University of Reading
Pauline Horne, Department of Psychology, University of Wales, Bangor
Rhiannon James, Consumer Sciences Department, Institute of Food Research, Reading Laboratory

Anne Keane, Department of Anthropology, Goldsmiths' College, University of london

Debbie Kemmer, Department of Sociology, University of Edinburgh

Mike Lean, Department of Human Nutrition, University of Glasgow

Diana Leat, Policy Studies Institute, London

Zara Lipsey, Department of Psychology, St George's Hospital Medical School, London

C. Fergus Lowe, Department of Psychology, University of Wales, Bangor

Sally Macintyre, MRC Medical Sociology Unit, University of Glasgow

Terry Marsden, Department of City and Regional Planning, University of Wales, Cardiff

David W Marshall, Department of Business Studies, University of Edinburgh

Lydia Martens, Department of Applied Social Science, University of Stirling

David W. Miller, Department of Film and Media Studies, University of Stirling

Marlene Morrison, Centre for Educational Development, Appraisal and Research, University of Warwick

Elizabeth Murphy, School of Social Studies, University of Nottingham

Georgina Oliver, Department of Epidemiology and Public Health, University College, London

Susan Parker, School of Social Studies, University of Nottingham

Christine Phipps, School of Social Studies, University of Nottingham

Tessa M. Pollard, Department of Anthropology, University òf Durham

Rachel Povey, Department of Psychology, University of Leeds

Jacquie Reilly, Department of Sociology, University of Glasgow

Richard Shepherd, Consumer Sciences Department, Institute of Food Research, Reading Laboratory

David Smith, Department of History, University of Aberdeen

Paul Sparks, Consumer Sciences Department, Institute of Food Research, Reading Laboratory

Andrew Steptoe, Department of Psychology, St George's Hospital Medical School, London

Ann Walker, Department of Food Science and Technology, University of Reading

Alan Warde, Department of Sociology, University of Lancaster

Jane Wardle, Department of Epidemiology and Public Health, University College, London

Anna Willetts, The Consumers' Association, London

Janice Williams, Department of Anthropology, Goldsmiths' College, University of London

Rory Williams, MRC Medical Sociology Unit, University of Glasgow

Judith Wright, School of Oriental and African Studies, University of London

Neil Wrigley, Department of Geography, University of Southampton

Trevor Young, CAFRE, School of Economic Studies, University of Manchester.

'The Nation's Diet' Research Programme Steering Committee

Dr Richard Munton (Committee Chair), Professor of Geography, University College London

Dr Robert Dingwall, Professor of Sociology, University of Nottingham

Dr Ronald Frankenberg, Emeritus Professor of Social Anthropology, University of Keele

Dr Alistair McGuire, Professor of Economics, City University, London

Dr Malcolm Anderson, Biological and Biotechnological Sciences Research Council

Dr E. Maureen S. Edmondson, Scientific Affairs Manager (Europe) Mars Confectionery

Dr David Lindsay, Ministry of Agriculture, Fisheries and Food (until 1996)

Dr Stephen Wearne, Ministry of Agriculture, Fisheries and Food (from 1997)

Dr Martin Wiseman, Professor of Health, Environment and Food, Department of Health

Acknowledgements

The first debt is to the UK Economic and Social Research Council (ESRC) for creating and funding 'The Nation's Diet' Research Programme. Both the editor and publishers are grateful to the ESRC for permission to use the Programme's name as the title for this book.

Among those whose contributions to the work of the Programme have been indispensable are members of the Programme's Steering Committee, especially its Chair, Professor Richard Munton; Pamela Janes, part-time secretary managing the Programme Director's office; colleagues, past and present, at ESRC's Swindon office; those who generously consented to assist the research projects in the collection of their data; and secretarial, computing, library and other technical staffs associated with each research project. Their work, commitment and advice over the Programme's six years is very gratefully acknowledged.

Sarah Caro, Social Science Editor of Longman, has been enthusiastic about this volume from the outset and patient ever since. Her advice has been invaluable.

CHAPTER 1

Food choice, the social sciences and 'The Nation's Diet' Research Programme

Anne Murcott

Introduction

This is a book about food choice in the 1990s.

It looks set to be a decade, so we tell ourselves, which has seen a veritable explosion of international public concern about food, a burgeoning of interest in diet and a growing fascination with eating. What may loosely be called the food economy appears more 'global' than ever, at the same time as North/South disparities in supply and accessibility threaten to worsen still further. Across the industrialised world people's interest in their own food has become intense. Cookbooks are reported to occupy a huge share of non-fiction sales. Elaborate television programmes on food are more numerous than ever; series that are game shows as well as cookery demonstrations, or travellers' tales of exotic ways of life as much as of unfamiliar cuisines. Full pages devoted to good eating and dining out are firmly established in broadsheet newspapers, never mind whole magazines in glossy full-colour.

People are not just more interested in what they eat: eating patterns and habits themselves are also held to be on the move – both cause and consequence. So-called 'ethnic' and theme restaurants and cafés have spread even to remoter regions. It is not just the cosmopolitanism of Mexican food in London, croissants in Sydney and English puddings that have crossed to Paris. Vegetarian and Indian cooking can be had in sparsely populated parts of Scotland; a Chinese takeaway is as likely, it seems, as the fish-and-chip shop in the heart of the South Wales valleys or the Yorkshire Dales.

Interest in other people's food is itself big international business: food and drink represent one of the largest UK exports (£8.2bn in 1993); exotic tropical fruits on sale in British stores now look quite ordinary. It is also competitive business. 'Cola wars', the siting of out-of-town supermarkets or genetically engineered tomatoes are among the more flamboyant current manifestations, strikingly representing the tip of the industrial iceberg. At the same time, from quite another quarter, interest in the whole population's eating habits has been integrated into public health policy and efforts to reduce heart diseases, the main cause of premature death in industrialised nations (Department of Health 1992). And the expression food scares has achieved a currency unimaginable a decade ago. Indeed, there is a strong impression that the mass media no longer need to add 'mad cow disease' in parentheses in items about bovine spongiform encephalopathy (BSE).

So, why do we eat what we do? Here is a key question for the 1990s, posed again and again in government departments, in sectors of the food industry, by professionals in health, in education and in catering, and many more. Here, perhaps, is a deceptively simple question. Here, certainly, is a question that is self-evidently open to social scientific investigation.

Coinciding with all this, the 1990s also look set to be the period in which, internationally, social scientists have at last begun to pay more sustained attention to food choice. Indeed, if the publication of textbooks, conference proceedings, new journals and research reviews is anything to go by, there are signs that their attention is becoming more firmly consolidated.[1]

In Britain, social scientists have been further enabled to attend to the topic by the Economic and Social Research Council (ESRC) which created a research programme on food choice – or, to give it its full title, ' "The Nation's Diet": the social science of food choice'. This book presents work from that Programme which adopted the key question posed above as its central theme. Indeed, it is *the* book of the Programme, hence sharing its name. As such, it has three main purposes.

First, it is designed to display the range of the Programme's research. As will be seen, one of the hallmarks of the Programme's research is variety – in the aspect of food choice studied, in the disciplines that are represented, as well as in the social group, geographic region or aspect of human affairs selected for special investigation. Setting out a selection of key research results, the book also provides an introduction to the constituent projects and sketches, where appropriate, the research designs, data collection and data-handling techniques they adopted. To these ends and for readers wishing to concentrate on just a few topics or on one discipline's approach, each chapter is written so that it may be read independently of the rest.

As well as offering a portrait of the Programme's work, this book has two other purposes. Both of these reflect the fact that, like all ESRC Programmes, 'The Nation's Diet' aims to exist as more than simply a checklist of projects. Each of these additional purposes derives from the two elements of the book's (and the Programme's) sub-title: 'the social science of food choice'. Being work on the *social science* of food choice allows the book to meet a second purpose. It aims to serve as a preliminary introduction to this group of sciences for readers who may have had little previous acquaintance with them. Almost six years' involvement with the Programme has taught that even as rudimentary a prelude to the social sciences as space allows here, anticipates questions born of unfamiliarity that are commonly asked about its work. This introductory aim is reflected in one of the bases for dividing the volume into parts, illuminating distinctive similarities and contrasts among the social sciences represented in the Programme. It is also integral to the whole book: the brief for each chapter in Parts One and Two requested that authors made plain their project's social scientific discipline's inheritance, indicating the inspiration in terms of theory, method and evidence on which they drew to set it up.

Being work in the social sciences on *food choice* serves as the occasion for examining what turn out to be quite varying interpretations and meanings in the way food choice is defined across the Programme. It was remarkable: all those working under its auspices were heir to the sub-title, yet they interpreted it in so many different ways. Was there anything in it? Did it matter? Or is 'food choice' merely a convenient expression, useful as a rough and ready designation of a general sphere of interest, and no more?

At times, it *is* to be no more than that. But the reader will not have to be particularly sharp eyed to detect one or two friendly differences of opinion lying below the surface of this volume, including varying degrees of enthusiasm for, and interest in, examining definitions of food choice. Indeed, Lowe[2] allows himself a moment of impatience; so forcefully is his attention riveted on what effects a change in the fruit or vegetables which children actually put in their mouths, that other considerations in conceptualising food choice, such as access to, or the supply of those fruits or vegetables, threaten an unwarranted distraction.

For some disciplines most of the time, and for all of us some of the time, reflecting on what anyone means by 'food choice' is liable to be reserved for another occasion. Bracketing the matter in this way presents no particular difficulties unless and until anyone proceeds on the assumption that the expression food choice is neutral, empty of connotations other than reference to a list of items between which selection is made.[3] Considering food choice in this fashion is, in important respects, the springboard for the whole volume.

In all, these three purposes combine to present as many disconti-nuities as commonalities between the chapters. But it is just such discontinuities that represent the state of the art whose nature is integral to the overall subject under discussion. If obliged to characterise 'The Nation's Diet' in a single word, then the word is 'diversity'.

Serving as both preface and introduction to the collection that follows, this opening chapter divides into three main sections. It starts with a description of the Programme itself, its origins, purpose and organisational character. Like all others supported by ESRC, the Programme consists of separate projects, in this case commissioned in two phases. Like all others too, it is multidisciplinary[4]: a theme pursued in the next section that turns to address the second of the book's purposes. Section two, then, consists of broad brush commentary on disciplinary differences and similarities in the social sciences and seeks to provide a reference point for this aspect of the Programme's diversity. Readers who already know about ESRC Programmes or who are familiar with the social sciences may well want to move straight to the third section of this chapter which concentrates on 'food choice' itself. Doing so springs from several puzzlements already hinted at above. How far is this ubiquitous expression tacitly treated as one that has achieved currency simply because of its brevity? Has it been adopted so readily as a convenient indication of a substantive held moderately stable while analysing other phenomena? Does the very expression 'food choice' and the manner in which it is used deserve analytic attention – i.e. as a topic of investigation rather than solely a resource for the investigator? The plan here is not to arrive at the answers, but to begin clearing the ground for future judgements about whether and in which directions to pursue the questions further. In order to do so, the intention is not to arbitrate between different definitions of food choice, but to expose, rather than leave concealed, the diversity that is a hallmark of the Programme's work.

The Programme's diversity is not solely evident in disciplinary terms. The chapters to follow consist of an equally diverse collection of substantive topics on which projects concentrated by way of addressing its question 'Why do people eat what they do?' Seeking to make its multiple diversities more manageable, the volume is divided into three parts. All three are prefaced by an editorial overview outlining the book's organisation, including a thumbnail sketch of the main features of each chapter. Chapters in Parts One and Two are based on research projects from both phases of the Programme and on one of the Programme's research fellowships. Much shorter, Part Three is made up of chapters that are amended versions of three reviews specially commissioned for the Programme when the second phase became imminent.

The reader will find that this introductory chapter repeatedly returns to the same point – the Programme's diversity – via different routes. And it will become apparent that in order to set the scene for the rest of the book, it is necessary, now and then, to stray some way from food choice. The second and third sections of this chapter have been written so that readers may consult them as free standing points of reference, after, or between, reading the chapters that follow.

In recognition of the extremely wide range of those interested in food choice, this volume has been prepared with a highly hetero-geneous readership in mind. As a result, this first chapter makes strenuous attempts to be non-technical and, along with the other contributions, has sought to make the diversity of the Programme's work accessible to a parallel diversity of expertise and experience, at the same time as aiming to steer a course that is neither mystifying or condescending. For the same reason, the book avoids being unduly burdened with footnotes and references. In any case, it can only be an introduction to the Programme and its constituent projects: each chapter presents only part of the study on which it is based. Readers wanting to pursue their more extensive write-ups are directed in the first instance to the consolidated list of references at the end of this volume and thereafter to the Programme's web page: http://www.sbu.ac.uk/~natdi.

Writing for so heterogeneous a readership brings with it a heightened awareness that selected chapters are concerned with analysing spheres in which, correspondingly, selected readers are highly expert. It is hoped that seeing their own specialty through social scientific eyes will be illuminating. Equally, it is anticipated that while some topics may thus be extremely well-known, other chapters will introduce thought-provoking coverage of hitherto altogether unfamiliar aspects of quite why people eat what they do.

'The Nation's Diet' Programme

In its own focus and internal organisation as well as in its broader academic, public and policy contexts, 'The Nation's Diet' has seen extensive evolution during its lifetime. The Programme was funded by the ESRC to run from 1992 to 1998. Its aims are to 'improve understanding of the processes of food choice' and to 'establish a clear and legitimate role for the social sciences in this field', aiming to remedy the comparatively low level of academic social scientific attention to the topic. At its core, it comprises 16 research projects and two research fellowships. Some of these are based on cross-institutional collaborations which means that more than 20 British universities are involved. By the end, well over 70 academic staff, one way or another, will have been associated with the work.

Partly by way of alerting the reader to what can be expected from this book, and partly because the word 'programme' (along with 'project' and even 'research') is so commonly used to mean widely differing tasks and working arrangements, some comment is needed on what an ESRC Research Programme is and is not. Above all, ESRC Programmes are geared to 'scientific and policy relevant topics of strategic and national importance'. It is to this extent that they represent 'directed' research. They do so, however, only in comparison with ESRC's 'responsive mode' funding, i.e. the competition for project grants on subjects chosen by academics themselves. Once a Programme's topic has been identified, however, the projects of which it is eventually composed are duly selected by the established system of scientific quality control, i.e. response to a call and peer review, where the more detailed version of the topic is worked up by the academics themselves. It is this set of procedures which in good measure creates a Programme's 'profile'.

Then, like all ESRC Programmes, 'The Nation's Diet' is multi-disciplinary (discussed further in the next section). And, like all

Programmes, it exists as a coordinated network of studies located in universities (or independent research institutes) across the country, led and supported by a part-time director and a steering committee. Though aligned with the aims of the Programme, each study is autonomous in that it is conceived, designed and carried out completely independently of the others. As a result, Programmes are not tightly regimented. Indeed, the Programme is probably best understood as a loose federation of projects with points of commonality that began to emerge only during the progress of their work and continued to evolve after they have concluded. So it is these institutional features, against a lively context of public and policy concerns, which have left their mark on the character of 'The Nation's Diet' and contributed to shaping the distinctive manner in which it is simultaneously selective and diverse.

Since a Programme's topic is originally determined in the light of policy as well as scientific timeliness, obviously the broader context also has a bearing on its inception. Equally obviously, much that has surrounded 'The Nation's Diet' is, and continues to be, highly dynamic. Over and above developments in the state of the art, there are two things in particular. Revisions to the UK national science policy is one. This underscored, but also required greater prominence of, selected features that were already built into the Programme, including attention to the public understanding of the social sciences. The other is the dramatic constellation of events associated with, and consequent on, mounting concern about the safety of the industrialised food supply, especially in Britain. These continue at sufficiently rapid a pace that report or commentary is almost bound to be out of date by the time it is published.

All three of these arenas of change are the subject of separate treatment (Murcott, forthcoming) – which is not, however, to disregard their importance as a backdrop to the chapters that follow. It would be facile to think that research conducted before some set of events took place, no matter how far-reaching they may be, was, as a result, less worthy of attention. Any effect of those events cannot be ignored and needs to be the subject of some suitably designed social scientific 'after' enquiry for which 'before' investigations are invaluable. Indeed, apart from constituting some of the evidence for future social and economic historians of 1990s Britain, the Programme's research retains its value, if anything, *enhanced* by the dramatic turn of events, in contributing to baseline studies against which later work can be compared.

One of the other distinguishing features of the Programme's research may contribute to its longer lasting utility. From the outset 'The Nation's Diet' was conceived as basic, rather than applied science, in keeping with the emphasis on its distinctive intellectual position.[5] For, as already indicated above, the original judgement was that a sustained contribution to the field from the social sciences was considerably overdue. It is a nice judgement, though. Far from disdaining any practical application, it is one that caters for an important, if less often expressed, view. This view holds that a solution of some problem is as well served, at times even better served, by investigation which concentrates on a social scientific characterisation of the phenomena in question, rather than the (quite properly partisan) version generated by those whose professional, practical, vocational or commercial interests keep them actively engaged in addressing what to them is a problem. Research that is non-aligned such that the various interests' opinion as to what is or is not a problem can be *included* as part of the field of study, may be poised to make as much contribution to the understanding of that problem as research which exclusively concentrates on it, or is expressly designed to find a solution. This often becomes more visible with hindsight as David Smith's selected exposition of some of the Programme's historical antecedents clearly illustrates in Chapter 19.

In any case, the designations pure/basic and applied need not be mutually exclusive; the distinction may be more a matter of emphasis. A project may have an obvious practical intent, with an immediate, workable application, yet still constitute basic research – Chapter 4 is an example. In all, though, remaining aware that the Programme consists of basic research should help place the following chapters in appropriate perspective.

Social sciences – and the question of multidisciplinary research

On the social sciences

It is very likely that there will be social scientists who would dissent from the previous section's view of basic and applied research. Equally, this section's selected observations on the nature of the social sciences may well fail to find agreement among colleagues. Properly this discussion requires expertise in, at least, the history and philosophy of the sciences: most ESRC programme directors are not polymaths, however desirable that might be. But there is a further reason why other social scientists may well disagree with the account of their field presented here. Even if it is agreed that, for instance, social anthropology and psychology, or sociology and economics are all social sciences, there are sufficient differences between the variants within each for it be highly unlikely for any one of their members to be sufficiently well versed in them all – at least to the satisfaction of their fellows in each discipline. This chapter's discussion of the matter is bound to be partial. For, despite the attempt to be even-handed, inevitably it is ignorant of critical areas and over-familiar with others. Undoubtedly, if 'The Nation's Diet' had had a director who was an economist or psychologist, rather than a hybrid social anthropologist/ sociologist, this discussion – and much else about the Programme – would look very different.

All of which is the first thing to say: the social sciences are not unitary. They exist firmly in the plural and consist of a plurality of intellectual and investigative perspectives. Whichever way they classify themselves, however, social scientists, some discontinuously more than others, are no different from natural and biomedical scientists or scholars in the humanities in as much as they early learn to live with a pre-eminence accorded to seemingly irresolvable argument, alternative standpoints, and the perpetually provisional nature of their enquiries. They are obliged to. They would not be particularly good at their research if they did not. They do not dwell on it all the time, and often, rightly, carry on working as if disagreements did not exist, suspending debate about alternatives in order to accomplish a particular task. But on occasion, and especially as members of a group such as an ESRC Programme that is explicitly designated 'multidisciplinary', they are acutely reminded of the fact – finding at times that no matter how cordial, so little is shared intellectually and professionally that talk is of something else altogether.

It is not solely that, in common with all scientific research, doubt or uncertainty are mainsprings to enquiry. There are good reasons, special to the social sciences, for their existence as collections of perspectives and provisional conclusions. These reasons are not to be treated as evidence, of the social sciences' immaturity, despite some (commonly non-social scientists') claims to the contrary along the lines of 'given time economics or sociology will grow up to be physics or chemistry'. Apart from a hint of mischief, such claims are also ignorant. The social sciences will *always* be different from other sciences, simply by virtue of their subject matter. Among other things, it means they can never proceed by strict replication.

In key respects, an experimental method tinkers with time; it puts the clock back to the first experiment or, rather, it stops the clock to create a place that is out of time, artificially suspending time's usual progress. Slavish conformity to this procedure is unavailable to the social sciences; it is, literally, impossible. Even in psychology where much non-animal work does proceed on an experimental basis, it is never going to be possible to remove from the human beings who consent to take part the (potential) awareness that they are indeed engaged in an experiment. Ultimately no one – not even, so the insights of much psychology teach us, the subjects themselves – has unimpeachable access to whether this awareness affects the outcome or not. Human beings have language and memory, capacities that provide for motivated originality; no one social circumstance is identical to another; no political configuration is ever reproduced exactly; no economic event is ever repeated precisely. In this sense, history is not just the past, it is also the present and future all in one; history is the passage of time.

The impossibility of replication and thus the irrelevance of a strict version of the experimental method (which, often as not, would also be unethical) is one of the reasons why a good many social scientists distance themselves methodologically from biomedical, physical or other (non-human) sciences. Correspondingly, some contrast themselves with 'scientists' *tout court* and refuse to name their (social scientific) work science. The persistent use of social *science* in this chapter is distinct, derived from a higher order. It depends on an older, broader meaning of science as knowledge – knowledge of a certain type that is always to be preferred above ignorance, guesswork, mere opinion and blind prejudice. Its use is intended to signal an insistence that any science integrally entails (aiming for) some mode of self-conscious devotion to theorising, i.e. rigorous, intentional analytic thought – in which, at times, some of the social sciences are closely allied to philosophy. Where they are distinguished from philosophy, however, is in the commitment to investigating what the world is *actually* like – an empirical focus, a requirement for evidence or some reality no matter how hard to pin down or define – which demands attention to methodology (in its original sense of the science and philosophy of method) and to research design and techniques of data collection, handling and analysis. It is in these last that the various disciplines included in the Programme are most particularly faced with the differences between them.

On multidisciplinary research in the social sciences

As the previous section indicated, the Programme, like all those funded by ESRC, is multidisciplinary. The particular collection of disciplines represented in it has been shaped by organisational as well as intellectual considerations. Those included are economics, human geography, psychology, social administration, social anthropology, sociology, as well as education studies, marketing (as a branch of business studies) and media studies – with the addition in a handful of projects of some collaboration with food science or nutrition science. Disciplines or subjects that are absent from the list of projects include social and economic history, political science and policy analysis, social studies of science, cultural studies and sociolegal studies. All could and should contribute to the investigation of human food choice. Correspondingly important substantive areas are not represented, for instance political scientific analysis of lobbies and pressure groups; contemporary historians' examination of the socioeconomic effects of competing nutritional claims of 'orthodox' and 'alternative' sciences; the reshaping of culinary cultures; the role and public consequences of chemical sciences in the social development of the food industrial sector. These and many more continue to be under researched by social scientists.

There is a strong impression, however, that across academic communities at large, as well, perhaps as beyond them, a devotion to multidisciplinarity is held to be a virtue over and above any even-handed catering for all types of university based research, or some concern for the equitable distribution of funds. If so, and if it becomes more than the rhetoric of diplomacy, there is an unfortunate possible side-effect. It risks creating wholly unrealistic expectations. It can foster an optimism that funding projects in a selection of disciplines under a single organisational rubric will, by itself, make for something more than it is – an assortment of disciplines. Such hopefulness is liable to founder and it is liable to do so ultimately because of the plurality of the social sciences.

The idea that, of itself, 'some' rather than 'one' guarantees superiority should be easily resisted. But it is harder to withstand an argument that since human food choice is so obviously multifaceted, its adequate study needs a multiplicity of disciplines. The Programme's original specification certainly looked in this direction. Concentrating on 'an examination of (human) food choice' would, it was held, permit 'complementary research from different academic perspectives' to be brought together. These perspectives 'resolve(d) into distinct social science areas which together reflect the many complex influences bearing on individuals . . . and determine their food choice and eating behaviour'.

The main thrust of the multidisciplinary research was to centre on four interrelated areas:

- the formation and impact on food choice of individual attitudes, beliefs and knowledge
- cultural definitions and the symbolic use of food
- social processes and food choice
- micro-economic influences on food choice.

A cynic running an eye down this list could easily tick off, in order, psychology, social anthropology, sociology and economics. But though there was indeed some appeal to the multifaceted nature of the topic's requiring provision for a multidisciplinary investigative approach, it remained programmatic. And in the event, more tightly specified aims for the Programme's multidisciplinary aspect were never developed. Despite enthusiastic claims made on its behalf (Fine, Heasman and Wright 1996: 3) the Programme had never been intended to create a new field of study or invent a new discipline such as 'food studies', nor was it meant to found an interdisciplinary social science of food choice; and it was certainly never set up to provide some synthesised *inter-disciplinary explanation* of food choice.

There was no special reason why it should have been. Multi-disciplinarity is one thing, interdisciplinarity, arguably, quite another. As proposed elsewhere (Murcott 1995) the latter can be considered to be a particular instance of the former, i.e. interdisciplinary research implies integration or synthesis, where multidisciplinary work need imply no more than a collection, group or assortment. In these terms, interdisciplinarity conveys something about the relation between the component disciplines, while multidisciplinary remains silent on the matter.

When introduced a little earlier, the disciplines represented in the Programme were carefully and even-handedly listed in alphabetical order. Rearranging them brings economics and psychology together (along with certain schools of sociology) as social sciences which rely on axioms, require operational definitions and entail measurement. On the whole, the theories on which these disciplines are founded revolve around the individual (even if the individual is not always the unit of analysis). Economists' theorising about human nature is familiarly based on an assumption of 'rational man' (and, presumably, woman); psychologists' attention to human nature commonly centres on assessing the relative contribution to human behaviour and response of the biological and genetic inheritance on the one hand, and nurture, learning, upbringing on the other. Each of these two disciplines' emphasis tends to be quantitative. By and large, economics is a social science highly likely to engage in secondary analysis i.e. to make extensive use of extant sources such as official statistics and data sets produced for routine monitoring or accounting purposes other than research. In general, psychology is the only social science to adopt experimental research designs· on any scale. The specialism 'experimental psychology' is long established: a specialism called 'experimental economics' or 'experimental political science' simply sounds impossible, absurd.

Of the remainder, social anthropology, certain strands of sociology and selected traditions in human geography, stand at an opposite pole (placing social policy, education, media studies, and marketing more as subjects rather than disciplines). Here the unit of analysis is unlikely to be the individual – rational or irrational. It is more likely to be phenomena that, in some fashion, exist between individuals; phenomena that shape the social positions they occupy and the social organisation of the relationships between them; phenomena that are supra-individual, such as power, its concentration and exercise, or social structures that shape opportunity and 'life-chances'. Specific examples of the unit of analysis range widely. For instance, one type may be social groups – the household as a food-sharing group, or friendship groupings at a slimmers' club. Another related type concerns social processes, for example, regularities of all manner of social relationships, from those between dietitians and their patients, to those among groups of colleagues be they environmental health officers (EHOs) or catering officers and their staffs. Different again is 'culture' – a phenomenon whose definition, whose very character even, is heavily contested by some social anthropologists and sociologists (see Chapter 16), but which analysts seem unable to dispense with, and which, if anything, albeit narrowed to refer to something like 'ethos', appears to be achieving widespread, non-technical currency. Though such supra-individual phenomena are the objects of study, their investigation still has to proceed via the actions, the behaviour of individuals and the reports they can provide.

Accordingly, this second grouping of disciplines inclines more heavily to the use of qualitative research techniques and the adoption of open-ended investigative strategies and flexible research designs. It is, though, a great, and regrettably common, mistake to draw rigid demarcation lines between quantitative and qualitative techniques and designs of research. The design and techniques adopted must bear a suitably thoughtful relation to the research question being investigated – and they may often enough mean either switching between types or

11

adopting a version of each in the same project. In any case, at a certain level, qualitative work is bound to be prior to all quantitative study: a phenomenon that has not been identified is not measurable. Equally, even the most qualitative of work in social anthropology, political science or social history is highly liable to entail a modicum of interest in frequency, size or amount.

Disciplinary difference in the Programme

This book duly displays the disciplinary diversity of the social sciences at large, of which 'The Nation's Diet' represents a selection. To convey something of the bases on which some disciplines are more and less like others in the terms just sketched, the volume is divided into parts. The chapters based on funded Programme projects are found in the first two. Grouped in Part One are those that tend to proceed from axioms, develop operational definitions and devise measurements. This includes contributions from psychology and economics. Part Two comprises chapters which come out of projects concentrating on sociopolitical processes and often quite fine-grained cultural variability. Contributions included are from social anthropology and selected approaches in sociology.

This division can only be rough and ready; disciplines (rightly) do not stand still, defying once and for all classification. Chapter 8, for instance, could equally be placed in Part Two in so far as the project on which it is based also adopted a qualitative data-collection technique as a precursor to their social survey in order to elicit meanings attributed to phenomena.

Part Three is short, consisting of just three chapters, all of which are revised versions of reviews commissioned by the Programme's Steering Committee. This was partly in recognition of gaps in the Programme's disciplinary and substantive coverage and partly to expand its reach in understanding this still underdeveloped field of study in the social sciences. Two disciplines/subjects are thereby 'added' to the Programme: a specialised branch of social policy and social history.

Though disciplinary diversity – contrast but also commonality – among the social sciences has to be a theme of this volume, it is left largely understated save for the considerations sketched in this chapter. So it remains for the interested reader to notice detailed differences in literary style and vocabulary (for the case of psychology, see Madigan, Johnson and Linton 1995) or differences in the type of data collected and in the mode of analysing them. The reader may also wish to reflect on the differences of emphasis conveyed by one or other term used to describe those who help provide researchers' data. Thus, many psychologists tend to refer to 'subjects', which social anthropologists would almost certainly never do. Instead they use 'informants' (Spradley 1979) or join sociologists in the use of 'respondents'. Economists are liable not to need such a term at all.

Equally, readers will realise that economists and psychologists are unlikely to need to refer by name to those who, giving informed consent, took part in the research, whereas some sociologists and social anthropologists quite commonly do. Where needed, confidentiality is preserved and anonymity assured by withholding identifying characteristics inessential to the analysis and by the use of pseudonyms for both places and people – as in all the chapters to follow. And the reader might also wish to keep an eye on the different usages of the word 'consumption'. The word is ordinarily used by economists to mean 'purchase', simultaneously conveying analytic potential in its contrasting consumption with production. Used by psychologists, however, it is no more than a formal way of saying 'eat'.

Noting detailed variation in style and mode of presentation favoured by the difference social sciences is one way of gaining the most out of the distinctive contribution made by each discipline. Putting a multiplicity of disciplines together is no guarantee of anything more than the simplest listing of the parts; it does not, of itself, add them together in any integrative sense. Amalgamating several disciplinary approaches in some seamless fashion is going to demand something far more. Intellectual mergers are not self-evidently on the horizon. If there is, though, some aspiration to transcend disciplinary differences and produce some as yet unim-agined novel synthesis, then requiring disciplines to rub shoulders is probably necessary as a beginning, even if of itself it cannot achieve that end. For there are certain differences between disci-plines which militate against much in the way of evolution from multi- to interdisciplinarity. Whether the aim is to transcend multi-disciplinarity and achieve interdisciplinarity or not, a corollary of pluralism among the social sciences is that aligning their *modus operandi* will not happen without some deliberate changes, some purposeful abandonment of certain principles and practices in favour of others – much like a set of takeovers.

Pursuing such a thought – and examining the politics and economics of the associated turf wars – has to lie well beyond present purposes. The moral of the tale for the moment, however, resides in appreciating, if not the detail, at least the fact, of the nature and extent of potentially mutually contradictory modes of procedure among the social sciences. As a result, care can more readily be taken to avoid dismissing work in one discipline that does not in all particulars proceed by the criteria for adequacy appropriate to another. If nothing else open-mindedness (as distinct, from empty-headedness) is afforded a worthwhile start, turning now to 'food choice' the central topic of the whole Programme.

'Food Choice'

Much has been made so far of contrast and disciplinary diversity in the work covered by this book. As much needs to be made of what might be shared, or any perspectives that are similar.

Perspectives in common across the Programme

One primary point of agreement among the Programme's constituent projects would seem to be so fundamental that it tends to be left tacit. This is the observation that 'food is not just something to eat' – an obvious remark that is not to be mistaken for a conclusion but adopted as a starting point. Each discipline can present an elaboration of this observation. A version might go something like this:

> Eating does more than keep the human organism going (or fail to do it sufficiently or optimally). Food brings the natural and the social (in its generic sense, i.e. to include the economic, psychological, cultural, etc.) into focus. Eating serves as one means of describing the manner in which human beings are simultaneously biological organisms and social beings. It is virtually impossible for people to live without sociality and remain describable as human (feral children, hermits, the lunatic are defining instances, respectively unsocialised, apart and disengaged physically or mentally and thus considered 'odd'). Without food at all an individual does not survive. Here and there failure to survive from want of food may be counted a personal tragedy, may be sanctioned as a means of achieving some culturally defined preference (e.g. infanticide as a locally accepted means of rearing males rather than females) or may be culturally favoured as humane (e.g. refraining from feeding the hopelessly congenitally disabled or the injured who are reduced to what is tellingly described as a 'vegetable'). If individual failures to survive for lack of food grow to a sufficient scale, the whole fabric of a society is affected. Food means more than biological survival; it also means psychological and cultural survival, and is some of the stuff of social and economic relationships.

Observing that food is not merely something to eat is not to deny that it is *also* something to eat, i.e. is fuel essential to the biological organism. On the contrary, the fact that it is simultaneously biological fuel – and the fact that both food and human beings are organic and perishable (Fine, Heasman and Wright 1996) – is ever present in the various social scientific viewpoints. Which fashion it may be represents and reflects the core of which ever social science is in question, If, for instance, scarcity is the core of economics, then scarcity – and its obverse, plenty or surplus – of food is liable to be the core of an economic approach to food, given its biological necessity.

The observation that food is not only something to eat is very closely related to another: 'all that is nutritious and non-toxic is not food'. This is the second observation that is the subject of mostly tacit agreement across the Programme. Any number of writings and commentaries testify to the monumentally familiar set of facts that, first of all, human beings do not eat indiscriminately. Second, the manner in which they discriminate is not simply and observably a matter of idiosyncratic individual variation, any more than, third, it is either uniform across the human species, or historically unchanging. A purely biological explanation is, then, most unlikely to suffice.

This is the line of reasoning that provides for the contribution of the various social sciences to investigating the non-biological bases for human discrimination in eating: reasoning that, in turn, gives rise to the question on which the Programme's work centres: 'Why do we eat what we do?'

All projects addressed this question. Similarly, all projects are heir to the Programme's other identifying paraphernalia, including the expression 'food choice' of its sub-title. This, as indicated in the opening section of this chapter, prompts further questions. Does 'food choice' have an agreed meaning? If not, does that signify anything? Maybe it is merely an administrative convenience, or nothing more than a shorthand born of expediency.

Various approaches to 'food choice'

Since posing the Programme's central research question resulted in the design of so intriguingly varied a set of projects, it was possible that an equally varying set of interpretations of 'food choice' implicitly underlay them. Initially projects tended to remain silent on the matter. But even if the different studies were not going to be able to move beyond the simplest version (the loose federation of projects) of multidisciplinary work within the lifetime of the Programme, exposing points of convergence and divergence might just lay the foundations for some future assessment of the likelihood of development towards something more integrated. Making explicit any differences in the interpretation of 'food choice' offered one way of starting. And it is at this point, unsurprisingly, that divergences between the disciplines do indeed re-emerge – at least as they are represented among those working under the aegis of 'The Nation's Diet'. In turning to introduce some of these divergences, it is essential to emphasise, incidentally, that the intention is not to adjudicate between interpretations of 'food choice' but, among other things, to illuminate differences – thereby serving as an additional device for portraying what makes the various social sciences distinctive.

Six definitions of 'choice' (omitting the two listed as obsolete) are given in the *Oxford English Dictionary*. Between them they represent several nuances which foreshadow if not contrasts, then certainly firm variations in emphasis that become apparent when comparing the chapters to follow:

1 the act of choosing; preferential determination between things proposed; selection, election
2 the power, right or faculty of choosing; option
3 that which is specially chosen or to be chosen on account of its excellence; the preferable part of anything, the 'pick'
4 abundance and variety to choose from; scope or field for choice

5 the person or thing chosen or selected
6 an alternative – used both in the exact and loose sense of that word, i.e. of the terms between which one may choose, or a term which may be chosen.

While not wanting to suggest that these half-dozen definitions exhaust, or wholly aptly characterise the matter, they provide a convenient point of initial reference for indicating how different chapters in Parts One and Two tackle 'food choice'. It allows, for instance, note that none of the chapters explicitly refer to the third definition, although Warde's and Martens' Chapter 8 on eating out brushes close. The reader will realise that, once again, it is a matter of chance rather than intention that the Programme includes no study of the relevance of good taste to the question 'Why do people eat what they do?' (but see Mennell 1985).

At the opposite extreme, checking against the *Oxford English Dictionary*'s list of definitions allows noting that, one way and another, all the chapters' use of 'food choice' embraces definitions (5) and (6). For the most part this usage is left unstated; referring to a broad, background state of affairs that, it can be assumed, is readily recognisable for anyone familiar with industrialised living. 'Food choice' acknowledges that foods are the things being selected and implies some sort of recurrence of alternatives. The chapters also have in common an assumption, admittedly at a high level of generality, that they are interested in what leads to food choice, i.e. the things selected. But they do so in such divergent and potentially conflicting ways that the initial shared assumption gets overshadowed.

So far, so unexceptionable. Potentially instructive differences begin to show up by realising that virtually all the chapters in this volume stray across more than one of the *OED*'s definitions. If there is an obvious exception it is Lowe, Dowey and Horne's (Chapter 4). Theirs is the only one explicitly aligned solely with definitions (5) and (6), firmly concentrating attention quite literally on the thing that is chosen. For Lowe, Dowey and Horne, the key investigative task is to identify and establish the causal factors that effect a change in the foods which are eaten – to this extent, 'food choice' becomes an outcome measure that is integral to the study design.

It is important, however, not to place too much weight on this aspect of differences in usage. Lowe, Dowey and Horne happen to exclude determining factors from their interpretation of food choice, whereas Steptoe *et al.* (Chapter 2) allow the inclusion of both 'attitudes to different types of food and patterns of purchasing' as well as the selection that is actually eaten. Similarly, Conner *et al.* (Chapter 3) include in their definition elements of human behaviour, notably the act of selecting, cognition ('e.g. the mental processes of decision-making') the food that is eaten *and* interrelations between all three. To this extent, both Conner *et al.* and Steptoe *et al.*'s interpretations echo aspects of the *OED*'s first definition. Only further discussion (beyond even what has been feasible in a coordinated Programme) would establish whether these variations have analytic or other implications over and above describing differences between specialisms in psychology. All the same, it needs to be remembered that exposing this type of (sub-) disciplinary difference is part of the rationale for the present discussion.

Psychologists' interpretations of food choice take the availability of an array of foods as given (although, at times, especially experimentally, they may well seek to manipulate the availability). The existence of 'the economy' is assumed. Economists' interpretations, on the other hand, build on a certain type of psychology. Proceeding on an axiomatic basis, these assume a psychology that has people perennially seeking the maximum benefit to themselves in selecting, out of a certain range of options, what they most want to eat. As Young, Burton and Dorsett point out in Chapter 5, this concept of 'rational man/woman' lies at the heart of the orthodox economist's approach to consumer choice, whether it be of food or anything else – an approach, they note, which operates within very confined limits. Where psychologists are interested in what affects – or, more stringently, causes – food selection, economists' interest tends to be narrowed to those factors, notably a limited budget which constrain selection. Once financial constraints are identified, the extent to which they operate can be compared with other types of constraint.

That, at the least, is what lies at the heart of an orthodox economics. Fine, Heasman and Wright, however, propose a break with its conventions (Chapter 6). They advance the idea that understanding consumer choice is to start with the things, the foods, being chosen, but then go on to examine not only the patterning of their consumption (roughly, the demand side) but also the systems of their provision (the supply side). In this fashion, the tie between consumption of a food (or groups of foods) and the way in which its (their) provision is organised, is not simply preserved but included in the analysis. At the same time, the consumption provision tie (what Fine, Heasman and Wright call the systems of provision) for foods, be they dairy products or sugar, meats or fruits, are seen as separated from one another. This makes comparisons between systems possible. Fine, Heasman and Wright's interpretation might thus be said to lock three *OED* definitions together: the thing chosen, the selections made and the scope/field from which to choose (respectively definitions 5, 4 and 1).

Two other chapters (9 and 7), by Flynn, Harrison and Marsden, and by Wrigley respectively, deal with the supply side. Each primarily representing recent developments in human geography, their interpretations of 'food choice' centrally encompass both the things chosen and the abundance and variety made available. In the process Wrigley offers a timely reminder not to confuse numbers of different brands of the same product with the availability of variety. Flynn and Wrigley's interpretations do not, however, solely turn on the array on offer. Their usage of 'food choice' also allows for the examination of social and political forces that, along with the economic, *create* the scope for shoppers' selections. By implication, they also cater for the act of choosing. Indeed, what Wrigley sketches in passing, Flynn attends to centrally. Among other things, his interpretation of 'food choice' makes a link between preferential determination and study of the consumers' rights in the expression of those preferential determinations – an element of *OED* definition (2) joined with that of definition (1). In this, Flynn's discussion is marked off somewhat from the other chapters considered so far, and aligns his usage of 'food choice' more closely with some of the others in Parts One and Two.

Interpretations of 'food choice' among these remaining chapters hover close to versions of *OED* (2) – power, the faculty, as well as the right of choosing. This is not to say that chapters already discussed in this section fail to consider these angles on the ability to select: as already noted, for instance, economists prominently concern themselves with financial constraints. Rather it is to point out that, as work in disciplines such as social anthropology and sociology, the remaining chapters in Part Two allow for analysing social processes along with aspects of culture that go toward fashioning the ability and capacity to select. Indeed, Murphy, Parker and Phipps (Chapter 15) are clear that interpretations of 'food choice' need to encompass not only *OED* (1) but also (2) and that neither is straightforward, either as a concept or as social phenomena associated with what ends up going into someone's mouth.

Common to these approaches is the concern plainly stated by Caplan *et al.* (Chapter 10). Their chapter interprets 'food choice' as a phenomenon that is not just a question of individual preference but of shared values, judgements and tastes which, however, loosely reflect everyone's various identities in terms of their ethnicity, age, gender and so on. Burgess and Morrison (Chapter 13) develop this view that examining 'food choice' needs to include the social and cultural context. Why people eat what they do reflects the degree to which they enjoy autonomy, the extent to which power and control over selections may independently be exerted. In turn this is linked to systematic practices of social inclusion and exclusion.

Interpreting 'food choice' to entail the collective and shared rather than individual expression of preference lies at the heart of Henson *et al.*'s Chapter 11 which regards the selection of foods as a shared, collective decision in the household. In parallel, Kemmer, Anderson and Marshall (Chapter 12) aim to reveal the negotiation, the give and take, liable to be operating between a young couple newly making a home together. For them, 'food choice' not only refers to what is selected but how that selection comes to be made. For Macintyre *et al.* (Chapter 14), many of the interpretations of 'food choice' already summarised are accounted for in their approach to the expression. Their concern, though, is not to focus only on the foods that people plump for when making their selection, but also to consider the opposite. For them, 'food choice' is to include the collective bases for people's (sudden, concerted) rejection of some foods, the omission of items from their selection.

In certain fundamental respects, Warde and Martens' Chapter 8 and also Williams *et al.*'s Chapter 16 interpretation of 'food choice' stand at a completely opposite pole to Lowe, Dowey and Horne's. Their interpretation resolutely fastens on to 'food choice' as the outcome of a great many factors determining what people select. By contrast, Warde and Martens rehearse what might be described as a very particular form of the *OED* definition (2) which completely rules out the power, right or faculty to choose. This is the sociological position which, in effect, denies the existence of choice. It does so in as much as it enshrines a preoccupation with analysing social forces and institutional arrangements that militate against anyone's being able to act utterly irrespective of other considerations. Among those other considerations, as both Warde and Martens, and Williams *et al.* note, are the social mechanisms that give people their identity, shaping them as members of social groups that share culturally inherited outlooks and ways of behaving.

Different types of society, however, at different periods of history are liable to vary in the extent to which shared outlooks and cultural conventions governing ways of behaving are tightly prescribed or left much wider open. The modern idea of a 'consumer society' may well be a candidate for the latter: much is often made of consumption as allowing, encouraging even, just such fluidity in outlook and just such imaginative inventiveness of self-expression. In any case, various modern political rhetorics have 'consumer choice' as pivotal: Warde and Martens comment on the political philosophy prevailing in the 1980s which was dominated by 'an equation between private ownership, markets and freedom of choice'. As their discussion suggests, care is needed to sidestep the risk of exaggeration posed by political rhetoric. The extent to which choice is free deserves to be examined rather than assumed.

Williams *et al.*'s interpretation of 'food choice' closely parallels Warde and Martens'. Also concerned with the collective, rather than only the individual, for Williams *et al.* the matter centres on whether choice is either limited or created by cultural conventions running right through the social organisation of eating, whole cuisines and the economic systems in which they are set. Attending to patterns of migration involving contrasting cuisines, cultures and their related types of economy, provides their chapter a comparative basis for revealing variations in the degree to which cultural prescriptions for outlooks and behaviours tighten or relax.

'Food choice': some implications of various definitions

All in all, the chapters that make up Parts One and Two of this volume offer an expanded appreciation of the expression 'food choice' in defining it over and above a minimum of 'the foods selected'. Certainly the minimum allows continuing to concentrate on interpreting it to refer to the act of choosing which results from the workings of individuals' psychological make-up; certainly the minimum allows examining the manner in which this is further subject to constraints external to the individual (notably financial) in being able to select from the extensive array of foodstuffs and products now on sale nationwide. Certainly that minimum does not rule out the effects on the foods selected of highly idiosyncratic variation between people – especially as an expanded appreciation of 'food choice' points to the extent to which inventiveness might have become culturally permitted, or even, dare it be said, promoted.

What the expanded range of interpretations of 'food choice' contained in this book also permits is recognising the evidence of counter-intuitive instances, which by the same token provides for understanding them. Take the case of people who suffer no particular physical or mental incapacity or infirmity, whose daily lives are not marked by circumstances out of the ordinary, who are not alerted by some source or another that there might be a difficulty with some item in the food supply, and whose diet is reasonably well aligned with current dietary guidelines. On the face of it, we are liable to discount the likelihood of such people fairly regularly both eating foods they do not much like and not getting to eat foods they prefer. But Williams *et al.* among others point to just such a sociocultural constraint on the satisfaction of preferences. This type of constraint is associated with selected social conventions of the food-sharing domestic group such that women are to cook according to others' preferences rather than their own. So doing is to be understood as part of a (marital) relationship of exchange – serving cooked food 'to order' in return for the raw materials deemed provided by men.

Warde and Martens' chapter reports parallel social constraints on 'food choice'. Those in their study very often claimed to have no say in the decisions whether or where to eat out. Possibly, this is even more striking an instance, since it might be assumed that eating out offers even fewer practical restraints on the satisfaction of preferences than does eating at home or at another's house. Warde and Martens' work suggests that here, too, the social complexities of decision-making, the negotiations among couples or the give and take between friends differentially affects the 'say' people have in what they actually get to eat, limiting the 'freedom' to choose.

In sum, this swift tour round different chapters' interpretation of food choice does more than illustrate the various topics covered by the Programme and goes beyond portraying disciplinary differences and similarities. First, it begins to specify the expanded reach for substantive enquiry. Second, it suggests that the expression food choice does indeed carry connotations over and above administrative convenience and a useful shorthand. It is probably no longer possible to confine the expression 'food choice' to some technical, neutral usage. It carries too many overtones. As a result, it can mould analytic thinking. Its abbreviated use may well mean that lines of enquiry may be closed off unintentionally, unnoticed, by default. If lines of enquiry are to be limited, it is self-evidently important to ensure doing so is deliberate. Its elaborated use, i.e. one that specifies what is and is not meant, may not simply sidestep unwanted overtones, but underscores the extended diversity for substantive investigation this discussion suggests.

Closing comment

This introductory chapter has sought to alert the reader to the breadth, variety and contrast in the work of 'The Nation's Diet' Programme, by providing a guide to the diversity which is its signature. It is that very breadth and diversity, however, which ensures that a single conclusion, ready answers or simple summaries are hard to come by. This is so not just for 'The Nation's Diet', but wherever evidenced reasons for human activities and practices are sought: the Programme reflects the state of the art.

Yet despite its variety, two important themes run right through the whole collection of studies presented in this volume. The first of these confirms that so many of the social, cultural, economic or psychological forces affecting human eating habits in industrialised societies, can have relatively little to do with hunger, nutrition and health, or even the food itself. The point may be obvious, especially once stated. But it deserves constant reiteration and requires regular research confirmation. This way, at the very least, it will support those whose craft, profession, or commercial interest leads them to focus on food, on nutrition and health, on eating itself, who must strive to bear in mind that not everyone shares their preoccupations.

The other theme of the chapters to follow returns to the original question which provided the springboard for 'The Nation's Diet' Programme. Although inclined to be left implicit, this second theme needs to be emphasised. For it endorses the initial suspicion that asking 'Why do people eat what they do?' is deceptively simple. Among other things, identifying new lines of enquiry testifies to the complexity of the answers. The Programme's work is, quite properly, open-ended. Its results combine to produce a unique portrait of 'The Nations' Diet'. Its distinctive federation of studies brings together a thought-provoking range of research techniques and theoretical analyses that invite more attention. In this fashion, the Programme duly represents a first, not a last, word on the social sciences of food choice offering a broad set of shoulders on which future researchers are urged to stand.

Acknowledgements

I am pleased to have this unusually comprehensive opportunity of thanking the award holders and their research staff for their energetic collaboration during more than six astonishingly busy years of 'The Nation's Diet'. Without it this book, and much more besides, could not have even been mooted. Elizabeth Murphy and Teresa Rees remain endlessly generous in making time for conversation and I am especially grateful to them both.

Notes

1   For textbooks, see for instance: in psychology, Booth 1994; in sociology, McIntosh 1996, Whit 1995, from the US and Bearsdworth and Keil 1997 in Britain. For examples of conference proceedings: sociology in the Nordic countries, Prättälä *et al.* 1991; social history in the UK, Smith 1997a. Examples of research reviews include pan-European history, Teuteberg 1992; in sociology, Mennell, Murcott and van Otterloo 1992; and for journals, the *Journal of the Association for the Study of Food and Society*, largely sociology, was inaugurated in 1996, complementing *Appetite*, founded in the 1970s to carry work in psychology and *Food and Foodways*, founded a decade afterwards to include the humanities as well as social history, social anthropology and sociology.

2   Details of each project's staffing is provided on the web page whose address is given on page 5.

3   Even that might pose problems. On occasion it does matter whether the items are reckoned in terms of nutrients, food groups, ingedients, commercially marketed products, dishes or even whole cuisines, e.g. the 'Mediterranean Diet' – as those who recollect the furore following the publication of a COMA report (Department of Health 1994) will recognise.

4   Thus bringing staff trained in different social science disciplines into research contact with one another – some, including those at senior level, for the first time in their careers.

5   ESRC provides the following definitions:

Basic research is original investigation undertaken to gain new knowledge and understanding but not necessarily directed towards any practical aim or application. *Pure basic* research aims to advance knowledge but has no orientation towards practical application. *Oriented basic* research aims to produce a broad base of knowledge which has some orientation towards practical applications which may have economic or social benefits. Applied research is original investigation undertaken to gain new knowledge and with practical aims or objectives. *Applied strategic* research should aim towards practical applications which are likely and feasible but cannot yet be specified in detail. *Applied specific* research has a clearly-defined, feasible application.

Part One

Social Science and Food Choice Proceeding from Axioms, Operational Definitions and Measurements

Overview to Part One

Grouped in this section is work from those projects in disciplines which, broadly speaking, rely on axioms and/or proceed by developing operational definitions and devising measures. Included here are chapters from psychology, economics, a sub-field each of human geography and of sociology. The section opens with three chapters in psychology. Although all three are concerned with understanding factors affecting dietary change in individuals, each concentrates on quite different angles, using completely different research designs.

In Chapter 2, Andrew Steptoe, his research team and their collaborators concentrate on changes that occur naturally, in the ordinary course of events. Studying the relationship between stress and food intake, they followed two groups over periods during which heavy and light workloads could be dated in advance – peak periods of examinations for university students and the sales or Christmas period for employees in department stores. They discuss the rationale for this type of research design and for adopting a suite of measures to assess not just food intake and perceived stress but also psychological well-being, smoking and other behaviours. Changes in food intake were registered, but the associations with stress were neither the same in each group nor straightforward. In anticipation of exams it was the students with greater measured anxiety and low levels of social support – vulnerable sub-groups – who tended to eat more in total as well as to eat foods yielding higher fat intakes. Among the shopworkers, however, changes in food intake were recorded across all those in the study, not simply among the more vulnerable.

Steptoe's concern with dietary change might be described as closely allied with the newly burgeoning field of health psychology. Mark Conner and his colleagues, on the other hand, approach dietary change as social psychologists. In Chapter 3 they provide a broader introduction to the sub-specialty against which to detail the commonly cited 'theory of planned behaviour' (TPB) and variants. Recent attention in the field has been turned toward improving the predictive power of

TPB, and their own interest revolves around the only too familiar human ability to hold positive and negative beliefs simultaneously: what Connor and colleagues call attitudinal ambivalence. They review measures of ambivalence that may be adopted, going on to confirm that at least some facets of eating do indeed generate, in some people, considerable levels of reported ambivalence, especially in respect of eating a low fat diet. They are obliged to admit, though, that models such as TPB incline to oversimplify. More refined models introduce the idea that there are different stages between initial intentions to change and finally succeeding in changing. And yet further complexities have to be proposed. People not only think about the business of changing their behaviour differently at successive stages, but the kinds of information and interventions needed to effect change also varies depending on the stage reached. Illustrating their chapter with reference to a number of separate studies they conclude that extending the understanding of dietary change may well be achieved by integrating established, more static, models with both stage models and, even, analysis of other health-related behaviours.

Fergus Lowe's concern with dietary change is unequivocally applied to reducing the burden of disease, by helping people adopt a healthier pattern of eating, preferably from childhood onwards. As experimental psychologists, he and his research group briskly point out that certain investigative modes of procedure are insufficient. Their Chapter 4 begins by stressing that it is no good relying solely on what people report about their preferences and attitudes to food; what they say has to be related to what they actually do. Similarly, it is not enough to study associations between responses to attitude measure and measures of dietary intake; correlation does not establish cause. It is necessary, they say, to identify the reasons responsible for changes in what people eat before it will be possible to achieve the required alterations in the general population's dietary habits.

Although the rationale for their work is applied, the research – in line with the Programme's character – is basic psychology. This is made clear when they turn to set out their theoretical background emphasising the assumption that eating is learned not innate behaviour, and thus amenable to alteration. Successfully achieving changes in what young children eat, they detail some of the factors affecting the variability to which these changes are subject. Able to continue their work after funding under 'The Nation's Diet' ended, they have gone on to confirm that the results presented in this volume look very promising.

With much in common by way of the underlying philosophy of their social sciences, a noteworthy practical contrast between psychology and economics is none the less evident in turning to the next two chapters. Studies in economics reported in both Chapters 5 and 6 are not based on specially collected evidence, but on the analysis of existing data-sets. As Trevor Young and his collaborators (Chapter 5) describe, this can then require a series of operational decisions reconciling the manner in which economic theory is based on the rational decision-making individual and the available data's being collected at household level. Drawing on the *National Food Survey* (described in MAFF 1991) they address 'a fundamental shift in consumer attitudes' seemingly faced by the meat industry; there is evidence that increasing numbers of people in the UK are deciding not to eat meat at all. In effect, their study of almost 20 years of data is able to confirm that reductions in meat purchase are associated with socioeconomic factors over and above the price.

Designed to last just 18 months, Young and colleagues' project was the shortest in the Programme (with just one research staff). Chapter 6 is based on a two year study, the most common project length in the Programme. Ben Fine and his two full-time colleagues, designed a more extensive study in economics which also drew on *National Food Survey* data, from four separate years during the 1980s. Their work departs from the more usual analysis that averages quantities of a food are purchased weekly by each household. Their approach aims to distinguish whether foods are or are not purchased (a matter to which Young and his colleagues are also sensitive) and to take account of whether purchases are distributed unevenly over time, i.e. 'bulk' purchasing. Combining the study of these data with other indicators of the food systems of provision, Fine's team illustrates the economic complexities that, for instance, underlie the simultaneous rise in the purchase of items such as low fat milks/yoghurts and the sales of butter-fat incorporated into newly marketed products.

Arising from his one-year, single-handed Programme fellowship, Neil Wrigley's Chapter 7 picks up on the supply of foods, focusing especially on the distributive aspects. His work derives from a branch of human geography that pays close attention to the economics of retailing location – a market refers literally to a place to go to buy and sell, but also to a set of complex politicoeconomic relationships regionally, if not potentially globally. Many of the dramatic changes in British food retailing in the 1990s will be more than familiar to most readers, even those whose specialist expertise does not lie in analyses of the food supply. Supermarkets' loyalty schemes rewarding regular customers or the readier availability of tropical fruits and out-of-season vegetables are but two manifestations that have rapidly become commonplace in the nation's weekly shopping trips. Wrigley demonstrates that several factors, including changed competitive conditions coinciding with more stringent land use planning regulation, have to be inspected in order to reveal the underlying forces that have not just reshaped the type and range of foods on sale, but contributed to Britain's internationally unique position in food retailing.

Rounding off Part One, Alan Warde and Lydia Martens (Chapter 8) move from their discussion of the sociological attitude to 'choice' that turns on constraint and on limits to freedom, to note some of the questions raised for attempts at understanding eating habits and to illustrate the manner in which constraints on choice may be operationalised for investigative purposes. Their chapter concludes by drawing on data from their project which, as far as is known, is the first sociological research on eating away from home. Eating out represents a strategic case for examining the balance between freedom and constraint in food selection. After all, eating out, as distinct from eating at home, is held to permit a greater degree of discretion in what, as well as where, to eat. Yet their study very clearly reveals circumstances and mechanisms that constrain individual discretion when eating out a good deal more than popular impressions would imply.

CHAPTER 2

The effects of life stress on food choice

Andrew Steptoe, Jane Wardle, Zara Lipsey,
Georgina Oliver, Tessa M. Pollard and G. Jill Davies

There are many different influences on food choice, a number of which are discussed in this book. There is a comparable diversity in the methodological approaches that can be taken to investigate the topic. This chapter outlines the background to our research into the effects of stress on food choice, and provides a rationale for the methods that were used. The data collected in this project are extensive, so they will not be presented in detail here. Rather, some findings will be outlined to give a sense of the associations between stress and food choice that we identified.

Since the relationship between stress and food intake in the general population (rather than patients with eating disorders) has not been extensively studied in the past, we decided that a broad approach would be appropriate, and that we would not restrict our studies to particular foods or macronutrients. We define food choice as the selection of foods made by individuals from the range of options available to them. In experimental settings the range is typically very limited, while in everyday life conditions more possibilities are available. Food choice in this framework may include attitudes to different types of food and patterns of purchasing as well as actual intake. However, since our interest is primarily in the potential effects of stress-induced choices on health and psychological well-being, food choice was measured in terms of food intake rather than other activities.

Why study stress?

The major objectives of this research project were to assess the impact of life stress on food choice under naturalistic conditions, and to identify the individual differences that might lead some people to modify their food choice in unhealthy ways when under stress. In comparison with some other social and cultural influences on food choice, the role of stress may seem rather obscure. However, there are several reasons why stress is potentially important. Perhaps the most important is the impact of eating on health, and the development of disorders with major socioeconomic consequences such as coronary heart disease, high blood pressure, diabetes mellitus and various types of cancer. There is ample evidence that food choices contribute to the risk of these disorders, with a high intake of dietary fat and salt and low consumption of fruit and vegetables being particularly significant (Tomatis 1990; Kesteloot and Joossens 1992). Psychosocial factors such as life stress and social support are also thought to contribute to the risk of disease (Steptoe and Wardle 1994). Consequently, it is important to discover whether the association between psychosocial factors and disease is mediated (at least in part) through stress-induced alterations in food choice, since this may have serious implications for the health of the population.

Second, emotional stress may play an important role in the development and maintenance of eating disorders and related problems. Bulimia nervosa is characterised by dietary restraint coupled with episodes of excessive consumption, and much binge eating appears to be triggered by emotional distress. It has been argued that obese people will increase food consumption when stressed, because they are not able to distinguish hunger from anxiety (Bruch 1961), although the evidence for this is inconclusive (Greeno and Wing 1994). Knowing more about the links between stress and food choice may be helpful in broadening our understanding of these clinical problems.

Third, food choice may be influenced by, and may contribute to, variations in mood. Some investigators have proposed that certain constituents of the diet have a direct influence on neurochemical pathways in the brain; thus carbohydrates may stimulate the synthesis of serotonin and thereby have an antidepressant and alerting effect (Rosch 1995; Christensen 1996).

These factors indicate that the study of the association between stress and food choice may be fruitful. However, it is important to put the influence of stress in perspective, and not to exaggerate its likely effect. Stress is only one of many influences on food choice; sociocultural, economic and motivational factors also play significant roles. The impact of stress may be limited, and perhaps confined to susceptible individuals.

Stress, coping and eating behaviour

A robust theoretical framework in which to investigate psychosocial stress is essential. Most research on psychological stress and health is carried out within the framework outlined in Figure 2.1 (for details see Steptoe 1991, in press). Stress is not simply a response to events and experiences, however aversive, since people's reactions vary with the psychological and social resources they can bring to bear on the situation. Even a potentially damaging event such as a divorce elicits a

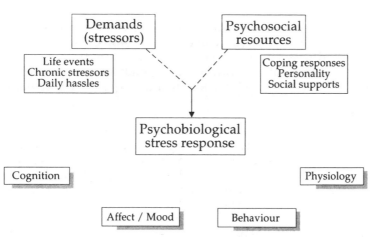

Figure 2.1 Outline model of factors stimulating psychobiological stress response

range of responses of varying intensity from different people. Stress responses arise when there is an imbalance between the demands and the coping resources of the individual. Demands (or stressors) that typically elicit responses include life events such as bereavement, assault or dismissal from a job, chronic stressors like sustained high workload or caring for a disabled relative, and minor stressors that are known in psychological literature as daily hassles. Hassles are events such as misplacing something, being interrupted or having an argument, that take place on a day-to-day basis. The interplay between life events and daily hassles is complex, but some of the effects of major events (for instance, marital breakdown) on psychological well-being are mediated through increases in hassle levels (Pillow, Zautra and Sandler 1996).

The psychosocial resources and vulnerability factors that are relevant to stressful transactions include temperamental dispositions, social networks and social supports, and psychological coping style. Thus a temperamentally stable individual who has strong social supports and a tendency to cope with stressors by taking a problem-solving approach, is likely to react to an experience like sudden illness in the family differently from a socially isolated person with a neurotic disposition. The psychobiological stress response itself is multifaceted, and includes changes in cognitive processes such as memory and decision-making, affective or mood responses, changes in behaviour, and physiological reactions in the neuroendocrine, autonomic and immune domains. Within this framework, food choice can be seen as one of the behaviours that may change during episodes of life stress. Other behaviours in this category are alcohol consumption, smoking, and self-care (Steptoe *et al.* 1996).

The method of discovering whether stress affects food choice might seem straightforward: assess food choice (in our terms, the amount of each type of food eaten during a specified time period), then either impose a stressor artificially or wait for a naturally occurring adverse event, measure distress or upset to check that the experience is actually stressful, then reassess food choice. Unfortunately, the issues are not so simple for the following reasons. First, different types of stressful experience may have different effects. The way someone copes with the breakdown of a significant relationship may be very different from their reaction to heavy demands at work. Uniform changes in food choice for different stressors are not therefore to be anticipated. Second, since responses vary as a function of psychosocial resources, it is necessary to take these factors into account. The availability of social support may be particularly important for food choice, since the purchase, preparation and consumption of food can be highly social activities, and will differ markedly between someone who is socially isolated and another who lives in a richly supportive milieu. The individual's habitual style of coping with threat may also be significant, since some people take an active problem-solving approach to their difficulties, while others distract themselves or avoid confrontation with the issues. Third, in addition to the general resources and vulnerability factors outlined in Figure 2.1, there are specific factors that moderate food choice. These include dietary restraint or the tendency to control eating and limit choice to foods low in calories. Dietary restraint is a relatively stable characteristic that can be assessed with standardised questionnaires, and varies substantially across the population. It is especially high among bulimics and those suffering from anorexia nervosa, but also characterises the eating behaviour of many people in the population, notably young women (Wardle 1987).

Finally, the relationship between changes in food choice and the emotional distress elicited by stressful experiences is complex, since at least three different patterns of response may occur:

1 Changes in food choice and in distress are separate but parallel components of the psychobiological stress response (as in Figure 2.1). If this is the case, no particular association between the magnitude of changes in food choice and increases in distress will be postulated.

2 Changes in food choice are stimulated by increased distress, and only take place among people who are very upset. If this is correct, changes in food choice occur not as a direct consequence of exposure to stressors but indirectly as a result of mood change, and a threshold of distress may exist beneath which no alteration of food choice will be elicited.

3 Changes in the type and quantity of food eaten may ameliorate emotional distress, acting to comfort or distract people from the problems that beset them. Consequently, the more that people alter their eating, the less upset they will become. A negative correlation

between distress and change in food choice can be predicted under these circumstances.

The possibility that all three of these patterns might be relevant in different situations greatly complicates investigations.

Methods of study

Assessment of the effect of life stress on food choice can be approached in a number of ways. One possibility is to carry out animal experiments in which exposure to aversive situations is precisely controlled and food intake is monitored exactly. Stressful procedures such as tail-pinching have been used in several studies, but results have been rather inconsistent (Greeno and Wing 1994). A second option is to ask people whether their choice of foods is affected by stress. We have used this approach to a limited extent in the development of a questionnaire measure of motives underlying food choice (Steptoe, Pollard and Wardle 1995). The strategy is predicated on people being aware of the links between their choice of foods and emotional state, and this may not always be the case. A third method is to carry out experimental studies in which eating is monitored when people are exposed to different types of acute emotional experience such as watching exciting or upsetting films (e.g. Wardle and Beales 1988). This paradigm has been extremely useful in the investigation of dietary restraint and other factors. It is, however, restricted to the study of short-term changes in food choice and food intake.

An alternative approach is to study food choice in naturalistic settings, examining the impact of emotional stress as it impinges in real life. The advantage of this method is that it has ecological validity, and there are few difficulties in generalising findings to the real world. The limitation is that many extraneous uncontrollable factors may contribute to changes in eating behaviour in such studies, and the randomisation of participants to different conditions is not possible.

Naturalistic studies do not conform to the premises underlying experimental scientific research, but come within the orbit of methods used in the social sciences. There are also practical problems in naturalistic studies, the chief one of which is that we do not know who is going to experience stressful events in their lives, or when these events are going to occur. Without this information, it is difficult to be certain that measurements will be taken at appropriate moments. Nevertheless, we were interested in carrying out a set of investigations of stress and food choice under naturalistic conditions, so as to discover whether some of the phenomena described in experimental studies also apply in everyday life. Within this framework, we were anxious to use objective measures as far as possible, not only for the assessment of food choice, but also to evaluate exposure to stressful events.

A quasi-experimental study: academic examination stress

The first study assessed the impact of the stress of anticipating academic examinations on food choice in a sample of university students. Assessments were made during a period of normal academic work (baseline session), and then during the two weeks preceding important end-of-semester examinations (exam session). The study was quasi-experimental in that it had some of the characteristics of a genuine experiment. There was a control group of students who were comparable to the exam-stress group in most ways, except that their courses were based on a different examination schedule. They therefore controlled for seasonal changes in food choice that might not be due to examination stress *per se*. Examinations have the advantages of being precisely timed events, and experiences that may be anticipated for days or even weeks, allowing systematic changes in food choice to emerge.

Previous research on examination stress has been inconclusive, with no reported changes in food intake taking place in some studies (O'Donnell *et al.* 1987; Niaura *et al.* 1991), and increases in energy intake (Michaud *et al.* 1990) and decreases in the 'nutritional quality' of diets in other studies (Weidner *et al.* in press). Two factors may account for this variability in response. The first is the nature of the measure of food choice and intake. Some studies have used rather imprecise self-report measures which may have limited accuracy. An alternative is to have participants complete dietary records. Although diaries are more accurate, there is a risk that the attention people are forced to pay to their food choice when keeping records may distort their pattern of intake. One person might, for example, become embarrassed about the amount of socially proscribed food (e.g. 'fast' food) they are consuming, while another may deliberately maintain a 'healthier' diet than normal when recording intake, so as to appear in a positive light. The burden of keeping detailed food records might also be excessively onerous for students prior to examinations. We therefore elected to use 24-hour dietary recall, and to embed the measure within a broader assessment of psychological well-being, smoking and other issues, so as to avoid placing undue emphasis on food choice. Twenty-four-hour food recall methods have been shown to have similar accuracy to food frequency and other techniques when assessed against computerised weighing (Bingham *et al.* 1994).

The second reason for variability in studies of examination stress is that few investigations have taken into account the psychosocial resources that people bring to the experience. Some individuals prepare for examinations much more calmly than others, and these differences may be significant for food choice. We therefore predicted that alterations in food choice would not be a general phenomenon, but confined to people who might be particularly vulnerable to stress.

The study involved 55 women and 64 men in the exam-stress group, and they were compared with 45 female and 16 male controls (see Pollard *et al.* 1995 for details). Students were taking an average of 2.83±1.1 examination papers, and the tests were generally rated as important or very important. Measures of anxiety-proneness (or trait anxiety) and perceptions of social support availability were obtained from participants. The impact of anticipating examinations was confirmed by ratings on the Perceived Stress Scale, a standardised questionnaire measure of the extent to which people feel under pressure (Cohen, Kamarck and Mermelstein 1983). There was an increase in perceived stress ratings of 9.8 per cent in the exam-stress group but no change among controls. Psychological well-being was assessed with the widely used General Health Questionnaire, and showed an average deterioration of 33.1 per cent in the exam-stress group and no significant change among controls.

The 24-hour food records were analysed for macronutrient composition using the Microdiet programme. There was no overall change in total energy intake or in the proportion of energy obtained from protein, fats, and carbohydrates (starch and sugars). However, significant interactions between trait anxiety and social support were observed. Anxious students with poor social supports showed an average increase of 19.7 per cent in total energy intake from the baseline to exam sessions, while the group with low anxiety and good social supports reduced intake by 14.4 per cent. Interestingly, there was also an increase in total fat intake of 28.5 per cent and in saturated fats of 32.1 per cent in the high anxiety/low support students in anticipation of examinations. This effect is important, because low anxiety proneness and good social support have both been shown to ameliorate the impact of life stress on subjective upset and other aspects of the stress response (Bolger and Eckenrode 1991). Food choice responses to examination stress would appear to conform to this pattern of results. The study therefore provided direct evidence for the impact of life stress on food choice in susceptible individuals.

Work stress and food choice

The second study evaluated the impact of stress associated with paid employment on food choice. We thought this type of life stress important to study for several reasons. First, work occupies a substantial portion of waking life for adults who are fortunate enough to have jobs. Some 14 million men and 12 million women are engaged in paid employment in the United Kingdom. If work stress adversely influences food choice, there is a strong possibility that effects will be of some significance to public health. Second, work has emerged as an important focus of health research over recent years, with investigations of the demand/control model of job strain, and studies of the impact of paid employment on women in a changing world of occupational roles (Long and Kahn 1993). Third, work load for many types of paid employment can be quantified objectively, thus conforming to one of the major themes underlying this project.

A study carried out with office workers in the USA suggested that work demands might indeed have an impact on food choice. McCann, Warnick and Knopp (1990) followed a small group of office workers over periods of high and low work load, utilising four-day food diaries to assess food intake. The energy value of the diet, total fat intake, and percentage of energy derived from fat were significantly greater during periods of high than low work load. Our study also involved assessment of a group of workers over periods of varying work load, and was designed to test the hypothesis that heightened work demands would be associated with increased distress and changes in food choice. So as to reduce the variability associated with different types of job, a group of working people were selected who had rather uniform tasks and who were available on several occasions. After considering a variety of occupations, we decided to carry out the study with shop-workers in the retail industry; according to the Central Statistical Office (1996), 8.6 per cent of working people in the UK are employed in sales activities. The relatively low educational and occupational status of shop-workers provided an interesting contrast with the university students previously tested.

The study was carried out in a large department store over a six-month period. Volunteer employees were assessed on four occasions with measures similar to those used earlier, including 24-hour dietary recall, blood cholesterol, the General Health Questionnaire and measures of perceived stress. In addition, saliva samples were obtained for the analysis of the stress hormone cortisol, and a metabolite of nicotine was assayed as an index of smoking. All sessions took place on weekdays and were preceded by a working day. Data concerning food intake were analysed for total energy intake and macronutrients.

There are several dimensions to work demand, including total paid work hours, shift pattern, how busy the staff are, the volume of turnover and so on. We used paid work hours as the measure of work stress since this is readily quantifiable, although we recognise that there are many other sources of stress within the work environment. The four sessions for each person were therefore ranked on the basis of paid work over the past seven days from highest to lowest work hours.

One of our concerns in the academic examination study was that unusual occurrences or events over the previous 24 hours may have distorted the representativeness of eating measures. It was therefore decided to average the two sessions that followed the longest working weeks, and the two sessions following the shortest working weeks, so as obtain more robust estimates of the impact of job stress. Data were provide by 90 employees of the department store, including 58 women and 32 men, with an average age of 37.7±11.3 years. The time worked over the past seven days averaged 35.1±7.4 hours on the low demand sessions, compared with

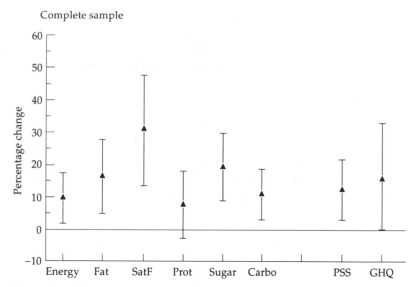

Complete sample

Figure 2.2 Increases in per cent between low and high work load sessions in energy intake (energy) and consumption of fat, saturated fat (satf), protein (prot), sugars and carbohydrate (carbo), and in scores on the perceived stress scale (PSS) and General Health Questionnaire (GHQ). The error bars represent 95 per cent confidence intervals

44.1±7.5 hours on the high demand sessions. This represents a large increase in work demand, and potentially in work stress.

Figure 2.2 summarises the percentage change between low and high work load sessions in total energy, macronutrient intake, self-reported stress and psychological well-being indexed by the General Health Questionnaire. Positive changes indicate an increase from low to high work load sessions, and the error bars are 95 per cent confidence intervals. It can be seen that there were significant increases in total energy intake (9.31 per cent), fat intake (16.2 per cent), saturated fat (30.7 per cent), sugars (20.4 per cent), and total carbohydrate (10.5 per cent, all p <0.01). The only macronutrient not to show a significant increase was protein. These changes in the amount of food eaten were accompanied by a significant increase in perceived stress and deterioration in psychological well-being.

This study therefore revealed general increases in food intake and in the amount of fat and sugars consumed under conditions of high work stress. People ate more during periods of high work stress, and the food they ate was especially rich in fat and sugar. The change in dietary saturated fat is particularly striking in view of its role in risk for coronary heart disease. Effects were observed across the entire sample, and not just in vulnerable sub-groups as was apparent in the academic examination study. The reasons for this difference are not clear, but they suggest that the pressure of work demands in a job may lead to pronounced changes in food choice. Interestingly, there was no correlation between the increase in perceived stress or deterioration in psychological well-being on the one hand, and food measures on the other. We did not find therefore that the changes in food intake were more prominent among workers who became especially distressed.

Individual experiences: a diary study

The results of the examination and work studies are intriguing. They suggest that people's dietary choices change during stressful experiences. Our studies had the advantages of objective measures of exposure to stressful events, and a rigorous approach to the assessment of food intake. The findings are, however, confined to a restricted range of life stressors. We do not know whether similar changes would occur in response to more emotionally upsetting events, or to experiences that generate sadness, anger and despair. Despite the overall increase in food intake and fat consumption shown in Figure 2.2, not all people respond to heightened work demands by changing what they eat. Perhaps those individuals who are unresponsive to increased work demands would alter food choice with other types of stressor. There is also the possibility that some people respond to stressors by an increasing intake of foods that are damaging to health, while others show a reduction in total consumption.

It is difficult to identify groups of people who undergo predictable emotional upsets in the future within an ethical framework of research. These considerations led us to formulate a study that permitted investigation of more idiosyncratic associations between food choice and stress. We carried out a diary study in which daily hassles and mood were monitored along with food choices. This technique entails a loss of precision and ability to quantify parameters, but has the benefits of allowing variations between people to emerge more clearly. Diary techniques have been used previously in a small number of studies, and have shown promising results. Stone and Brownell (1994) analysed ratings from 158 adults over 84 days, looking at associations between stressful events each day and responses to the question 'Did you eat more/less/same as usual?' The predominant pattern was reporting eating less than usual on stress days, although a proportion of individuals consistently stated that they ate more. MacDiarmid and Hetherington (1995) described a study of self-defined 'chocolate addicts' and controls, with ratings of hunger, mood and craving for chocolate over 20 days. The chocolate addicts did indeed consume more chocolate, and were more depressed, guilty and less relaxed before eating chocolate than controls. However, they remained guilty and no less depressed after eating chocolate, suggesting that mood did not improve with consumption. Another investigation tested the notion that depressed people might 'self-medicate' by eating a high carbohydrate diet to reverse serotonin depletion in the central nervous system, but failed to show supportive effects (Schlundt et al. 1993).

We decided to involve employed people in this study, so that daily hassles associated with work and domestic life could be assessed. Participants were drawn from two professions that have been shown in other research to experience high levels of work stress: schoolteachers and nurses (Tyler and Cushway 1992; Travers and Cooper 1996). So as to increase the chances of observing substantial variations in daily hassles, the study continued for an eight-week period. The requirement to complete diaries daily for this length of time was quite demanding, so those who agreed to participate in the study may not have been representative of these professions in general.

Every evening for the study period, the volunteers completed ratings of mood using methods based on the Profile of Mood States (POMS: McNair, Lorr and Droppleman 1981). Measures of smoking and alcohol intake were also taken, together with consumption of 30 common foods (e.g. fruit, chocolate bars and sausages). Amounts were assessed on a scale ranging from 'none' to 'five or more servings'. The measure was not intended to be comprehensive, but rather to assess classes of foods that might be particularly relevant to health and mood. At the end of each week, a more extensive set of measures was obtained, including assessments of physical symptoms, anxiety, depression and perceived stress. Respondents were also asked about the occurrence over the past seven days of ten work-related and ten home-related hassles. These were derived from the Hassles and Uplifts scale (Lazarus and Folkman 1989), and were rated as 'Did not occur', 'Occurred, but was not stressful', 'Caused me some stress', and 'Caused me a lot of stress'. The items were the top ten most frequently endorsed hassles from an earlier study of 250 nurses, and from pilot work with teachers. Work hassles included items such as 'I had too many interruptions', and 'I worried about career plans'. Non-work items included 'I worried about unexpected expenses', and 'I was concerned about the health of a family member'. Participants were also able to add personal experiences of their own: examples of these items are 'I had to take the day off work as my youngest child was ill' and 'I had abnormal smear results'.

There are several approaches to the analysis of diary data, and the information provided here is just illustrative of findings. The food records were averaged into weekly consumption levels for each item. This was done because many types of food are unlikely to be eaten every day, so aggregation across the week allows direct comparison with life-stress measures. One method of analysis was to compute within-subject correlations between consumption and hassles across weeks. Each participant provided eight pairs of data points (week 1 hassles, week 1 number of portions of fruit, etc.), and these were correlated to assess the covariation between measures. Figures 2.3a and 2.3b illustrate the pattern for two foods, the number of packets of crisps consumed and the number of portions of fruit and vegetables. Each has been correlated with the number of hassles (work and home combined) that were reported that participants rated as stressful. Figures 2.3a and 2.3b illustrate the distribution of correlations. Positive correlations

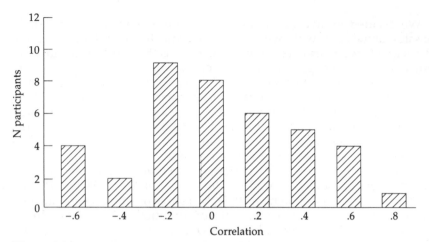

Figure 2.3a

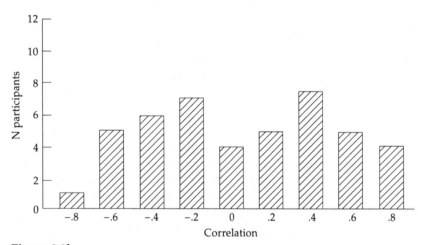

Figure 2.3b

Figure 2.3 Correlations between hassles and weekly consumption of crisps (2.3a) and fruit and vegetables (2.3b). The figure shows the distribution of correlations, which range from negative to positive.

indicate that the number of packets of crisps or the number of portions of fruit and vegetables was consistently greater on weeks during which more stressful hassles occurred, and that consumption was lower on low stress weeks. Negative correlations indicate the reverse, with more consumption during low stress weeks and fewer crisps or fruit and vegetables when stressors are more frequent.

Several points emerge from these analyses. The first is the wide range of correlations in both sets of analyses. Participants did not act in a uniform manner, and the distribution of correlations is not statistically normal. Second, some individuals showed high positive correlations while others showed high negative correlations (a perfect correlation is +1.0 or −1.0), indicating that consistent covariation between the consumption of these foods and hassle levels was present in some members of this sample. Associations were strong but varied, with some people increasing their consumption of crisps during high stress weeks, while others showed the reverse. Still others displayed an inconsistent pattern, with no discernible association between stress and food intake. Interestingly, there was no similarity between the behaviour of individuals in the two analyses. Thus the likelihood of eating more fruit and vegetables when stressed was just as high, whether or not the person ate crisps on weeks when there were hassles.

Figures 2.3a and 2.3b show just two of the associations that have emerged from our diary study, and many other relationships between hassles or mood and food intake have been identified. The task now is to characterise those individuals who show consistent associations between stress and types of food that may be health-promoting or health-damaging.

Reasons for stress-induced changes in food choice

The studies carried out in this project provide evidence that food choice may be affected by life stress. However, the results stimulate as many questions as they answer. One of the most pressing is why these changes in food choice take place. In considering this issue, several possible reasons can be put forward. One is that there is no direct link between stress and food choice, but both depend on a third unmeasured factor. For example, there are seasonal changes in food choice, and episodes of festive overeating (such as Christmas), and these may coincide with periods of life stress. This factor is unlikely to have accounted for the results of the examination study (since a control group was included), the work stress study, or the idiosyncratic patterns recorded in the diary study. We are nevertheless left with a number of other plausible alternative explanations:

1 Changes in food choice may emerge through a biological mechanism. Life stress is known to be associated with a range of autonomic and neuroendocrine responses that have effects on glucose utilisation and on fat metabolism (Brindley et al. 1993). Psychobiological stress responses may also have an impact on appetitive mechanisms (Castonguay 1991).
2 Changes in food choice may be the result of psychological processes of which the person is unconscious or only dimly aware. Eating certain foods may provide comfort or may mask dysphoria and distress (Polivy, Herman and McFarlane 1994). Eating could act as a distraction from stressful preoccupations.

3 Some people may make deliberate decisions to change the type of food they eat during periods of life stress. They may, for example, have beliefs that certain foods give them energy or keep them alert. Others may choose to reward themselves for hard work, or to cheer themselves up by eating foods that are normally proscribed.

4 There may be a stress-induced disinhibition of restraint and restrictive eating. Many people limit their food selections for health reasons (e.g. eating fruit and vegetables instead of fatty foods), or in order to reduce weight. During periods of life stress, these concerns may appear less pressing and exert less influence, so fat intake rises.

5 Food choice may be altered as a matter of convenience, without any particular conscious preference for different types of food. When people are preoccupied with work or other stressful events, they may consume more fast or convenience foods which are typically high in fat. If people eat what comes to hand and chose foods that require little or no preparation, it is likely this will lead to a bias towards high energy/high fat foods rather than other products.

These possibilities will be explored in future studies.

Acknowledgements

Additional support for this work was provided by the Biotechnology and Biological Sciences Research Council. We gratefully acknowledge the contribution of Lynn Canaan and Rachel Mills to the project, and assistance in data collection from Kate Wrightston, Rebecca Lewis, Pauline McGlone, Suzanne Owen, Caroline Mulvihill and Helen Lightowler.

CHAPTER 3

Understanding dietary choice and dietary change: contributions from social psychology

Mark Conner, Rachel Povey, Paul Sparks,
Rhiannon James and Richard Shepherd

Introduction

Psychologists have long been interested in dietary (or food) choice and its determinants. Much of this research was originally carried out from a physiological or learning perspective, giving rise to insights into the influence of physiology and learning processes on food choices. More recently social psychologists have contributed to the understanding of dietary choices and dietary changes, principally through the study of what people think about food and diet (e.g. through cognitive factors such as peoples' attitudes and beliefs). Their major contribution has been in the development of theories of the determinants of such choices.

In this chapter we review the contribution of social psychologists. We begin by examining the approach to studying dietary choice taken by social psychologists. We then go on to outline psychological theories of dietary choice. Some general theories are presented first, before we focus on recent social psychological theories and present some contributions from our own research. In a subsequent section, we examine social psychological contributions to the understanding of how people change their diet (dietary change), again focusing on psychological theories of the determinants of successful change and including our own research findings. Finally, we summarise the arguments presented.

Dietary choice

Social psychological perspectives on dietary choice

Social psychologists are interested in understanding and predicting behaviour in its social context. Over the past 25 years, the most widely applied approach has assumed that social behaviour (such as dietary choice) is best understood as a function of people's perceptions of reality, rather than as a function of the actual situation. This has been called the 'social cognitive' approach (Schneider 1991). Thus, as social psychologists using this approach, we are interested in the person's cognitions or thoughts as processes which intervene between objective stimuli (e.g. foods) and responses (e.g. eating) in specific real-world situations (Fiske and Taylor 1991). In relation to food or dietary choice, we are interested in choice in terms of behaviour (e.g. the act of taking), in terms of an object (e.g. that which is taken, the food), and in terms of cognition (e.g. the mental processes of decision-making), and especially the interrelationships among these three elements. The behaviour might be the purchase, selection, rejection or consumption of a food. The object might be, for example, a particular food (e.g. low fat milk), a group of foods (e.g. low fat foods) or even a whole diet (e.g. a low fat diet) and might be one of a very limited or very broad set of choice options. The cognitions might be beliefs about a food (e.g. about its health properties), attitudes toward a food (e.g. an overall evaluation), preferences for a food (e.g. desires for a food), or intentions to consume a particular food (e.g. plans to purchase or consume).

The approach taken to understanding dietary choice by social cognitive psychologists has a number of important components. A first component is the development of theories relating cognitions about the object and behaviour in relation to the object. Such theories describe the important abstract concepts (e.g. attitudes) and the nature of their interrelationships (e.g. how they combine to predict behaviour) in mathematically testable formulae. A second component is the operationalisation of these abstract constructs into concrete, measurable variables which can be assessed for reliability (i.e. stability over time) and validity (i.e. demonstration that they measure the construct of interest). By their nature many of these variables can only be assessed by various self-report measures (e.g. through questionnaires) and hence assessing the reality of these self-reports has been a matter of considerable interest. A third component concerns the empirical testing of these theories to confirm or disconfirm the hypothesised relationships among concepts and the power of the theory in predicting behaviour. Evidence from empirical studies is used to further refine and develop the theory. In the next section we describe one such social cognitive theory, its application to understanding dietary choice and possible extensions to the theory.

Determinants of dietary choices

Several different models of the determinants of food or dietary choice have been proposed which it might be helpful to review to give context for our subsequent review of social psychological models. Early attempts by nutritionists (e.g. Yudkin 1956) split the factors influencing food choice into three categories: physical factors included geography, season, economics, and food technology; social factors included religion, social class, nutrition education, and advertising; and physiological factors included heredity, allergy, and nutritional needs. On the other hand, more recent conceptions by psychologists (e.g. Booth and Shepherd 1988; Shepherd 1989; Conner 1993a) generally split the influences into those factors related to the food, to the external environment and to the individual. External factors linked to the food and the environment (the social and cultural context in which dietary choices take place) are assumed to influence sensory, psychological and physiological factors within the individual and together these produce food choices. As we have noted earlier, the social cognition approach favoured by most social psychologists focuses on the psychological factors within the individual.

Let us first examine the external influences on food choice in a little more detail. The first external factor – the physical composition of food – will have effects on food choice through three routes: via sensory attributes of the food, via physiological effects of the food, and via psychological effects of the food. Aspects of the food, such as its chemical and physical composition, give rise to properties of the food which are perceived by the individual as sensory characteristics (e.g. its appearance, taste and smell). In addition to producing sensory effects, the chemical composition of the food includes nutrients such as protein, carbohydrates, fat, minerals and vitamins which are vital to physiological functioning. Indeed many theories of food choice emphasise the life-sustaining aspect of food ingestion over all others. Ingestion of the chemicals in foods will have other physiological effects. For instance, the consumption of high-energy food will lead to satiation and the reduction of subsequent food consumption (Blundell and Rogers 1991). Similarly, if the food leads to vomiting and sickness it will probably be avoided in the future (Rozin and Vollmecke 1986). Thus, the chemical or physical properties of the food have an influence on subsequent food choice and intake through post-ingestional effects. The third way in which the chemical and physical properties of the food will affect food choice and intake is through the post-ingestional effects of consuming particular foods on psychological functioning. For example, some foods affect mood or alertness and it is possible that association between these effects and a particular food might influence the subsequent selection of the food under appropriate circumstances.

A second set of external factors which influence food choice are the general social and cultural environment (Rozin 1990). Food choices differ between cultures and the social milieu surrounding the individual may have an impact on their food choices. Religion, for instance, may require that certain dietary choices are made regardless of personal preferences. The availability of food, its price, and aspects of advertising and marketing can all have a further influence on individual food choices.

In addition to the external influences on food choices, there are also influences located within the individual which interact with these. They include physiological, psychological and sensory factors which are likely to interact with physical aspects of the food and the environment to produce food choice. Physiological factors within the individual which are likely to influence food choice include hormone levels, disease, intolerance to particular food constituents, and a range of other factors. Psychological differences between individuals such as personality also affect food choices (Pliner and Hobden 1992; Raudenbush, van den Klaauw and Frank 1995). Sensory differences between individuals in terms of sensitivity to and acceptability of differing levels of the constituents in food will also influence food choices.

In summary, while the above factors are all likely to be important in a broad overview of food choice, social psychologists have tended to focus on cognitive factors as more immediate determinants of dietary choices. This is based on the assumption that the above factors influence dietary choices principally via their influence on these cognitive factors. For example, a physiological intolerance to particular foods is likely to be translated into a negative attitude or belief about eating that food and it is these attitudes or beliefs which are likely to influence future avoidance of this food. In the next section we describe these cognitive factors and present a theory of how they mediate other influences on food choice.

Social psychological theories of dietary choice

Social psychological research on the processes whereby the above factors influence food choice has frequently reflected the importance of cognitive factors such as attitudes and beliefs in predicting food choice (e.g. Shepherd and Stockley 1985; Tuorila 1987; Sparks, Hedderley and Shepherd 1992). These cognitions are often held to be of central importance because they mediate the effects of other variables on food choice (Conner 1993a). However, the link between attitudes, beliefs and behaviour is by no means simple (Schuman and Johnson 1976). Here we examine the nature of these cognitions, before presenting models of how they relate to food choices. A small percentage of human beliefs and attitudes towards foods result directly from our interaction with foods (e.g. taste aversions). However, most beliefs are derived from socially transmitted information. These include beliefs about which foods are healthy and which foods are generally acceptable (e.g. some concerns in Western culture with eating too much are clearly linked to widespread cultural notions of an ideal slim body shape).

One view is that our attitudes consist of three distinct components (Eagly and Chaiken 1993). These are emotional or affective reactions to objects ('gut' reactions or preferences for particular foods, e.g. liking ice-cream); our behavioural tendencies towards objects (intentions to consume or avoid a food, e.g. planning to avoid eating ice-cream); and thoughts or cognitions, including what we believe about the consequences of consuming a particular food (that eating a particular food will lead to particular outcomes, e.g. eating ice-cream will make me fat). The extent to which components are consistent with one another will vary considerably as a function of the object which is the focus of attention (i.e. the attitude object), the context, and the individual (Zanna and Rempel 1988). Across studies, when differing influences on food choices are compared within an individual, the major determinant of food choice tends to be the flavour or taste of the food, with physiological factors like tolerance and satiety sometimes important, but health beliefs of much less importance and factors such as price and convenience having little or no effect on consumption (Shepherd 1989). Moral commitments (e.g. embodied within certain forms of vegetarianism) may also have an influence (Sparks and Shepherd 1992).

How might these differing components of attitudes interact to produce food choice and consumption? Several models relating affective, behavioural and cognitive components of attitudes to behaviours (e.g. actual food consumption) have been developed and extensively applied in social psychology (e.g. see Conner and Norman 1996). Most such models emphasise the rational accounts people give of their behaviour. Behaviour is predicted on the basis that these rationales reflect the underlying decision-making processes. Most assume that behaviour is based on elaborate analysis of the subjective costs and benefits of the outcomes of differing courses of action. This assumption has roots going back to expectancy-value theory (e.g. Peak 1955), which takes people to be favourably disposed towards objects or issues where they believe there would be benefit to them, and to dislike those objects or issues that might damage the chances of reaching their goals. This is similar to many economic models of choice. Outcomes of behaving in a particular way are assumed to have differing (subjective) probabilities of occurring and to be of differing cost or benefit value to individuals. Comparison of costs and benefits of the expected outcomes of alternative behaviours leads to the preference for and subsequent choice of that behaviour with the greatest balance of benefits over costs. Perhaps the most widely used such model has been the theory of reasoned action (TRA) (Ajzen and Fishbein 1980), recently extended to a theory of planned behaviour (TPB) (Ajzen 1991). This approach to attitude research continues to attract a great deal of attention in social psychology (Sheppard, Hartwick and Warshaw 1988; Olson and Zanna 1993).

Theory of planned behaviour

The theory postulates that behaviours such as food choices are best predicted from an individual's intention to perform the behaviour, with intention determined by three sets of factors. Intention is regarded as a plan to act in a particular way. The first determinant of intentions is the attitude towards the behaviour. Attitude is here described as the affective reaction to the behaviour (i.e. the affective component of attitude described earlier) and is measured by a positive–negative semantic differential scale (e.g. a 'good–bad' scale). The overall attitude is held to be based on the individual's beliefs about the salient outcomes or attributes of the behaviour (i.e. the cognitive component of the

attitude described earlier). Such outcomes include behavioural outcomes (e.g. the food will fill me up) and emotional outcomes (e.g. this
food will taste pleasant). For each outcome, an expectancy (i.e. a rating
of the likelihood that the behaviour will lead to that outcome) and a
value (i.e. a rating of the evaluation of that outcome as 'good' or 'bad')
are obtained and the two ratings multiplied together. According to
the model, the sum of these expectancy-value calculations across the
individually salient outcomes should predict overall attitude.

The second determinant of intention is the subjective norm (i.e.
sometimes described as the perceived social pressure to perform the
behaviour in question). The subjective norm reflects the social
psychological assumption that our intentions to perform a behaviour
are shaped by expectations that others hold for us as well as by our
personal attitudes. The subjective norm is assumed to be a sum of the
normative beliefs about what salient groups or individuals believe
about the individual performing the behaviour, each weighted by the
motivation to comply with the relevant people (i.e. desire to do what
others want us to do).

The third determinant is the amount of control that the individual
perceives him/herself to have over the behaviour in question – referred
to as perceived behavioural control (PBC). Ajzen (1991) suggests that
the control component will predict both behavioural intention and,
where the individual is correct in perceiving that they have control over
the behaviour, it will also predict behaviour. Perceived control is
estimated from evaluations of the power of factors to facilitate or inhibit
the performance of the behaviour, each weighted by their frequency of
occurrence. These factors include both internal control factors (e.g.
personal deficiencies, skills, abilities, emotions) and external control
factors (e.g. opportunities, dependence on others, barriers). The recent
inclusion of this component reflects the fact established by other models
(see Conner and Norman 1996) that intentions are. determined by
perceptions of control over performance of the behaviour as well as by
attitudes and social pressures.

So, according to this theory, individuals are more likely to form a
preference for, choose and consume a particular food if they believe (all
other things being equal) that consumption of that food will lead to
particular outcomes or have particular attributes which they value
positively, if they believe that people whose views they value think they
should engage in the behaviour, and if they feel that the action is easily
brought under their own control. The theory combines all three aspects
of attitudes: the affective element is reflected in the attitude component,
the behavioural component in the behavioural intention, and the
cognitive component in the outcome beliefs and control beliefs. Other
influences on dietary choices are assumed to operate via changing
beliefs about outcomes, normative pressure or control factors (i.e. the
other influences are more remote determinants of behaviour).

Food choice has been the target behaviour investigated in a number
of TRA and TPB studies. For example, using the TRA, Manstead, Plevin
and Smart (1983) investigated infant feeding, while Brinberg and

Durand (1983) looked at visiting fast-food restaurants. The TPB has also been applied to food choice by a number of authors (Beale and Manstead 1991; Towler and Shepherd 1991; Sparks and Shepherd 1992; Sparks, Hedderley and Shepherd 1992; Lloyd, Paisley and Mela 1993). Strong relationships between food choice and attitudes have been demonstrated using this theory (e.g. Shepherd and Stockley 1985; Tuorila 1987; Conner and Sparks 1996). For instance, in a study of snack-food consumption (Conner 1993b), attitudes, subjective norms and PBC accounted for 65 per cent of the variability in intention to consume snack foods and 60 per cent of the variability in previous snack-food consumption in a sample of English adults. The major factors distinguishing heavy snackers from infrequent snackers were attitudes and beliefs. In particular, heavy snackers held more positive attitudes towards consuming snack foods and these attitudes were supported by a greater belief in the positive taste of snack foods and their value for money. Normative beliefs and control beliefs appeared to play only a minor role in determining intention and actual consumption of snack foods. The theory does, however, assume that the determinant which will be most predictive depends upon the dietary choice being investigated.

Among social psychologists working in this area, recent attention has focused on other variables which might improve the predictive power of this model. This is because it has become clear that in some instances the TPB only accounts for a modest amount of the variance in behaviour (i.e. much behaviour is unexplained by the theory). For example, Sheppard, Hartwick and Warshaw (1988) noted that about 10 per cent of studies they reviewed reported weak relationships between behavioural intentions and behaviour (i.e. correlations below .20). Ajzen (1991) reports the relationship between intentions and attitude, subjective norm and PBC to be strong (multiple correlation of .71) across the 16 studies he reviewed. Ajzen also reports the relationship between intentions, PBC and behaviour to be moderately strong (multiple correlation of .51). Similar findings are reported by Godin and Kok (1996) across a larger number of studies. While these values are comparatively high for social science models, a variety of additional variables which might improve this predictive power have been investigated, including need to change (Paisley and Sparks forthcoming), descriptive norms (e.g. Cialdini, Reno and Kallgren 1990), moral norms (e.g. Sparks 1994; Parker, Manstead and Stradling 1995), anticipated affective reactions (e.g. Richard, van der Pligt and de Vries 1995, 1996), self-identity (e.g. Sparks and Shepherd 1992), and past behaviour or habit (e.g. Bentler and Speckart 1979; Fredricks and Dossett 1983). One variable we have investigated in this regard is the concept of attitudinal ambivalence.

Attitudinal ambivalence

Attitudinal ambivalence is based on the idea that we may simultaneously hold both positive and negative beliefs about, or affective reactions towards, an attitude object (Eagly and Chaiken 1993) (e.g. I may believe that chocolate cake will both taste nice, but also be bad for my health). Typically, psychologists tend to average such evaluatively inconsistent ratings to give a mean response, which is likely to be near to the mid-point of a bipolar attitude scale. However, such averaging loses potentially important information and prevents us from distinguishing individuals who have these inconsistent affective reactions or beliefs, *the ambivalent*, from those who simply hold a set of affective reactions or beliefs which are consistent and at the mid-point of a bipolar scale, *the indifferent*.

It is possible to distinguish a number of forms of ambivalence: inconsistent beliefs, inconsistent emotions (mixed feelings), inconsistent emotions and beliefs (the heart versus the mind), and inconsistent evaluations. While each of these forms of ambivalence may be important to understanding food choice, here we discuss only the last and the first of these in relation to measuring ambivalence. In relation to ambivalence as inconsistent evaluations, Kaplan (1972) modified a widely used measure of attitudes (the semantic-differential technique) by separately assessing the positive and negative attributes ascribed to an attitude object; one measure assessed the positive attributes (e.g. My feelings about food X are . . . not at all *favourable* to extremely *favourable*) and another measure assessed the negative attributes (e.g. My feelings about food X are . . . not at all *unfavourable* to extremely *unfavourable*). Generally, the two measures have been found to show low negative correlations with one another. We could then recombine these two scores to obtain separate measures of overall attitude and ambivalence. Kaplan (1972) suggested that in a measure of ambivalence, scores should increase as these two judgements become more polarised and the more equal they are in absolute value. A variety of measures of ambivalence has been proposed to capture these conditions in a measure of ambivalence. The one we use is associated with Thompson, Zanna and Griffin (1995): ambivalence is calculated as half the polarisation of the two positive and negative judgements, minus the absolute difference between the two.

An alternative, belief-based measure of ambivalence would obtain evaluations of different beliefs about the attitude object and combine the positive and negative evaluations into an index of ambivalence. Instead of providing a standard set of modal beliefs such as is commonly done with the TRA/TPB, a self-generated list of salient beliefs is used, which may more accurately reflect feelings of ambivalence. In our belief-based measure of ambivalence we used a method associated with Bell, Esses and Maio (1996), where respondents write in likely outcomes of a behaviour (beliefs) and then evaluate each on a scale from 'bad' to 'good'. So, for example, in relation to eating ice-cream, a respondent might write down 'tastes nice' (evaluated +3 or *extremely good*), 'fills me up' (evaluated +1 or *good*) and 'fattening' (evaluated −2 or *very bad*). These positive and negative evaluations are then separately summed and put into the same ambivalence equation.

What differences might we expect between individuals high and low in ambivalence on such measures? If we assume that attitudinal ambivalence is a measure of attitude strength (Petty and Krosnick 1995; i.e. ambivalent attitudes equate to a weaker attitude), then we might expect ambivalent attitudes (weaker) to be more easily changed, less related to behaviour, and less stable over time. To date, only the last of these hypotheses has been demonstrated empirically (Bargh *et al.* 1992). In our own research we wished to test if ambivalent attitudes about dietary choices were indeed weaker predictors of such choices than non-ambivalent attitudes, as this might have important implications for understanding dietary choice. However, in relation to dietary choices it was first important to demonstrate that attitudes towards diet were indeed characterised by ambivalence in at least some individuals.

Hence, we first investigated the extent to which ambivalence was likely to occur for food choices compared to other behaviours. In an initial questionnaire study, we obtained self-report measures of positive and negative attitudes towards 12 different behaviours from a group of 143 students. The results are shown in Table 3.1 (scores standardised to values between 0 and 1). There were clearly considerable differences in the extent to which different behaviours produced feelings of ambivalence. Eating a low fat diet produced the second highest level of ambivalence, while increasing fruit and vegetable consumption produced one of the lowest. Hence, we were encouraged that at least some eating behaviours produced considerable levels of ambivalence in some people. The reasonably large standard deviations (a measure of variability between people) for dietary choices also showed that people differed on our measures of ambivalence. We next examined the extent to which such feelings of ambivalence might moderate the relationship among variables in the TPB.

In a separate study we investigated attitudes towards the consumption of a low fat diet among students (N = 158). In an initial questionnaire we used measures from the TPB and also positive/ negative attitudes and belief-based measures of ambivalence and then in a later questionnaire measures of the extent to which respondents actually consumed a low fat diet (based on a food frequency measure). It was thus a prospective design. The sample was split at the median on the two ambivalence measures (half respondents then classified as low ambivalence, the other half as high ambivalence). We then calculated the correlations between measures of beliefs, attitudes, intentions and behaviour (subjective norm and perceived control measures were not included in this analysis because we expected the impact of attitudinal ambivalence to be on the attitude component of the theory) separately for the half of the respondents with higher levels of ambivalence and the half with lower levels. As expected, the correlations among components were significantly higher in the lower ambivalence group than in the higher ambivalence group. This difference was particularly pronounced for the split based on the belief-based measure of ambivalence. The research thus demonstrated that ambivalent attitudes were more weakly related to actual behaviour. This implies that for the average person with a positive attitude toward eating a low fat diet, that attitude will be less predictive of subsequently eating a low fat diet in those whose attitude is ambivalent compared to those whose attitude is not ambivalent. This represents good evidence that attitudinal ambivalence moderates the relationship between the beliefs, attitudes, intentions and behaviour in the TPB. This finding has been replicated in several of our studies with different food choices.

Thus, models of behaviour such as the TPB might usefully incorporate measures of ambivalence to improve their predictive power. It is only among those with non-conflicting beliefs and attitudes (non-ambivalent) that good relationships hold between beliefs, attitudes, intentions and behaviour. For those who report ambivalent attitudes, food choice may not be strongly related to intentions, attitudes or beliefs. Ajzen (1996) argues that salient beliefs are the basis of cognitive responding and the basis of behaviour. Hence, one interpretation of this effect of ambivalence would suggest that those who report ambivalent attitudes have many conflicting beliefs on which to base both responses to cognition and behaviour questions. Thus, inconsistencies between cognitions and behaviour are more likely because different beliefs become salient in the two situations in which cognitions and behaviour are elicited. Those who do not hold ambivalent attitudes in contrast have evaluatively consistent beliefs and no matter which beliefs become salient in different situations, the outcome should be the same (i.e. positive cognitions and approach behaviours, or negative cognitions and avoidance behaviours).

Thus, in summary, the TPB appears to provide a good description of many of the more immediate determinants of behaviours such as dietary choice. Other variables' influences upon behaviour are assumed to be mediated via the variables in the model and there is reasonable evidence to support this contention (Conner and Sparks 1996). However, there is also research investigating the role of additional variables which might usefully be added to the model. One promising variable we have presented findings on is the idea of attitudinal ambivalence. Our research would suggest that only individuals with lower levels of ambivalence show good relationships among the cognitive variables in the TPB and dietary choices.

Dietary change

Social psychological perspectives on dietary change

Theories such as the Theory of Planned Behaviour (Ajzen 1991), take a relatively simplistic view of behaviour change. They assume that the adoption of a new behaviour is based on subjective expected utility (or expectancy-value) considerations of the differing costs and benefits of adopting the behaviour, with a behaviour being likely to be adopted if it possesses a greater balance of benefits over costs (i.e. greater utility) compared to alternative behaviours (Ajzen and Fishbein 1980). In more sophisticated applications of the TPB, a new behaviour is adopted if its expected utility exceeds that of the salient alternative behaviours. This is assumed to occur through the development of intentions to perform a new behaviour. However, little attention is given to how such intentions are transformed into action, and how this action, if performed, comes to be maintained. A single linear equation indicates the individual's likelihood of action.

More sophisticated 'stage' theories have also been developed by psychologists and applied to dietary change. These try to describe the process of change in behaviour or adoption of a new behaviour in more detail and do not assume a linear relationship between intentions and behaviour change. They describe the factors which might influence behaviour change at different stages (see Norman and Conner 1996). Stage theories suggest two things: that people at different stages think about behaviour change in qualitatively different ways, and that the kinds of interventions and information needed to move closer to action or adoption of a new behaviour vary from stage to stage (Weinstein 1988).

One of the first stage theories was put forward by Prochaska and DiClemente (1984) in what they call the Transtheoretical Model of Change. Their theory has been widely applied to analyse the process of change in a variety of behaviours including dietary change (e.g. Curry, Kristal and Bowen 1992; Greene *et al.* 1994). In its most recent form, Prochaska, DiClemente and Norcross (1992) identify five stages of change: pre-contemplation, contemplation, preparation, action and maintenance. Individuals are thought to progress through each of the stages in order to achieve successful maintenance of a new behaviour. Taking the example of changing to eat a low fat diet, it is argued that in the pre-contemplation stage the individual does not consider that this part of their behaviour constitutes a problem and therefore has no intention to change. In the contemplation stage, the individual starts to think about changing their behaviour, but as yet is not committed to try to reduce the fat in their diet. In the preparation stage, the individual intends to change in the near future and starts to make plans about how to do this. The action stage is characterised by active attempts to change, and once the initial problems of successfully eating the new diet are overcome, the individual moves into the maintenance stage which is characterised by attempts to prevent relapse and to consolidate the newly acquired behaviour. While relatively widely applied, the evidence in support of the theory and the different stages is at present relatively weak (see Sutton 1996). Our own research would support the idea that individuals classified at each of the different stages are behaving in different ways with respect to the target behaviour (food choice). For example, the study of low fat diets mentioned earlier found a difference in the number of calories and percentage energy derived from fat in the diet between individuals in different stages of change (i.e. this was lower among those in the action and maintenance stages). We also found differences in beliefs, attitudes, intentions and attitudinal ambivalence. Beliefs and attitudes towards eating a low fat diet became more favourable across stages, intentions to eat a low fat diet became stronger, while ambivalence showed an inverted U-shaped relationship, peaking in the preparation stage. The biggest differences were between people who had not formed an intention to change (those in the pre-contemplation and contemplation stages) and those who had (those in the preparation, action and maintenance stages). Such findings are 'necessary, but not sufficient' evidence to provide unequivocal support for the idea that all the stages are truly distinct. It may be that these variables change in a linear fashion across some stages and that a theory with fewer stages may be more appropriate (e.g. a pre-decisional and post-decisional stage).

Heckhausen (1991) has similarly identified phases in the initiation and maintenance of behaviour change; these are the 'pre-decisional', 'post-decisional', 'actional' and 'evaluative' phases, which follow a similar progressive sequence as that outlined by Prochaska and DiClemente (1984). Heckhausen further suggests that different types of cognitions are important in each of these phases. So in the pre-decisional phase, cognitions about the desirability and feasibility of the behaviour are thought to be important determinants of an intention to perform the behaviour in question. This phase ends with the formation of an intention to change. In contrast, the decisional phase focuses on the development of plans and ends with the successful initiation of the behaviour. In the actional phase, the individual focuses on effectively achieving performance of the behaviour and this ends with the conclusion of the behaviour. In the final, evaluative phase the individual compares achieved outcomes with initial goals in order to regulate and maintain behaviour. While this four-phase theory of behaviour was not developed specifically for the prediction of food choice, the potential of its application to this area is clear. Other research also demonstrates the utility and applicability of this theory (see Gollwitzer 1996). The data we have collected to date might be interpreted as being consistent with such a theory.

Intention–behaviour 'gap'

As we noted earlier, applications of the TPB predict intentions better than they do behaviour. Consideration of the cognitive variables important in translating intentions into action may considerably improve our understanding of the basis of behaviours such as food choice. In relation to stage theories of behaviour, this involves consideration of the factors important in the action and maintenance stage of behaviour change. At present, relatively little detailed attention has focused on the cognitive processes underlying the successful initiation and maintenance of behaviour. Research mentioned earlier would suggest that intentions are more likely to be translated into behaviour if the individual has non-ambivalent attitudes. Bagozzi (1992) suggests another way we can help implement our intentions is through the formulation of detailed plans. One way in which plans are more likely to be acted on is through the development of 'scripts', or cognitive rehearsal, whereby the individual imagines themselves performing the instrumental act (Anderson 1983). Another is through the use of 'pre-committing devices' whereby performance of the behaviour is made more likely by pre-committing oneself to it (e.g. eating low fat spread rather than butter at home by only having low fat spread in the house).

Schelling (1992) and Ainslie (1992) have produced important work focusing on how people may act to ensure particular choices are enacted. For example, Ainslie describes a number of pre-committing devices that people may use to influence their future motives or place 'physical limitations on future behaviour' (1992: 126). Four such pre-committing devices appear to be important in behaviour change: 'extrapsychic devices' serve to constrain a range of future choice options or employ 'external' methods to influence future motivations (e.g. appetite suppressants, keeping certain foods out of the home); 'attention control' devices serve to divert attention from thoughts that might promote impulsive behaviours; 'emotion control' devices involve taking steps to avoid certain emotional states that might precipitate impulsive behaviours; 'personal rules' are rules that a person sets up which serve to categorise certain actions as proscribed (such a categorisation system may be bolstered by private 'side bets' which involve the person forfeiting something of value if they break the rule). All these devices essentially serve the purpose of 'impulse control'. These ideas overlap with Kuhl's (1985) theory of action control which identifies the processes by which individuals attempt to control their actions and achieve their goals. These processes may be particularly important in allowing individuals to overcome temptations to revert to their old behaviour (see Loewenstein 1996). Such pre-committing devices may be useful in helping to understand how people make successful changes to their own diets.

In order to assess people's use of pre-committing devices readers of *Healthy Eating* magazine who had made changes to their diets, were asked about the strategies they found useful in attempting to eat a healthy diet or in making change to their diet. The responses showed a variety of barriers matched by a variety of strategies that might be used to overcome them. Pre-committing devices were in evidence: examples of 'attention control' (e.g. where respondents described focusing their attention on things other than tempting foods) and 'extrapsychic devices' (e.g. getting someone else to do the shopping in order to avoid temptations) were offered. Some respondents showed evidence of a belief in the importance of 'personal rules' (e.g. rewarding oneself for overcoming eating urges) but also an awareness of the problems of rigid 'restraint'. A number of people, even those who did not mention pre-committing devices directly, recorded their view of the importance of 'willpower' in overcoming temptations. Many strategies that people reported did not relate to motivational conflicts but rather to external social barriers that influenced whether or not they were able to act on their preferences. Other responses implied that the motivational barriers did not relate primarily to temporary shifts in preference, but to the issue of carrying out actions to ensure that non-motivational barriers did not occur at crucial times in the future. For example, 'planning' was frequently cited as an enabling device – a necessary step in the process of being able to make and maintain changes; it was frequently noted as a requirement in order to enable certain preferences being realised in the future (it was particularly used in relation to planning meals, shopping and cooking). Whereas some of the extrapsychic mechanisms used as pre-committing devices serve to restrict the range of choice options at a future point in time, such enabling devices seem to serve the opposite function: of increasing the range of options available at some future time point (see Schelling 1992).

Thus, in summary, social psychologists have devoted some attention to the development of models of behaviour change that can be applied to dietary issues. It would seem that at least a pre-decisional and post-decisional stage of behaviour change can be distinguished. While many of the cognitive variables identified in models of dietary choice are relevant to the pre-decisional phase, it may be that additional variables (such as pre-committing devices) are also relevant when considering the post-decisional phase of behaviour change. Further research is needed to tackle which factors are important in ensuring good intentions are translated into successful dietary changes.

Conclusion

Social psychologists have contributed to the understanding of food choice and dietary change particularly by the development of models of the cognitive determinants of these behaviours. They treat intention as key variables linking various cognitions (e.g. beliefs, attitudes) and behaviour (e.g. dietary choice). Broader social influences on food choice are regarded as being mediated by these cognitive variables. One important model linking cognitions and behaviour was described (the TPB) and possible extensions (e.g. attitudinal ambivalence) considered. In order fully to explain dietary choice and changes in dietary choice it may be necessary to develop a more dynamic model that examines different stages or phases in the contemplation, initiation and maintenance of behaviour. An integration of current models (such as the TPB) with stage models of behaviour change may considerably further our understanding of dietary choice and dietary change. Several authors have also recommended such an integration in relation to other 'health' behaviours (e.g. Marcus et al. 1994; Godin et al. 1995; Courneya, Nigg and Estabrooks forthcoming) and such integration may increase our understanding of how cognitive factors influence behaviours such as dietary choice and dietary change. We also need to devote further attention to the relationships between cognitive and affective influences on dietary choices and the social conditions which promote the development of such influences.

CHAPTER 4

Changing what children eat

C. Fergus Lowe, Alan Dowey and Pauline Horne

Introduction

While there could be endless academic discussion revolving around the concept of 'food choice', most agencies concerned with the health of the nation are primarily interested in improving people's diets. This is hardly surprising given the ever-accumulating evidence that eating fruit and vegetables confers major health benefits, including lessening the risks of various forms of cancer and cardiovascular disease, and lowering overall mortality rates (see Gillman 1996; Key *et al.* 1996). The goal of helping people to change to healthy diets or, even better, of ensuring that they adopt healthy eating habits from childhood onwards, is also central to our research strategy. Such an enterprise requires an understanding of the psychological determinants of human food preferences set within the broader context of general psychological theory. Though this may in part entail studying what people say about their food choices or preferences (i.e. what might be called their 'attitudes' to food), it is critical to relate what they say to what they do: that is, to what they *actually* eat. And it is not sufficient merely to describe correlations between people's performance on attitude scales or questionnaires and their real or reported dietary intake: it is essential above all to establish the *causal* factors that bring about changes in people's food consumption. Only thus will we be able to effect significant changes in the eating habits of the general population. Experimental psychology has a central role to play in this endeavour.

Theoretical background

Many factors combine to determine which particular foods an individual will select and consume at any given developmental stage. A great deal of research has focused on the interaction of two broad domains of influence: the biological and the sociocultural. Among biological factors may be included whether a particular substance can be safely ingested and is digestible (Logue 1991: 118), innate preferences for sweet tasting substances (Desor, Maller and Turner 1973; Crook 1978) and for salt (Denton 1982; Beauchamp 1987), innate rejection of bitter tasting substances (Geldard 1972; Steiner 1977), other genetic contributions to taste sensitivity (Fischer et al. 1961; Glanville and Kaplan 1965; Jefferson and Erdman 1970; Hall et al. 1975; Davis 1978) and genetic influences on metabolic processes (Simoons 1969, 1970). Because biological factors are involved in every situation where food is selected and consumed, any comprehensive analysis of food preferences must clearly take account of them. On the other hand, the factors that determine which of the vast array of possible foodstuffs any one individual habitually selects are, it has been argued, mainly sociocultural. As Rozin has observed:

> there is no doubt that the best predictor of the food preferences, habits and attitudes of any particular human would be information about his ethnic group . . . rather than any biological measure that one might imagine. (Rozin 1982: 227)

The sociocultural practices that surround individuals serve to eliminate the need for protracted trial-and-error sampling, and establish for them which substances are 'foods'. These practices vary widely. Thus, for example, South American Indians eat monkeys, grubs, bees and headlice and Australian Aborigines relish insects (Farb and Armelagos 1980), all of which foodstuffs are absent from the European diet. Similarly, it is cultural practice that indicates acceptable combinations of foods (e.g. Europeans do not eat cake with steak), appropriate consumption times of particular foodstuffs (e.g. cereal for breakfast not lunch), and particular methods of preparation. It would clearly be very useful if we could harness the processes involved in achieving such cultural influence to enable children to eat healthy diets. For example, instead of restricting their consumption to only a few of the range of food items available to them (as is often the case in Western society), children could learn to eat a wide variety of foods and thereby maximise their opportunity for healthy development.

Our theoretical perspective

Out of a theoretical perspective combining contemporary work on learning and cognitive processes with the sociocultural perspectives of L. S. Vygotsky (1934/1987) and G.H. Mead (1934) we have sought to provide a new account of the social origins of language and its impact upon human learning (see Lowe 1979, 1983; Lowe, Horne and Higson 1987; Horne and Lowe 1996; Lowe and Horne 1996). According to this view, while we should expect Pavlovian and operant conditioning processes such as those that govern animal learning to also influence human behaviour, language is a social influence unique to human beings that transforms cognition and brings about a higher-order regulation of human behaviour through, for example, naming, verbal propositions and rules. We have recently (Horne and Lowe 1996; Lowe and Horne 1996) attempted to show how this higher order verbal regulation of human behaviour is established in young children.

A child born into a particular culture learns first to comprehend or respond in a culturally specified manner to the 'names' of culturally salient objects and events spoken by others; later, when control of the vocal musculature develops, the child learns to produce or vocalise those names herself upon encountering those specific objects. Thus, learning a name in its totality entails not only being able to make the appropriate vocalisation (e.g. 'spoon' on seeing a spoon) but also responding to one's own vocalisation in the sense of being able to reorient to the object and perform the particular culturally given behaviour that is apposite to it (e.g. picking the spoon up and bringing it to the mouth). Moreover, since the culture teaches the use of a particular name (e.g. 'vegetables') for a variety of objects (cabbages, beans, carrots), in learning a name a child learns a generalising relation between a class of objects and a particular spoken word. And, most important, thanks to this generalising relation the child, on being taught a new behaviour for one category member or exemplar, can *without being directly taught* extend that behaviour to all the other category members they have learned to call by the same name.

So it is that although food preferences may initially be established directly by Pavlovian or operant conditioning processes, once children become verbally adept they no longer respond directly to particular foods but, instead, to named 'classes' of foods. Although it may not be immediately obvious, this is as true of a food named, for example, 'a tomato' as of one named 'a vegetable', for tomatoes come in a wide variety of shapes, sizes, colours, varieties, degrees of sweetness, texture, etc., and can be prepared for eating in many different ways. But a child who, once verbally adept, has eaten a particular tomato that is named as such and has not liked the taste, or who, as often happens, has heard a friend say 'tomatoes are awful', may thenceforth reject all instances of that 'class' of food items, infinitely varied though they be. If an entire overarching class of important foods such as 'vegetables' is indicted in a similar vein the effects on a child's diet can clearly be dire. If we are to counter any such negative effects of the generalised relation inherent in children's verbal constructions about foods and eating it is essential that we learn how to harness that same generalising property to enable children instead to like and to eat a wide variety of healthy foods.

Changing food preferences

Confronted with the problem of how to change the food preferences of young children, our 'naïve' working assumption initially was that *almost any child can learn to eat almost any food*. That is, although there are some biological constraints, *eating is fundamentally learned behaviour*. Given that such is the case, children's food preferences should be malleable and subject to the influence of many of the verbal and other cognitive and learning factors intensively studied in experimental psychology over recent decades. Our series of experiments on food preferences, illustrated here by some of the studies we have conducted with five to seven-year-old children, sought to address these issues.

In brief, our initial strategy was (1) to select children who consistently refused to eat a range of vegetables and fruit; (2) to have their parents present to them at home a video featuring peers who extolled the virtues of eating these foods and promised rewards for eating them; and (3) to have parents deliver those rewards if the foods were eaten. In designing this video intervention we drew on an extensive psychological literature that shows that observational learning or 'peer modelling' can affect behaviour, particularly when (1) the models are perceived by the observer to be similar to them (Bandura 1977); (2) the models are of similar age or slightly older than the observer (Brody and Stoneman 1981); (3) the model's behaviour is rewarded (Bandura 1977; Deguchi 1984); and (4) the observer's imitation of the model is rewarded (Bandura 1989, and see Gewirtz and Stingle 1968; also Baer and Deguchi 1985). Although previous studies have sought to examine the impact of peer-modelling on children's food preferences, these have mainly been concerned with effects on children's verbal statements, rank ordering of preferences, and measures other than the amount of food consumed *per se* (Duncker 1938; Marinho 1942; Harper and Sanders 1975; Birch 1980; Brody and Stoneman 1981; but see Greer *et al.* 1991).

Television as a potentially important source of modelling and information about food preferences for young children has also been studied. This research has shown that television can be effective in increasing children's knowledge about which foods they should eat and in altering their stated preferences for particular foods (Goldberg, Gorn and Gibson 1978; Stoneman and Brody 1981; Gorn and Goldberg 1982, 1987; Peterson *et al.* 1984). Again, however, most of this work has not directly investigated the effects on their food consumption of what children have seen on television. One study which did explicitly set out to record food consumption as well as other measures of preference and attitudes (Peterson *et al.* 1984) showed that television programmes designed to teach children the nutritional value of particular foods were effective in changing five to six year-old children's nutritional knowledge but had no effect on what they ate or even on their stated preferences. In their study of groups of children aged four to five and nine to ten years, Jeffrey, McLellarn and Fox (1982) also reported that advertisements that promoted foods deemed to be of high nutritional value were ineffective in changing consumption of those foods; on the other hand, advertisements directed at foods considered to be of low nutritional value had a small but statistically significant effect on consumption of the latter. In summary, however, most previous studies have failed to address seriously the question of whether children's established eating habits can be altered to incorporate healthier options (e.g. fruit and vegetables) by the modelling of either real-life or televised peers and, certainly, none have reported long-lasting changes in food consumption as a result of such interventions.

Research on the role of rewards in altering food preferences has come up with conflicting results and conclusions. For many years the effectiveness of contingent rewards and other consequences in altering behaviour has been acknowledged in the general psychological literature. Although the processes governing these effects are complex (Lowe 1979; Lowe, Horne and Higson 1987), there is a substantial corpus of research, both in experimental and applied settings, that testifies to the efficacy of reward contingencies (Skinner 1969; Bellack, Hersen and Kazdin 1985). It is therefore surprising to read in much of the food-preferences literature that providing rewards for children's eating of a particular food results in a decrease, rather than an increase, in preference for the food in question (see, for example, Birch 1987; Rogers and Blundell 1990; Rozin 1990; Logue 1991: 110–111; Booth 1994: 78; Koivisto, Fellenius and Sjoden 1994). This view arises from relatively few experimental studies directly concerned with food preferences (see particularly Birch *et al.* 1982; 1984; Mikula 1989; Newman and Taylor 1992) but is linked to a broader literature on the 'detrimental' effects of rewards (e.g. Deci 1971, 1975; Lepper and Greene 1978; Lepper *et al.* 1982; Deci and Ryan 1985). Such research and the conclusions drawn from it have recently come under critical scrutiny (Dickinson 1989; Bernstein 1990; Flora 1990). The main charges are that not only is the work in question conducted under highly artificial circumstances, but it yields only weak and transient detrimental effects, if any at all, and uses procedures in which reward contingencies are poorly managed.

Within the context of the food-preferences literature, Horne *et al.* (1995) have argued that it is vital to consider not only the rewarding effect of presenting a food item (Food B) as a consequence for eating another food item (Food A), but also what the consequence may 'say' to the child about the experimenter's expectations and evaluations (i.e. that Food B is obviously 'better' than Food A). Indeed, under some circumstances, any reward for eating a particular food, particularly perhaps if it is given by a parent, may be construed negatively. The child may, for example, think that since they are not normally rewarded for eating the things they like, there must be something dislikeable about the food they will be rewarded for eating. Or perhaps they may resent the parent/reward-giver controlling their behaviour. As these arguments suggest, however, the conclusion that rewards *qua rewards* necessarily have detrimental effects on preference should be treated with some caution, especially in the light of findings from a wide range of studies conducted with children, some in 'real-life' clinical settings and others in laboratory contexts. These show that rewards can, in other circumstances, be a very effective means of increasing consumption of particular foods (Bernal 1972; Hatcher 1979; Siegal 1982; Riordan *et al.* 1984; Handen, Mandell and Russo 1986; Stark *et al.* 1986; Baer *et al.* 1987). However, it should be noted that the studies by Stark *et al.* (1986) and by Baer *et al.* (1987) also show that school nutrition campaigns, or rewarding children's promises to eat nutritious food, increase children's knowledge of what foods they should eat and declarations of intent to choose nutritious foods, but have little or no impact on which foods they actually eat.

This debate in the literature (for a review see Dowey 1996) does, however, provide some pointers as to how rewards should be used in interventions designed to alter children's food preferences. These are that (1) studies should as far as possible be conducted in real-life contexts; (2) rewards should be potent; (3) reward delivery should be criterion-based (i.e. related tightly to behavioural outcomes); (4) effects should be observed over time and not, as in most studies, just on one or two discrete occasions before and after the intervention; (5) instructions or rules given to the children should clearly specify the reward contingency; and (6) what children actually eat should be recorded rather than just what they tell an experimenter they might eat or prefer.

How rewards affect food preferences and how rewards interact with the effects of peer-modelling, either in real life or via television, clearly remain empirical questions. The series of experiments we next briefly summarise were directed at exploring these issues and incorporated all the design features outlined above.

The effects of a video-based peer-modelling and reward intervention on children's food preferences: Experiment 1 – Specific food names

This study was designed to investigate the relative impact on children's consumption of previously refused foods of (1) repeated visual exposure to those foods; and (2) a video-based peer-modelling and reward intervention in which child actors modelled consumption of specifically named foods, instructed the viewer to eat those foods, and offered them rewards for doing so.

Method

Design
Much of our work employs single-subject research designs (see Sidman 1960; Kazdin 1982). These designs require, for each subject, repeated measures of dependent variables (e.g. amount of target food eaten) before and after the introduction of experimental interventions. A particular strength of such designs for research on the psychology of food preferences is that they provide, for every experimental subject, repeated measures of preferences for specific foods throughout the time-course of their acquisition and maintenance. In the multiple-baseline design used here, the introduction of interventions is staggered over time between each subject and across different foods. The design thus controls for the amount of pre-intervention visual exposure to the foods presented in the context of the study and for order effects of the intervention across three different categories of foods, yielding several

replications of the effects of the independent variables on the dependent variable, namely, the children's eating of the foods they have previously refused.

Subjects and Setting

There were four children (three girls and a boy) in Experiment 1. The children (as in all the studies reported here) were between five and seven years old and were recruited, via local schools, on the basis of parental responses to a written request for children to participate; only children with a reported history of consistently refusing to eat several fruits and vegetables were selected. The studies were conducted in each child's home where, to enable naturalistic observation of behaviour during mealtimes, video cameras were installed out of the view of the child. To maintain the real-life quality or 'ecological validity' of the study, the children never directly encountered any members of the research team; both the operation of the video at mealtimes and the reward presentations were implemented by their parents.

Foods

With parental assistance, six reliably refused foods (two vegetables, two fruits and two pulses) were identified for each child. These foods included celery, broccoli, coleslaw, cauliflower, Brussels sprouts, kiwi fruit, guava, mango, lychee, blackeye beans, butter beans and chickpeas. Parents were asked not to present these foods at times other than those specified by the experimenters and were trained to estimate the amount of target food eaten using an observational scale graduated as follows: (1) 0; (2) up to 25 per cent; (3) >25 to 50 per cent; (4) >50 to 75 per cent and (5) >75 to 100 per cent. The video recordings enabled these measures to be validated by the experimenter and also permitted inter-observer reliability to be established.

Procedure

Baseline 1: In the first baseline phase of the experiment (see Figure 4.1), each child was presented daily with a different food pair drawn from the six previously refused foods (i.e. either two vegetables, two fruits, or two pulses) for five days per week. These foods (approximately 30 ml of each) were presented to the child, and to any other members of the family present, as part of the regular family evening meal. One food in each pair served as the 'target' food (i.e. was subject to the interventions) and the other served as a control food. The order of presentation of the three pairs of foods was different across the four children, but remained constant for each child throughout the study. The duration of Baseline 1 also differed across children, lasting for between six and ten presentations of each pair of foods, following which the first intervention phase was introduced.

Intervention 1: Before the evening meal on day 1 of the video peer-modelling and reward-intervention phase, each child was shown one of a series of short video films in which a group of older children, the 'Food Dudes', enthusiastically ate one of the specifically named target

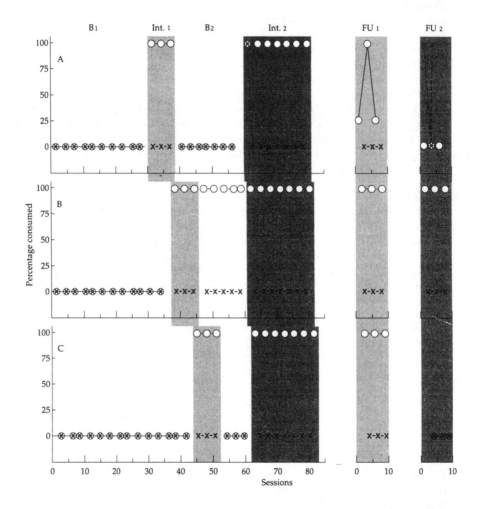

Figure 4.1 For child SR in Experiment 1, percentage consumption of each of the three pairs of foods, vegetables (A), fruit (B), and pulses (C), when presented at each evening meal. This shows consumption during the main phases of the Experiment: Baseline 1 (B1), Intervention 1 (Int.1), Intervention 2 (Int.2), two-month Follow-Up (FU1) and six-month Follow-Up (FU2). Target foods (i.e. celery (A), kiwi (B), and blackeye beans (C)) are indicated by open circles, and control foods (i.e. coleslaw (A), lychee (B), and butterbeans (C)), by crosses. For details of experimental procedures and phases of the experiment, see text, Experiment 1.

foods and exhorted the viewer to do likewise in order to help the Dudes in their struggle against the evil 'Junk Food Junta'. In return, the children were promised gifts (e.g. Food Dude caps, lunch boxes, T-shirts) and membership of the prestigious Food Dudes' Club. After the video, during the evening meal, each child was presented with the target food featured in the film (e.g. celery), and its control pair member (e.g. broccoli). Reward was contingent on the child eating 75 per cent of the target food. How much of the control food was eaten was also monitored. On subsequent intervention days, before watching each target food video, the child was given a reward if 75 per cent consumption of the target food had occurred during the previous session in which that food was presented. Each pair of foods was presented to each child in this manner on three separate occasions.

Baseline 2: Baseline conditions (food presentation in the absence of the Food Dude videos) were then resumed for at least three further presentations of each food pair.

Intervention 2: Following this a second intervention phase was introduced. Presentations of each food pair occurred only once per week and the children were notified by the Food Dudes that if they ate the target foods over the following seven weeks they would earn a special family outing of their choice. The children monitored their own progress by placing a sticker on a monitoring card provided by the Food Dudes whenever they ate the target food; parents checked the accuracy of their child's record. The promised reward was given if the child ate 75 per cent of the target foods during the seven weeks. Since all the children succeeded in achieving this, they all received tickets for their chosen outing within days of completing this phase.

Follow-ups: The long-term effects of the experimental interventions were investigated in two follow-up phases, after two-month and six-month intervals, during each of which baseline conditions were reinstated; that is, the children were simply presented with the three food pairs, each of which was presented on three occasions over three weeks as part of the usual evening meal. There was nothing to indicate to the child that a 'test' of any kind was in progress.

Results

To illustrate the general findings we present consumption data, for a single child, SR, over the course of the study (Figure 4.1) and for the group of children averaged across each phase (Figure 4.2). Figure 4.1 shows that, following several presentations of all six foods to SR in Baseline, the video-based intervention was first (Section A) introduced for celery, with coleslaw as the control food, and second (Section B) for kiwi fruit, with lychee as the control food, and third (Section C) for blackeye beans, with butter beans as the control. These data show that none of the six previously refused foods, target or control, was eaten during the baseline sessions. As

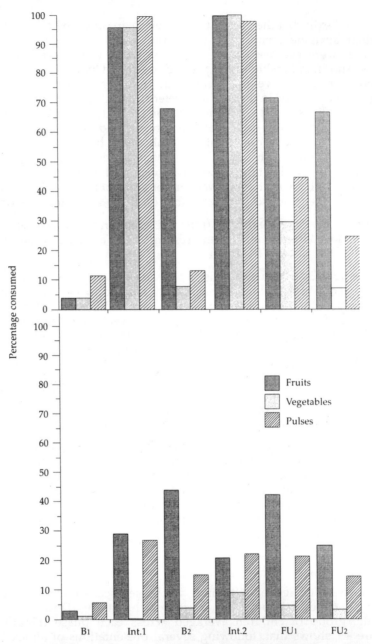

Figure 4.2 Summary data for consumption of target foods (upper section) and control foods (lower section) during Experiment 1. This shows group mean consumption of fruits, vegetables, and pulses during Baseline 1 (B1), Intervention 1 (Int.1), second Baseline (B2), Intervention 2 (Int.2), two-month Follow-Up (FU1) and six-month Follow-Up (FU2).

the first intervention was introduced for each target food in turn, consumption of each rose immediately to 100 per cent for the duration of this phase; none of the control foods were ever eaten. When the intervention was withdrawn in the second baseline, consumption of celery and blackeye beans fell to zero but consumption of kiwi fruit remained at 100 per cent. When the second intervention was introduced the child once again ate all of the target foods on every occasion they were presented during this seven-week phase. With the exception of the first session, when coleslaw was eaten, no control foods were consumed.

At the two-month follow-up the child ate all the kiwi fruit and blackeye beans and averaged 50 per cent consumption of celery. At the six-month follow up, while the child still ate all the kiwi fruit, consumption of both of celery and blackeye beans was at baseline levels; for reasons that remain to be explained, the child ate 100 per cent of the control vegetable, coleslaw, in two of the three sessions of this follow-up.

Figure 4.2 (top panel) shows that for all four children consumption of the target foods in Baseline 1 was uniformly low, but rose to almost 100 per cent throughout the first intervention. Withdrawal of Intervention 1 resulted in a marked decline in the amount of vegetables and of pulses eaten but mean fruit consumption remained high. When Intervention 2 was introduced, consumption of all three target foods rose again to almost 100 per cent and remained so throughout the seven weeks of this phase. At the two-month follow-up, consumption of target foods was highest for fruits (79 per cent), followed by pulses (50 per cent) and then vegetables (33 per cent). After six months, fruit consumption remained high (75 per cent) while that of pulses and vegetables declined to 31 per cent and 10 per cent, respectively.

Levels of consumption of control foods were also low in Baseline 1 (Figure 4.2, bottom panel) and rose during Intervention 1 in the case of fruit and pulses, but not vegetables. Fruit consumption remained up in Baseline 2 and the follow-up phases, though not at levels comparable to those observed for the target fruits. Consumption of the control pulses remained above 20 per cent through to the final follow-up while that of the control vegetables remained at relatively low levels throughout.

The children's behaviour at evening meals was recorded on video in most phases of the study, including their spontaneous comments and expressions of preference. Thus, for example, in the first baseline phase when SR (see Figure 4.1) was presented with kiwi fruit, she said 'I don't like kiwi . . . I hate kiwi, it's really horrible' and she pushed the bowl of kiwi fruit away. This contrasts with SR's reactions to kiwi fruit following the introduction of Intervention 1 when she remarked that 'These (kiwi) are nice' and was caught trying to take extra kiwi fruit for herself from her mother's fruit store. Similar changes in spontaneously expressed liking for some of the target foods were recorded for other children.

Discussion

The most striking finding of this study was that the interventions resulted immediately in the children's eating all targeted foods at close to maximum levels. These foods were vegetables, pulses and fruits which the children had consistently refused to eat over many previous weeks despite their regular presentation during the family evening meal. Repeated visual exposure therefore had little or no effect on the consumption of these foods. However, once they had seen the modelling and reward video for a target food the children proceeded to eat that food: this was true on all ten occasions that any one of the target foods was presented over the nine weeks of the intervention phases.

The effectiveness of the video-modelling and reward intervention was clearly demonstrated in the marked difference in consumption during Intervention 1 as compared with that in Baseline 1 and Baseline 2.

It should be noted that, although in the first intervention phase a video was presented each evening prior to target-food presentation and performance was directly rewarded (i.e. by T-shirts, caps, etc.), in the second intervention phase no video was shown and the only immediate rewards for food consumption were the self-monitoring stickers used by the child; the main reward was the Food Dudes' promise of a family outing some time in the future should the child meet the food-consumption contingencies. Nevertheless, this second intervention was extremely effective, demonstrating that as long as they are instructed about the relationship between a particular behaviour and its reward, linguistically competent human beings, unlike other animals, are able to perform that behaviour even when the consequence is delayed, as in this case, for several weeks (Lowe 1979; Horne and Lowe 1993).

Another notable feature of these results was that although all the foodstuffs had similar baseline consumption levels, the after-effects of the interventions on levels for fruit were much stronger than for either pulses or vegetables (Figure 4.2, Follow-ups). Thus, although consumption of fruits was rewarded in only three trials in Intervention 1, this was nevertheless sufficient to establish very high levels of consumption when the intervention was removed; similarly, fruit continued to be eaten at high levels in the follow-ups. Why particular foods should be differently affected by the interventions in this way and, indeed, what governs the maintenance over time of changes in consumption patterns, are the obvious questions raised here.

One clue comes from the literature on 'taste exposure'. Findings from a number of studies have indicated that if subjects repeatedly taste a particular food this leads to enhanced preference for that food (Birch and Marlin 1982; Pliner 1982; Birch et al. 1987). The main challenge, however, is to bring about that repeated tasting. If, as a result of an intervention such as ours, children do repeatedly taste particular foods, this repetition may enable the *intrinsic* rewarding properties of these foods to maintain consumption even in the absence of *extrinsic* rewards. This may depend on the number of taste exposures provided and some foods may require different amounts of taste exposure. If, for example, as some have argued, children do have an innate preference for sugar (Desor, Maller and Turner 1973; Crook 1978; Logue 1991: 120), then fruits, with their higher sugar content, may well have enhanced intrinsic reward value over pulses or vegetables for this age group. Vegetables and pulses may therefore require more taste exposures than fruit before the inherently rewarding consequences of consuming them take effect and the children 'acquire the taste'. To our knowledge, no systematic studies have been conducted to investigate with human beings the number of taste exposures required to establish preferences for different types of foods.

We return to these issues in discussing the remaining studies and to the more general question of how permanent changes in food preference can be established. In the present study only ten tastings of each of the target foods were rewarded, which appeared not to have been sufficient to maintain high levels of consumption of some of the foods up to the six-month follow-up (see Figure 4.2). In the next study to be reported, we increased the number of taste exposures.

Another limitation in the effectiveness of the interventions employed in this study was that although the impact on consumption of the target foods was great, there was little 'generalisation' (i.e. spread of intervention effects) to consumption of the control foods, particularly vegetables and pulses. To have maximum practical utility, it would be highly desirable if the interventions could be designed to alter preferences, not just for a few specifically named foods, but for the broader named categories 'fruit' and 'vegetables' that together embrace the many different foods that form the basis of a healthy diet. This was the goal of our next study.

Experiment 2 – General category names

The procedure was the same as in Experiment 1, except that (1) in the video and modelling interventions, the Food Dudes referred to general food categories (e.g. 'eat all *vegetables*', 'eat all *fruit*') rather than to specifically named food (e.g. 'eat broccoli', 'eat guava'); (2) there was a longer intervention phase, designed to provide more taste exposures; (3) the number of foods was increased to test for the generalisation of intervention effects across the categories of 'fruit' and 'vegetables'.

Method
Four new children (three girls, one boy) participated in the study. Each was presented with 12 foods. For three children these were eight vegetables and four fruits; for the fourth these were 12 vegetables.

Procedure
Baseline 1: The duration of this phase varied across children. At the evening meal each child was given a randomly determined selection of three of the 12 target foods (two vegetables and one fruit, for three of the children; and three vegetables for the fourth), until each of the target

foods had been presented on at least three occasions (i.e. a minimum of 12 sessions took place).

Intervention 1: The video-modelling and reward intervention was then introduced, targetting, for two of the children, fruits first and then vegetables, and vice versa for the others. During this phase, rewards were contingent on the child's eating 75 per cent or more of the total target foods presented each evening. This phase was continued for each child until criterion consumption in each of the target categories (vegetables or fruits) had been achieved in four sessions.

Baseline 2: Baseline conditions were reinstated for a minimum of five sessions.

Intervention 2: From the 12 foods, four vegetables and two fruits (or, for the fourth child, six vegetables) were randomly selected, with replacement if one of these foods had not been consumed on at least one occasion during Intervention 1; these six foods were assigned to a 'high-exposure' food group. The remaining six foods constituted the 'low-exposure' group. Then, in each of 30 successive sessions, the six-high-exposure foods (three each session) were presented to each child; a token reward system was employed as in Experiment 1 (Intervention 2).

Generalisation test: Once Intervention 2 was completed, the six low-exposure foods were presented under baseline conditions for six sessions. This enabled a comparison to be made of consumption of the six low-exposure foods pre- and post-Intervention 2 (which was targeted at the other six foods).

Follow-ups: As in Experiment 1, the long-term effects of the experimental interventions were investigated after two-month and six-month intervals.

Results

Figure 4.3 shows one child's (JK) consumption of vegetables throughout all phases of the experiment. Consumption was minimal throughout the 25 sessions of Baseline 1 but when Intervention 1 was introduced, increased to 100 per cent on four of the six sessions of this phase (and was 50 per cent or more in the remaining two sessions). When Intervention 1 ended, consumption declined to Baseline 1 levels over the course of five sessions. The token reward intervention introduced for the six high-exposure vegetables resulted in above criterion levels of consumption on all of the 30 occasions in this phase. During the following Generalisation Test phase, consumption of the low-exposure vegetables (under baseline conditions) averaged 58 per cent, as compared with 25 per cent in the Baseline 2 phase for this child. Consumption of the high and low-exposure vegetables was similar during the two-month (means 42 per cent and 44 per cent, respectively) and the six-month follow-up (63 per cent and 52 per cent, respectively).

Group mean consumption of all 12 foods during Baseline 1, Intervention 1 and at follow-ups is shown in Figure 4.4. During

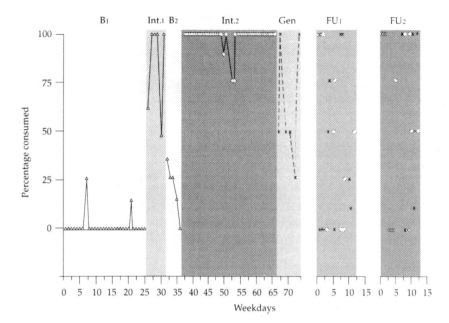

Figure 4.3 For child JK in Experiment 2, percentage consumption of vegetables during Baseline 1 (B1), Intervention 1 (Int.1), Baseline 2 (B2), Intervention 2 (Int.2), Generalisation Test (Gen), two-month Follow-Up (FU1) and six-month Follow-Up (FU2). Open triangles indicate consumption of any two of the eight previously refused vegetables; open circles indicate consumption of any of the four "high exposure" vegetables (i.e. those presented during Int.2); crosses show consumption of any of the four "low exposure" vegetables (i.e. those not presented during Int.2). For details of experimental procedure and phases of experiment, see text, Experiment 2.

baseline, very little fruit or vegetables were eaten. When Intervention 1 was introduced, consumption increased to 70 per cent for fruits and 65 per cent for vegetables. At the two-month follow-up, fruit consumption was 75 per cent while vegetable consumption was 40 per cent. At the final (six-month) follow-up, fruit consumption was maintained at 75 per cent and vegetable consumption was 50 per cent.

A breakdown of consumption for the foods designated 'high-exposure' (upper panel) and 'low-exposure' (lower panel) during the main phases of the study, is shown in Figure 4.5. Comparison of the group means across Intervention 1 and Baseline 2, shows that the allocation of foods to each of these two groups (following Intervention 1) was such that consumption was greatest for the foods that were later to be given high-exposure in Intervention 2. Throughout Intervention 2 consumption of fruit in the high-exposure condition was at maximum levels and this was maintained after two months and then six months had elapsed since the intervention. Intervention 2 boosted vegetable consumption to 83 per cent, and it was still at 58 per cent six months later.

71

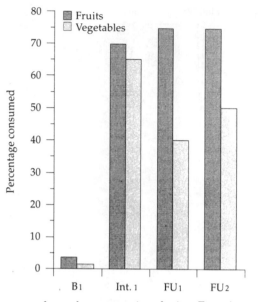

Figure 4.4 Summary data of consumption during Experiment 2. This shows group mean consumption of fruits and vegetables during the Baseline 1 (B1), Intervention 1 (Int.1), two-month Follow-Up (FU1) and six-month Follow-Up (FU2).

When, following Intervention 2 with the high-exposure foods, the remaining low-exposure foods were presented in the Generalisation Test phase (lower panel), levels of consumption of fruit and vegetables were 50 and 43 per cent respectively, compared to 44 and 18 per cent respectively in Baseline 2. This suggests that there was a strong generalisation effect with vegetables.

At the final six-month follow-up, much of this improvement was sustained. Because of the differing initial rates of consumption (e.g. in Intervention 1 and Baseline 2), direct comparison of the effectiveness of the high-exposure and low-exposure conditions is difficult. However, if we take increase in consumption at final follow-up in relation to performance in Baseline 2, the gain in consumption of high-exposure fruit and vegetables was 36 and 33 per cent respectively; this compares to 6 and 24 per cent respectively, for the low-exposure foods.

Discussion

This study confirms and extends the findings of Experiment 1; video-based peer-modelling and rewards are, in combination, a very potent means of increasing children's consumption of fruit and vegetables and effect long-term changes in eating practices. This study shows that the intervention need not entail a laborious successive targeting of individual foods; changes in children's level of consumption of a

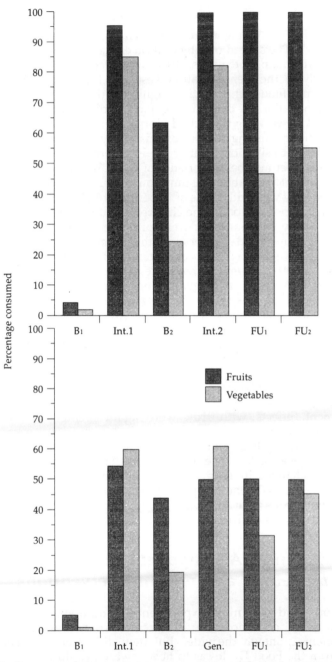

Figure 4.5 Summary data comparing consumption of the high-exposure foods (upper panel) and low-exposure foods (lower panel) in each phase of Experiment 3: Baseline 1 (B1), Intervention 1 (Int.1), Baseline 2 (B2), Intervention 2 (Int.2), Generalisation Test (Gen), two-month Follow-Up (FU1) and six-month Follow-Up (FU2).

whole category of foods can be effected simultaneously if the children are rewarded for eating foods that share a *generic* label (e.g. 'fruit', 'vegetables'). The spread of intervention effects across the foods in each of the two main categories, fruit and vegetables, was indicated particularly in the Generalisation Test and follow-up phases for the low-exposure foods. This finding highlights the importance of naming and categorisation in determining food preferences in humans (see Horne and Lowe 1996; Lowe and Horne 1996).

Another encouraging feature of this study was the maintenance of the effects up to six months after the interventions. For example, even though a greater number of varieties of vegetables was presented in this study, levels of vegetable consumption at final follow-up (50 per cent) compared very well with those of Experiment 1 (10 per cent). In the case of the high-exposure foods, the children's 100 per cent consumption of fruits on every occasion they were presented over the many months of Intervention 2 and follow-ups (the latter conducted without an intervention of any sort) obviously could not be bettered.

The findings also suggest that increased numbers of rewarded taste exposures may result in longer lasting intervention effects, the high-exposure foods in this study showing a greater gain in consumption levels by the final follow-up than the low-exposure foods. Clearly, further research is required to confirm this suggestion and to unpack the factors (e.g. taste, rewards, and children's observations of their own eating behaviours) that may contribute to the effect.

In Experiment 1 it was found that the enduring effects of the interventions were greater with fruit than with vegetables. Though long-term effects with vegetables were substantial in the present experiment, effects with fruit were again greater, confirming the findings of Experiment 1.

Though the modelling and reward procedure was highly effective, the particular aspects of the intervention that were critical in bringing about the changes in food consumption remained to be identified. Could it be that only one component, either peer modelling or rewards, is sufficient on its own to establish the effects that we observed here? This question was addressed in the next study.

Experiment 3 – A component analysis of the video peer modelling and reward interventions

This study had two main experimental conditions. In the first, the 'reward only' condition, the children were not, as they were in Experiment 2, shown the video but they did receive instructions by letter from the Food Dudes as to how rewards could be earned. In the second, 'video only' condition, the children were shown the video of the Food Dudes, as in Experiment 2, but without the brief sequence which promised rewards, and no rewards were given to them.

Eight new children (five boys and three girls) participated, with four being assigned to each condition. For all children the Baseline 1 phase was similar to that in Experiment 2; the foods selected for each child were eight vegetables and four fruits. For two of the children, the Reward Only intervention which incorporated a reward contingency similar to that of Experiment 2 (Intervention 1) was introduced following Baseline, first for vegetables and then for fruit; this order was reversed for the other two children in this condition.

Similarly, for the remaining four children the 'video only' intervention was introduced following Baseline, the order of targeting of fruit and vegetables being counter-balanced across the children.

Results

To enable comparisons to be made of the effectiveness of reward only, video only, and combined reward and video interventions respectively, Figure 4.6 presents group mean consumption in the Baseline and Intervention phases of each condition in Experiment 3, together with the consumption data from the combined intervention in Experiment 2 (Baseline 1 and Intervention 1). This shows that the children ate virtually none of the fruit and vegetables throughout the Baseline phases of either Experiments 2 or 3. Although the Reward Alone intervention had substantial effects on fruit consumption, the effect on vegetable consumption was small (9 per cent) compared with the large effects (65 per cent) achieved with the combined intervention in Experiment 2. The video alone intervention was the least successful of all, with consumption levels of 3 per cent during the intervention compared with 2 per cent in Baseline. Thus, video-modelling and instructions without rewards appear to have little, if any, impact on the consumption of previously rejected foods.

Of the three interventions represented in Figure 4.6, it was the combined video modelling and reward procedure that produced the greatest amount of behaviour change. Clearly, these differences between procedures need to be further investigated with larger groups of children.

General discussion

We began this programme of research with what we thought would turn out to be a naïve working assumption: that is, that almost any child can eat almost any food and that we could use known learning principles to bring about major shifts in eating behaviour. In the light of the studies reported here and others we have conducted subsequently, that assumption remains remarkably intact. All children who experienced either form of the combined video-modelling and reward intervention (i.e. Specific Food or General Category Names) showed major increases in consumption of foods that previously they had consistently refused to eat. Particularly in the General Category Names

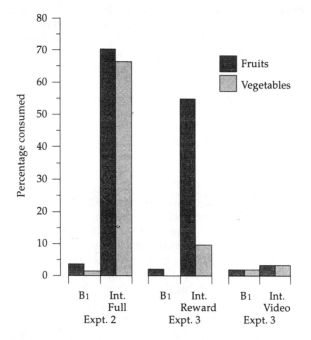

Figure 4.6 Summary data for consumption of fruit and vegetables during baseline and intervention phases of Experiments 2 and 3. Consumption is shown for Baseline 1 (B1) in each of the experiments, and for Intervention 1 (Int.Full) in Experiment 2 (Expt.2)), the Reward Only intervention (Int.Reward) in Experiment 3 (Expt.3) and the Video Only intervention (Int.Video) in Experiment 3.

intervention (Experiment 2), the effects were immediate: almost all of the previously refused foods were eaten and this continued over several weeks of the intervention; the effects generalised across a range of fruit and vegetables and, to a large extent, were maintained after six months had elapsed since the end of the intervention. Effects of this magnitude and duration on food consumption, established within the naturalistic context of the home environment, have not been reported previously in the literature. The findings indicate that the eating practices of children, at least in the age range five to seven years, are extremely malleable and subject to strong influence by sociocultural factors.

How these factors operate and how they interact with biological determinants is a central issue. The present studies showed that although, in the case of fruit and vegetables alike, the children's levels of baseline consumption were low, it was easier to establish long-term increases in consumption of the former. As we noted in our discussion of Experiment 1, this may be partly the result of innate biologically driven preferences for the sweetness characteristic of fruit. Nevertheless, vegetables, like other foods, do have intrinsic rewarding properties of their own, which children may come to appreciate given sufficient taste experience of them. What is critical is that we devise effective strategies to overcome children's initial refusals or reluctance to taste so that the innately rewarding characteristics of fruit and vegetables come to be, in the long term, determinants in themselves of children's eating habits.

Such 'educating of the taste buds' may be the result of a concatenation of biological and sociocultural factors. For once a child comes repeatedly to eat particular foods, not only do they gain access to the biologically rewarding characteristics of those foods, but regular eating of them cannot but have repercussions for 'commentaries' consequent on their behaviour. Thus, a child formerly described by parents and themselves as one who 'does not like vegetables', is now one who 'eats vegetables'. This new 'self-construct' consists of new verbal rules to govern their eating behaviour and they are likely to bring about long-lasting behaviour change (see Lowe 1979; Lowe, Horne and Higson 1987; Horne and Lowe 1996).

That verbal factors are potent determinants of preference is supported by the results from Experiment 2 that indicated good generalisation and maintenance of effects via category names (i.e. 'fruit' and 'vegetables'). Following Intervention 2 with the high-exposure foods, the low-exposure foods were consumed at high levels in the absence of any reward for doing so. Given that each of the low-exposure foods was generally not tasted more than once or twice in Intervention 1, and in the Generalisation Test was not even presented accompanying the high-exposure foods, then transfer of the Intervention 2 effects almost certainly occurred via the category names (cf. Experiment 1). Thus, though in Intervention 2 reward was procedurally contingent on the consumption of particular foods, it was in fact the consumption of named classes of foods (i.e. 'fruits' and 'vegetables') that was rewarded. This is an efficient means of extending preference to foods that have hardly ever been tasted but have the same category name as those that have.

It follows that to effect a wide-ranging change in diet it is important to ensure that children have enjoyable and rewarding experiences with exemplars of broad classes of foods and that rewards operate on the explicitly named categories. But how can such experiences be brought about? Clearly, if we wish to influence children to try fruits and vegetables that they normally refuse to eat, then simply providing peer modelling as in the video only condition of Experiment 3 may have little or no effect. Nor, as we indicated in the introduction, is there any good evidence in the literature that shows otherwise.

In the light of the psychological literature on food preferences, though not of more general psychological research, perhaps the most surprising outcome of the present series of studies has been the demonstrable effectiveness of rewards. Even in the reward only condition of Experiment 3 in which the modelling video was absent there were substantial effects on fruit consumption, though much less with vegetables. However, as indicated in the introduction, it is the context in which reward is delivered, and what it 'means' to the individual that may be critical in determining its effectiveness. In most cases, rewards to verbally competent human beings are not merely 'rewards' but events that are categorised and incorporated into that individual's cognitive and linguistic framework (Luria 1961: 22; Lowe 1979). Indeed, it is possible to envisage a range of situations when attempts by parents, psychologists and others directly to 'bribe' or persuade children to eat a food may have counter-productive effects, particularly if the reward carries with it the implication that eating the food is not of value in and of itself. This may have been the case in previous research on this topic (Birch *et al.* 1982; Birch, Marlin and Rotter 1984; Newman and Taylor 1992). The context in which rewards were employed in our study differed markedly. In the combined video-modelling and reward interventions, the intrinsic virtues and enjoyment of eating the target food were described by the Food Dudes who also provided additional incentives, such as Food Dude Club membership and prizes, for success in eating these foods. Even in the reward only condition, rewards were prizes won from a group calling themselves the Food Dudes. The 'symbolic' context of reward delivery was, thus, invariably positive and could not easily be construed as indicating that eating the target foods was a low-value activity.

Our finding that the effect of the combined reward and video-modelling intervention was greater than the sum of its parts is consistent with this analysis and has major implications for how television and rewards can be most effectively used to alter children's food preferences. Clearly, each of these two elements potentiates the other. In our study, television-modelling unsupported by rewards was found to be largely ineffective, a finding that concurs with other researchers' observations in this domain (Baer and Deguchi 1985). The video sequences, on the other hand, set the context in which rewards occurred and gave to them and to the behaviour in question (i.e. eating fruit and vegetables) *positive value*. In the light of our findings, it is imperative that the role of rewards in altering food preferences should be reassessed by researchers in the field. It is, after all, an odd irony that the field has largely ignored one of the most potent social influences on what children will eat. (In this regard it is also essential that any future work on reward effects be conducted by researchers who are fully acquainted with the principles and techniques of contingency management. See Kazdin 1982; Dickinson 1989; Bernstein 1990; Flora 1990.)

Another key issue for future work concerns measures of food choice or preference. A great deal of existing research in the field has not directly observed or measured what people actually eat over time but instead has relied on asking them about their preferences or to report what they eat. This may be easier research to conduct than recording consumption but it makes assumptions about a correspondence between what people say and what they do that other investigators have shown to be unwarranted (Nisbett and Wilson 1977; Baer *et al.* 1985; Deacon and Konarski 1987). The problem is compounded by the fact that so much of the work is obviously an 'experiment' in which the researcher conducts a specific intervention (e.g. providing information about why Food A should be eaten) and then asks questions or conducts a preference-ranking test of the foods in question. In such contrived situations children may, for example, (1) deliberately mislead the researcher, (2) provide the response they think the experimenter would like to hear (e.g. 'I would choose Food A'), or (3) respond as they would wish themselves to respond. Thus, if the message is 'eat Food A because it is healthy', then they may want to believe that they will indeed eat Food A. Whether they will or not, is the crux of the question and the one on which a great deal of health education and other research in this domain has foundered. A number of studies has shown that while interventions may succeed in altering children's knowledge of what is healthy to eat or what they say they will eat, this may bear little relation to what they do (Jeffrey, McLellarn and Fox 1982; Peterson *et al.* 1984; Stark *et al.* 1986; Baer *et al.* 1987). Thus, indices of food preference that exclude direct measures of consumption may be of little value; what people actually eat must be the basic datum. It is also important that behaviour is measured unobtrusively and, as far as possible, under naturalistic conditions while maintaining methodological rigour. We believe this was a distinctive merit of the procedure employed in the present studies where mealtime behaviour was video-recorded and the children never encountered the researchers.

To focus on what is eaten as the basic datum is not, however, to ignore the importance of people's intentions or what they say about food. Indeed, we have argued throughout that verbal rules and categorisations of foods are critical determinants. The task for researchers and agencies concerned with bringing about improvements to diet, however, is to forge a close correspondence between 'good intentions' or what people say to themselves (and others) about what they are going to eat, and what they will actually eat.

Future directions

The scope and opportunities for future research that adopts this perspective are great. The work reported here had relatively few children in each study and larger-scale replications are required. First, these could test the reliability of the present findings. (It is also possible that for some individual children with, for example, specific allergies or other clinical disorders, the present procedures may need to be adapted or used within an overall therapeutic framework.) Second, if a video and reward intervention, such as that employed here, is to be used to effect large-scale changes in the eating patterns of children, then it must be adapted for use with greater numbers. We (along with Michael Bowdery and Christine Egerton) are currently conducting research along these lines in local schools, the initial results of which are in agreement with those obtained from the home-based research reported here. It will also be necessary to investigate similar procedures with children of differing ages, as well as teenagers and adults. For example, using a video and reward intervention modified for this age group, we (with Janette Woolner) have conducted studies with three to four year- olds, which show similarities, but also some differences, with the results from five to seven-year-olds, suggesting that interventions need to be carefully tailored to suit the level of psychological development of the children. Another area that merits investigation, and in which we (with Paul Fleming) have conducted several studies, is the development of food preferences in early infancy and how they are affected by increased taste exposure to a range of novel fruit and vegetables. This work should reveal much about the genesis of eating habits and how they are affected by social and cognitive factors.

Practical implications

We believe that it is all too easy for researchers to get lost in the conceptual fog of what 'food choice' means. It might also be easy for government and other agencies to throw up their hands in despair at their inability, through health education and other measures, to have any significant influence on the nation's diet. In this regard perhaps one of the main contributions of this chapter is that it serves to demystify food choice. We accept that there is a complex interplay of factors involved in any one individual's food preferences and aversions, and that there is a vast array of psychological, sociological, anthropological, technological and economic evidence that can usefully be brought to bear on the question of how people come to eat the foods they do. However, what our studies show is that, if we focus on what children actually eat and some of the key cultural 'drivers' of this behaviour, it is not difficult to devise the means to get children to eat a range of healthy foods as a matter of routine. It is because there are so many other agencies at work, acting either wittingly or unwittingly, to influence children to eat diets which are not nutritious, that this approach is so desperately needed. The basic methodology exists; it is now a matter of further development and application on a wider scale to enable parents, schools and others concerned with children's diet to be effective in this domain. The aim of such a programme should be to influence the nation's children to eat a wide variety of fruit and vegetables. The benefits that this would yield in terms of health gain and quality of life could be very great (Gillman 1996; Key et al. 1996).

Acknowledgements

The research reported in this paper was co-funded by Unilever. We are indebted to Pat Barron, Christine Egerton and Gareth Horne for their help in the preparation of the manuscript, and to Pat Lowe for her editorial skills. We are particularly grateful to the school staff, parents and children themselves who participated in these studies.

CHAPTER 5

Consumer theory and food choice in economics, with an example

Trevor Young, Michael Burton and Richard Dorsett

Introduction

Economics is about scarcity, and consumer theory addresses how scarcity affects the individual consumer's choices. The theory focuses on the purchase decision, the outcome of the consumer trying to attain the most preferred selection of goods, given a set of constraints. For the most part no distinction is drawn between purchase and consumption. Indeed the distinction is only important for the economist when dealing with a durable, storable good (such as a refrigerator), in which case we distinguish the purchase of the good from the consumption of its services. We are also not concerned with desire or need *per se*, but rather with effective demand in the market place, i.e. the quantities of goods and services that the individual consumer is willing and *able* to purchase per unit of time under given market conditions. As will become clear, the economist's approach to consumer choice, of food or other products, is defined within very narrow bounds. This lends the theory predictive ability but at the expense of some generality and perhaps of meaningful interaction with the other social sciences.

The economic analysis of food choice has a long history, dating back at least to the work of Ernst Engel in the mid-nineteenth century. This chapter provides a brief overview of the theory and application of demand analysis, with specific reference to the demand for food. First, the important distinction is drawn between preferences and constrained choice. We then review how economists approach empirical work on demand, with particular attention to the way preferences are handled in applied work. Finally, we present an example of empirical analysis in this area, drawing on our own work in 'The Nation's Diet' Programme.

The theory of consumer behaviour

Rationality

The economist's approach to choice is based on the concept of a 'rational' individual attempting to maximise their welfare by choosing the most preferred outcome from a limited set of options. Rationality in this context can be viewed as 'action well-suited to achieve one's goals'. That is to say, it presupposes the prior existence of goals aimed at, as well as systematic, purposeful action by the consumer in their pursuit. Importantly, consumers' choice is *constrained*, principally by a limited budget but also by other factors such as time availability, and the legal and institutional framework.

Rationality can be interpreted in a number of ways but two forms have received particular attention in economics (Frank 1994). Under the 'present-aim standard' consumers act efficiently in pursuit of their goals *whatever these goals happen to be*. In this very broad approach all sorts of behaviour (e.g. altruistic, selfish and even self-destructive) may be viewed as rational, provided only that the consumer strives to meet these objectives at minimum cost. Alternatively, a more restrictive interpretation is adopted by many economists, namely the 'self-interest standard' in which it is assumed consumers behave opportunistically and their motives accord with their material interests. This view is exemplified by Adam Smith's well-known assertion: 'it is not from the benevolence of the butcher, the brewer, or the baker, that we expect our dinner, but from their regard to their own interest' (Smith 1904, Book I, Chapter 2: 16). The distinction between the two standards can become somewhat blurred, however, when we admit 'enlightened' self-interest, in which case the welfare of others might also be taken into account in assessing our own well-being.

For many applications the particular stance on rationality is unimportant; a formal theory of rational choice in economics can be developed under either standard. All that is required is that the consumer's behaviour is conformable with a systematic set of preferences with certain desirable properties. But before expanding on that point, we should note in passing that in the economist's approach to choice it is not being claimed that individuals always behave rationally. For the economist, rationality is merely a simplification, the usefulness of which rests on the extent that it provides satisfactory predictions of social phenomena.

Consumer preferences

In the main the economist is not overly concerned with what the particular goals or motivations of the consumer might be. Usable predictions of consumer behaviour can be generated provided we can presume that a *preference ordering* can be defined. This is a scheme that enables the consumer to rank different bundles of goods in terms of their desirability or order of preference. Given the choice between different consumption bundles (e.g. two slices of pizza and a small salad versus one slice of pizza and a large salad), the consumer can say whether one bundle is preferred to the other or whether they are indifferent between them. It is important to stress that we do not require that the consumer can say *by how much* one bundle is preferred to another; a simple ranking is sufficient.

Utility and utility function.

In the analysis of consumer choice, economists continue to make use of the term *utility*, first introduced by Jeremy Bentham in the nineteenth century. However, although it was once considered a quantifiable measure of satisfaction or well-being, it is now taken to reflect nothing more than the rank order of preferences: in finding the most preferred position, the consumer maximises utility. For some forms of analysis it is useful to have a function which provides a numerical representation of the preference-ordering and this is known as the *utility function*. This function assigns a number to each possible bundle of commodities such that if bundle A is preferred to bundle B, the number associated with A is greater than that for B, and if the consumer is indifferent between the two bundles, the numbers assigned by the function are the same.

The utility function is simply an analytical device to express a preference-ordering. Utility is not being measured in an absolute sense (c.f. traditional utilitarianism); the numerical representation is arbitrary, only the ranking is important (Hargreaves Heap *et al.* 1992).

Constraints on choice

The consumer's choice is constrained by their limited resources. The consumer's purchasing power or *budget constraint*, the ability to translate preferences into purchases, is governed by the consumer's income and prices in the marketplace. The consumer's problem then is to find the most preferred affordable commodity bundle, i.e. to maximise utility (defined over all market products) subject to the constraints imposed by the limits of the budget. The solution which emerges indicates that the demand for, say, a particular food product in a given time interval and *given tastes and preferences*, depends on:

1 the price of the product,
2 the prices of all other food and non-food products
   and
3 income.

A precise mathematical specification of the relationship between demand and prices and income is not provided by the general solution. However, the theory does suggest certain 'general restrictions' on the way in which the consumer's responses to prices and income changes are interconnected. Strictly, an empirical model of consumer demand must be consistent with these general restrictions if observed behaviour is to fully accord with the theory of demand (for the technical details, see Deaton and Muellbauer 1980).

The budget constraint is the constraint which receives most attention in the economic analysis of choice. However, it may be appropriate to adapt the analysis in order to incorporate other constraints:

1 *Time*. Following the work of Nobel Laureate Gary Becker (Becker 1965), time can be seen as an important input in the consumption process and as a scarce resource limiting consumption choices. The enjoyment of food, for example, requires expenditure of time, in purchasing, preparation and cooking, as well as money expenditure on the raw material. As time is limited, the consumer must decide on its allocation between labour market and consumption activities. The consumer problem in this approach is thus specified as one of utility maximisation given the budget *and* time constraints.

2 *Technical constraints*. How commodities are converted into goods which provide satisfaction or utility to the consumer is governed by the laws of biology, chemistry and physics. For example, the pleasure gained from food consumption may depend on the colour, taste and nutritional content of the food prepared, which in turn will be determined by the characteristics of the raw product, the household technology and the skills of the cook.

3 *Legal or institutional constraints*. A range of constraints arise as a result of macroeconomic policy and the need to protect the consumer or the environment. For example, consumer-purchasing decisions may be constrained by controls on credit or foreign exchange availability, by import bans, by controls on the use of food additives or drugs, by age limits on alcohol and cigarette purchase. These all restrict the consumer's choice in the market place, irrespective of underlying preferences or purchasing power.

4 *Sociocultural constraints*. To some extent, consumption patterns may be governed by social norms and customs. For example, the consumption of horsemeat is not considered proper in the UK; orthodox Jews and Muslims do not eat pork. Social norms may also be enshrined in the legal and institutional framework of the country.

The analysis can be modified to take account of these other constraints, but most empirical work tacitly assumes that these constraints are invariant over the period of analysis. In other words, it is founded on the basic model of consumer choice with which we started: taking prices and incomes as given, the consumers' task is to allocate their budgets to best serve these well-defined preferences.

Given the limits of space, we are able to give only a brief outline of the orthodox approach in economics to the problem of choice. Nevertheless it should be clear that the bounds of the analysis are narrowly defined. Namely, the set of determinants of consumer choice is mainly confined to prices and income and we are concerned primarily with the purchase decision. This is in stark contrast with other approaches, such as the 'behavioral approach', which attempt to encompass the whole decision process (problem recognition, information search and evaluation, purchasing processes, purchase and post-purchase behaviour) and which try to incorporate a wide range of influences, both individual determinants (learning and memory, attitude) and external factors (cultural, family, social).

There are a number of extensions to the basic economic model which could be considered – incorporating risk and uncertainty, for example – and a number of dissenting views to the orthodox approach (see, for example, Young 1996), including the Austrian school with its emphasis on ignorance and the discovery of knowledge. However, we now turn to a review of the representation of preferences in empirical work, and a brief example drawn from our recent work within 'The Nation's Diet' Programme.

Preference formation and preference change

The process by which individuals decide on their goals is, in the main, regarded as outside the economist's sphere of competence, and much of neo-classical economics takes preferences as given. Milton Friedman provides a succinct precis of this view:

> The economist has little to say about the formation of wants; this is the province of the psychologist. The economist's task is to trace the consequence of any given set of wants. The legitimacy of and justification for this abstraction must rest ultimately . . . on the light that is shed and the power to predict that is yielded by the abstraction. (Friedman 1962: 13)

This reflects Friedman's stance on economic methodology: that assumptions underpinning theory need not be realistic, as long as they provide useful predictions.

There are, however, alternative points of views. In part these have arisen from the relatively low predictive power of empirical models based on the abstraction, and we return to these in the following section. There are, though, alternative 'radical' views of preference formation. The significance of these alternative views is not merely that they address the determination of preferences, but that the determinants are assumed to lie within the realm of conventional economics (i.e. they are endogenous to the economic model). Thus:

> individual preference structures are products of economic activity. Or more precisely, individual preferences develop and change according to variables *endogenous* to the economic model: prices, quantities, and availabilities of consumption goods, jobs and social institutions conditioning the supply of labour. (Gintis 1974: 415)

This formulation does not necessarily involve straying far into the province of the psychologist, but it does have profound implications for much of economic analysis that is underpinned by the concept of consumer sovereignty (by which the allocation of resources in the private economy is held to respond primarily to consumers' demands for goods and services). If consumer preferences are formed within the economic model then the position of conventional welfare analysis is made untenable, as the latter involves the evaluation of changes in the economic system on consumer welfare. If the measure of consumer welfare itself is determined by economic variables then any *ceteris paribus* assumption is void. Examples of this process may be habit formation, where current preferences depend on previous expenditure, or where consumer preferences are interdependent (Pollak 1978), the effects of advertising (Chang and Green 1989), or education (Gintis 1974).

An alternative representation of preferences is given by Stigler and Becker (1977), who argue that preferences *do* lie outside the economic system and, what is more, are constant across individuals and across time. In order to sustain this position they argue that the basic units that enter the utility function (what they term 'Z' goods) are non-market goods (e.g. 'nutrition') that are produced by the household rather than individual commodities (e.g. 'meat'). There are, then, 'household production functions' which describe the process by which commodities, combined with time, physical capital and human capital (defined as human skills and knowledge), are converted into Z goods. Consumers maximise utility subject to the household production functions and a time constraint as well as incomes and prices. Differences in observed expenditure behaviour may then be attributed to differences in the constraint set. An example of this process may be given by reference to the acquired taste for fine wines: drinking wine of any type generates Z goods via the household production function, and requires time and money but also a level of appreciation (or palate) which may be considered as a stock of human capital. This stock will change over time because of education, or exposure to different types of wine, and hence there is a shift in consumption patterns, but with no change in the fundamental preference structure. Note that this argument does not depend on any psychological or physiological addictive qualities of alcohol, and has been applied to 'acquired tastes' for products such as classical music.

Doubts have been raised as to whether the Stigler and Becker model has any more explanatory power than the conventional view of changing tastes but it does represent a polar view of where to draw the dividing line between preferences and constraints as factors affecting consumer choice. It has also brought to the fore the importance of factors such as time in the process of consumption, and hence provides a framework for analysing some factors that are ignored from the standard approach (e.g. changing employment patterns on demand for products such as convenience foods).

The empirical analysis of food choice

The empirical analysis of food choice can be based on the theory outlined in the earlier section in a number of ways, depending on the data available. It is important to note that the vast majority of studies are based on secondary data: either large-scale surveys (covering thousands of consumers) or aggregate market data recorded over long periods of time. There are some studies utilising primary (survey) data (e.g. Smith and Goodwin 1992) and some based on experimental results, using human or even non-human subjects, that draw directly on the economic models outlined earlier (e.g. Kagel *et al*. 1981; Knetsch 1992), but these tend to be the exception.

Cross-section analysis

The statistical analysis of food choice has a long history, and probably started with Ernst Engel's analysis of household budgets in 1857. Based on family budgets for 153 Belgian families Engel proposed that 'The poorer the family, the greater the proportion of its total expenditure that must be devoted to the provision of food' (cited by Stigler 1954, who gives an overview of the historical development of the area). Although at first identified in a quite casual manner, and with no recourse to any theory, this 'law' has proved remarkably robust, both over time and space (Houthakker, 1957).

Many studies have extended the approach taken by Engel, based on a data-set collected at a point in time and applying regression analysis, either at the aggregate level of food expenditure, or to disaggregated commodities. Here the theory is relatively unrestrictive in so far as the prices paid for products do not vary significantly across households and hence cannot provide any basis for explaining variations in consumption (or expenditure, which is often used as the dependent variable where commodity aggregates are under investigation). When prices are found to vary there is the question of whether this is due to differences in the quality of the product (Cox and Wohlgenant 1986). This leaves us with income as the only variable derived from theory. This may suggest that these studies are relatively straightforward, but there have been a number of extensions to the basic analysis of expenditure as a function of income.

One of these relates to conducting the analysis at the level of the household rather than the individual. The operational design of most surveys employed by economists is such that data are collected at household level. As a result, in subsequent analysis there is no possibility of identifying individuals' consumption decisions, even though the economic theory is based on the individual. If we proceed with the analysis we have to assume that the household generates a well-behaved preference-ordering analogous to that of the individual. Putting aside the whole issue of how that preference-ordering may emerge from the interpersonal dynamics of the household, the composition of the household will affect preferences as a result of the different physiological and psychological needs of individuals of different ages and gender.

The way that this is often dealt with is to include variables describing the size and composition of the household explicitly in the estimated demand function, and these are often highly significant in explaining food choices (Chesher 1991). Essentially this is saying that the preference-ordering of the household depends on the demographic features of the household but there is seldom any formal theory employed to explain how this occurs: regularities in the data are simply captured by the statistical analysis.

What is more, if the data are available, researchers frequently extend the list of explanatory variables to include other 'non-economic' factors which may affect preferences. Such factors include type of employment and geographical location (Thomas 1972), race, education and sex of food purchaser (Cox and Wohlgenant 1986), health status (Jones 1989) and perceptions of food safety (Lin and Milon 1993). There is no appeal to any formal economic theory as to how these variables should enter the demand function, nor perhaps any strong *a priori* idea as to how many of them will affect demand, apart from the view that preferences may be heterogeneous across households and the inclusion of these socioeconomic factors is intended to capture the effects. In passing it should be noted that many of these factors were mentioned earlier as constraints to choice. This highlights one aspect of the applied work: empirically it is difficult, if not impossible, to distinguish models that include such factors as constraints and those that include them as part of the preferences structure. Furthermore, although crosssection studies may be able to give some indication of factors that may determine preferences at a point in time, they cannot identify changes in preferences over time. The methods by which this may be attempted are dealt with in the following section.

An additional problem with the approach is the use of purchases rather than consumption. Even if the data are collected for a single individual, there is no guarantee that consumption over the (usually short) period in which the data are collected will be equal to expenditure on the good. The most obvious difficulty is in cases where there are no purchases of the good recorded, but there is consumption out of stocks, or where the survey happens to take place when there has been substantial expenditure to rebuild stocks. To some extent it can be hoped that the use of large sample size will allow the true relationship to be uncovered, although non-purchase does present a particular difficulty (see Gould, 1992). Nutritional surveys (such as the Dietary and Nutritional Survey of British Adults 1986–87, OPCS – see Gregory *et al.* 1990) are exceptions, in that they contain detailed records of individuals' consumption, but are lacking in much of the socioeconomic data needed for this type of analysis.

Time-series analysis

The use of time-series data, which record price and income variations over time, permits greater consideration of the power of demand theory: all of the 'general restrictions' on estimated parameter values are relevant. The data used are normally aggregates for the entire population in the market, usually at an annual periodicity, although quarterly data are sometimes available.

There have been numerous studies of food demand based on time series data. They can be broadly categorised into three groups. In the first, a mathematical form of the utility function is assumed explicitly and hence the derived demand relationships will also take a mathematical form which must conform to theory. However, these tend to be very restrictive in their representation of preferences,[1] a disadvantage which led this approach to fall from favour in recent years.

The second group is based on demand systems that are much more flexible, and could potentially satisfy the general restrictions of theory although this is not imposed on them.[2] In practice, when these demand systems are estimated, the restrictions implied by theory are often rejected statistically by the data. This suggests that the data do not support the theory: the hypothesis of food choice being determined within a utility maximisation framework is incorrect. But other explanations are possible – the form of the empirical model is misspecified, there are measurement errors in the data, or the data have been aggregated across commodities or individual consumers incorrectly.[3] However, a more common response to a rejection of the theory is to explore the possibility that consumers are utility maximisers, but within a framework of changing preferences. This brings us to the third group of models.

In the third group, the consumer is still assumed to be a utility maximiser, but the underlying preferences change over time. This leads to specifications which are consistent with demand theory but at the same time include variables that represent the changes in preferences (a complementary approach in cases where there are no violations of theory is to ask whether the explanatory power of the model can be improved by allowing for changes in preferences). The question of how to represent the changes in preferences within the model then raises itself. One purely mechanistic approach is to allow the estimated parameters of the model to vary systematically over time (say, by the inclusion of simple time trends). A number of studies have taken this approach, especially in the demand for meat, and these have indicated significant shifts in preferences for different meat types, especially away from red and towards the white meats (see, for example, Chavas 1983; Martin and Porter 1985; Thurman 1987; Eales and Unnevehr 1988; Burton 1989; Moschini and Meilke 1989 and Burton and Young 1992a, 1992b). Although these studies identify changes in parameter values which they attribute to changes in tastes there is no real explanation of what may be causing them, although there is an appeal to changing lifestyles, health awareness, etc. One circumstantial piece of evidence that these trends may be identifying something real (as opposed to a statistical quirk) is the consistency of the results obtained across countries in the movement away from red towards white meat which appears to have occurred around the mid-1970s.

An alternative is to include variables that may represent the causes of these changes in tastes directly. Thus Dono and Thompson (1994) include the percentage of employed women in the population as a variable in a study of meat demand in Italy, which is identified as having a significant positive impact on the demand for chicken. This is justified on the basis of opportunity cost of time and the convenience embodied in chicken. Chang and Kinnucan (1991) include a cholesterol-information index into their model of fat demand in Canada and find that negative information about the relationship between butter and cholesterol was found to affect butter demand four times as much as positive information. Chang and Green (1989) included advertising in a demand system that covered five food categories, and found that there were significant effects, especially for meat and dairy products. They also found that increased advertising led to reductions in the response of demand to changes in the product's price.

Finally, there have been alternative approaches that correspond to 'endogenous' taste change. Thus there have been attempts to include past consumption levels as the determinants of the parameters of the utility function, to represent habit formation (see Houthakker and Taylor 1966; Pollak 1978).

An example of empirical analysis of food choice

Our project in 'The Nation's Diet' Programme (called 'The decision not to eat meat: an analysis of changing preferences') provides an empirical example of consumer-demand analysis which combines both cross-section and time-series elements. This section gives only a brief outline of the approach and indicative results. Further analysis and exposition of the research design and method are reported in Burton, Dorsett and Young (1996a, 1996b).

The meat industry appears to be faced with a fundamental shift in consumer attitudes, as evidenced by an increasing number of consumers in the UK deciding not to eat meat at all. The aim of our study is to gain an insight into meat demand through the analysis of cross-section (household) data over a number of years so as to better understand this trend. In particular, by explicitly accounting for some individuals' non-purchase, we can more accurately examine demand for those people who do eat meat.

The study begins from the the position that the decision whether or not to eat meat and the decision of how much meat to consume are distinct phenomena with different determinants and that the influence of these determinants is likely to vary over time. We therefore adopt an analytical technique (known as the 'double hurdle' model) which allows us to capture the household's two-stage decision process, namely:

- the participation decision, and if the consumer does participate,
- the expenditure decision.

Our approach is applied to the *National Food Survey* (NFS) data[4] over the period 1975–93. The NFS is a continuous sampling enquiry into the domestic food consumption and expenditure of private households in Great Britain. Approximately 7000 households cooperate each year. Each household in the survey keeps diary records for one week of the cost and quantity of all food bought. Socioeconomic characteristics of the households, such as age, sex, occupational class of householder, geographical location, and household composition, are also recorded (see Ministry of Agriculture, Fisheries and Food 1991, for further details). The bulk of our empirical analysis has concerned households comprising one adult, with or without children (this reduces our sample to approximately 1800 each year). This is because the NFS records *household* expenditure on food products, not the consumption of individual household members, and there is a more direct link between the personal preferences of the single adult and their recorded household expenditure. In particular, this approach avoids the problem of dealing with a household of several adults which records meat expenditure while some members of that household are vegetarian. The decline in participation of single adult households in the meat market is particularly marked, from 95 per cent in 1975 to 83 per cent in 1993 in our sample.

With this data-set we are able to quantify the influence of the following variables on household decision-making: *economic determinants* – the average prices paid per unit of meat, of dairy products, of fish, and of all other food products, and the total food budget; *characteristics of the household* – age of householder, sex of householder, number, age and sex of children in the household, occupational class of the householder, geographical location of household, and freezer ownership.

The model is first estimated for individual years and then for a pooled data-set comprising data from all years. The types of quantitative outputs which may be obtained from the analysis are:

1 the estimated probability that a household with specific socio economic characteristics will participate (i.e. decide to buy meat)
2 the contribution of each socioeconomic characteristic to the overall probability of participation
3 the influence of each socioeconomic characteristic (as well as the standard economic factors, prices and income) on the decision of how much to spend on meat.

For example, Figure 5.1 illustrates the estimated effect of gender and the

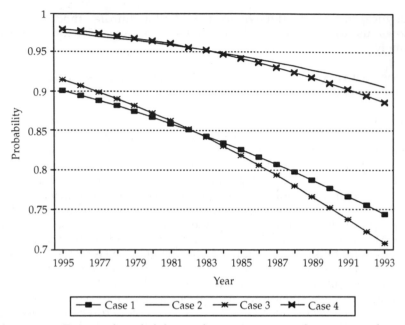

Figure 5.1 Estimated probabilities of participating in the meat market: the impacts of sex and children.

Case 1: Male householder, no children   Case 2: Male householder, with children

Case 3: Female householder, no children Case 4: Female householder, with children

The maintained characteristics are: Householder's age is 30, living in a non-metropolitan area, with no freezer

Source: Authors' calculations, using NFS data

presence of children on the probability of participation over time. In this figure there are two reference households corresponding to male – and female-headed households. In both cases these households are headed by a 30-year-old male or female, with no children, no freezer and located in a non-metropolitan area. Considering, first of all, these reference households, we can see that there has been a downward trend in participation for both males and females, although this has been particularly noticeable for females. From females being more likely to participate at the start of the period, this difference disappears by the early 1980s and subsequently reverses, with males becoming more likely to participate. Turning next to the influence of children on household decision-making, it is evident from Figure 5.1 that the presence of children in the household increases the probability of participation.

Other results, not illustrated, are that (1) having a freezer has a negative effect on participation, although this decreases over time so that by the end of the period the difference between those households with a freezer and those without has narrowed to the extent that a male-headed household with a freezer is more likely to buy meat than a female-headed household without; (2) living in a metropolitan area increases the probability of meat purchase across the whole period; (3) adding an extra ten years to the age of the head of the household serves to increase the probability of participation.

In terms of the level of meat expenditure, for those households which do buy meat, the meat budget share is smaller when the head of household is female, but larger in households with freezers and more purchasing power, as well as in those located in metropolitan areas. On the other hand, the presence of children of five years and over reduces the meat budget, but the effect of younger children is negligible.

In sum, our project illustrates one particular approach to the economic modelling of food choice, based on individual household records. The nature of the data dictates that economic theory plays a relatively small role in imposing restrictions on the estimated model, but it does allow us to incorporate in the analysis both economic determinants and the characteristics of the household, such as education, age and sex. Fine and Leopold (1993) argue that the conventional economist's approach 'isolates economics from other disciplines and renders it incapable of finding a partner for an interdisciplinary marriage'. Our approach may not be the basis for a successful marriage but perhaps we may be able to offer at least a casual affair.

Conclusion

There is now a large body of empirical work within economics concerned with the analysis of food demand, at various levels. At its most abstract, it is based on a model of an optimising consumer who can generate a preference-ordering over alternative bundles of goods. The source of these (constant) preferences is not specified, their structure is implicit in the empirical results. However, in much applied work this abstraction is relaxed to some extent. The inclusion of variables other than prices and incomes in cross-section work is a recognition that preferences are heterogenous across individuals, but systematically formed by other influences: the inclusion of variables such as employment and age are attempts to proxy the source of that variation, if only crudely. Time-series analysis allows us to investigate changes in preferences, but the use of aggregate or market-level data means that we have to use indicators of changes in the attributes of the consumer body as a whole. Often these are simply deterministic time trends which may indicate shifts in preferences but give no guidance as to the cause. The challenge for economists is to integrate their analysis

93

of food choice based on fixed preferences with a better understanding of how those preferences are formed.

Notes

1. For example, in the Linear Expenditure System (see Thomas 1987), a commonly used demand system, the demand for all goods has to rise as income rises, but in fact this may not be the case for some goods such as potatoes.
2. Within this group we could include 'dynamic' models such as Anderson and Blundell (1982) that have allowed the theory to be maintained in the long run, but suggested that consumers may deviate from it in the short run as they adjust to changes in prices. An application to GB meat demand indicated that the rate of adjustment to equilibrium is quite fast, with over 98 per cent of the adjustment occurring within a year (Burton and Young 1992a).
3. The latter is a very powerful argument to apply: only if individuals have very particular forms of utility function it can be expected that the aggregate will behave 'as if' generated by a representative consumer (see Kirman 1992; Lewbel 1989, for a discussion of the representative consumer and exact aggregation).
4. NFS data were made available through the Ministry of Agriculture, Fisheries and Food and the ERSC Data Archive.

CHAPTER 6

What we eat and why: social norms and systems of provision

Ben Fine, Michael Heasman and Judith Wright

Introduction

Although our project originated within the discipline of economics, its motivation represented a considerable breach with its standard treatment of choice, whether for food or otherwise. The orthodoxy is associated with neoclassical economics. It is familiar to legions of students and researchers, varying only in degree of technical sophistication, rather than conceptual content which tends to be reproduced unquestioningly, even axiomatically. The foundations of consumer choice are as familiar to economists as they are alien to other social scientists. An overview of all our work, and a detailed account of, and justification for, our points of departure from the economic orthodoxies is to be found in Fine, Heasman and Wright (1996) and Fine and Heasman (1997). This chapter sets out how we attempted to develop an interdisciplinary approach to an understanding of what we eat and why.

Our starting point, then, was the weaknesses of the theory of choice offered by orthodox economics. In brief, the latter is characterised by the reduction of food choice to the demand for physical objects by each individual consumer and, by extension, to society as a whole by aggregating over all individuals. Each individual's preferences or tastes are also taken as given, and individual motivation is confined to the single-minded satisfaction of those preferences. Our approach set out to be entirely different, in part as a response to the unreasonable assumptions of orthodox economics but without wishing to set aside the importance of economic factors. It drew on earlier work on consumption, Fine and Leopold (1993), which had critically reviewed the literature across the social sciences and had drawn some more positive general conclusions (and see Fine 1995b), especially in conjunction with empirical work on the ownership of consumer durables – see especially Fine and Leopold (1993) and Fine and Simister (1995).

In this light, consumer choice is understood in terms of what Fine and Leopold (1993) dubbed systems of provision – as in the housing, energy, fashion and transport systems, for example, or, most pertinent here, the food systems. A system of provision is interpreted as an integral or unified set of structures and processes that determines the way in which consumption is socioeconomically and culturally organised. Each system of provision will incorporate different elements along its vertically integrated chain, and the way in which that integration is constructed will vary from one system to another and over time. While each system is structurally differentiated from others, there can be interactions between them – the dependence of food on transport in a number of ways does not negate their constituting separate systems of provision.

In contrast to the economics orthodoxy, this opens the way for an interpretation of, and approach to, consumer choice that draws on insights from across the various social science disciplines. These too, like economics, have tended to focus on specific factors rooted within their own disciplines and to generalise across consumption – as in emulation and distinction or stratification, for example – to provide horizontal analyses. Fine and Leopold (1993) suggest that this has proved a barrier to the interdisciplinary study of consumption since the factors considered, as well as the corresponding theories associated with them, cannot be readily integrated. The assumption of fixed preferences and individual utility maximisation from economics, for example, is inconsistent with the socially interdependent and shifting preferences attached to emulation. Our approach has sought to overcome these incompatibilities by recognising that the determinants of consumption are differentiated from one commodity to the next by the system of provision to which they are attached. Thus, we do not begin with a bundle of theories of consumption and fit them together to provide an all-embracing general theory. Rather, we must begin with specific items of consumption and examine how they are provided and consumed, drawing appropriately from the various social sciences (Fine 1993b).

In examining food systems from this perspective, our work begins by seeking to identify 'food norms', i.e. systematic patterns of consumption, by socioeconomic variables. This is in order to pose one aspect of what has to be explained: what are the sorts of similarities and differences across groups of consumers in consumption of one food as opposed to another. We have then sought to provide answers by reference to the food systems (of provision). The notion of food system is already used in a variety of discourses, not least because of concern over where food has come from, how it has been made and whether it is healthy, safe and reasonably priced (e.g. Tansey and Worsley 1995). Interest has been stimulated to trace the journey to food consumption back from its origins in agriculture. Drawing on the academic literature for the separate components of the food system, we have attempted to formalise the study of particular food systems. This has led us to emphasise a particular aspect of food systems, the extent to which they are disproportionately dependent on what we have called their organic content. Precisely because it is ultimately destined literally for human consumption and has its origins in agriculture, food begins and ends its journey with processes that are necessarily biological. Although these may be controlled through the 'industrialisation' of food or whatever, the food system necessarily incorporates an organic content throughout its system of provision. This sets it apart from other consumption items.

So far, discussion has been careful to avoid discussion of a single food system, for the ways in which different foods are provided are themselves often quite separate and distinct from one another. The reasons why we indulge ourselves in ice-cream, and the socioeconomic patterns by which we do so, may be very different from the choice of convenience meals or low fat milk. Nor will this simply be a matter of consumer preferences but it will also reflect the different processes by which these foods have found their way into our refrigerators. In short, just as for consumption more generally, our interpretation of food choice is in terms of food norms which are themselves explained by reference to differentiated food systems, each of which, however, is distinguished by the way in which it incorporates the organic content of food throughout its vertically integrated chain of processes and structures.

Food norms

It is one thing to hypothesise the existence of food norms, it is another matter to devise statistical techniques in practice to measure them and to find an appropriate data-set on which to employ the techniques. Our own method for measuring food norms is extremely unusual, both in the context of food and even for consumption more generally. For food, it is common, if implicit, to discuss food norms in terms of average levels of consumption across the population, or a sample, as a whole or for particular socioeconomic groups within these. This might either be for economic purposes or in order to provide some estimate of the excessive or deficient levels of nutritional intakes. Drawing on previous work on the ownership of consumer durables, we focused on whether a food was consumed at all or not, rather than on how much was consumed if at all.

Put simply, our technique involved taking the sample of consumers as a whole (in our case, from the *National Food Survey* [NFS] discussed below) and finding how it ranked a selection of foods by popularity, defined as whether each food had been purchased or not. The proportion of the sample purchasing the food was described as the (absolute) frequency of purchase, which is not to be confused with how many times an individual purchases the food. It is simply the proportion of the sample purchasing the food at least once during the survey period. As mentioned, the foods are then ranked by this measure of popularity, or by relative frequency. This is then taken as the first step in defining food norms for the set of foods included. It is simply a matter of how popular they are by ranking of frequency of purchase.

A second component of the norm is to measure how much the sample violates or conforms to the initial ranking. For example, if one consumer purchases five foods out of 20 considered, then there is perfect conformity to the norm if the top five foods are the ones selected. Otherwise, a measure can be made of the number of 'mistakes' made by the consumer relative to the norm and, for the sample as a whole, it is possible to devise an overall measure of the extent of conformity to the norm. Now, we have a norm for the sample as a whole that also incorporates a measure of the uniformity of choice across the sample as a whole.

The third aspect of the norm is to partition the sample by some socioeconomic characteristic, such as age, social class, income or household composition. For each of the sub-samples, a norm can be constructed as for the first and second components outlined above for the sample as a whole. It is then possible to discern how particular socioeconomic variables lead to variations around the norm. Rankings of particular foods may consistently move up or down with age, for example. It is also possible to examine, irrespective of the extent to which sub-sample norms vary from the sample norm, whether sub-samples exhibit greater or lesser deviation from their own or from the sample norm than the sample itself.

Finally, the norm can be refined even further and, subject to sample size, more or less indefinitely. For sub-samples by one socioeconomic characteristic can themselves be sub-sampled by another characteristic to examine the interaction of the two variables, as in the impact of income and age, for example.

In practice, a particularly convenient way of presenting the results was found in terms of a table that we have named the dramatrix. Before giving an example, it is worth presenting a brief discussion of the data-set we used. This was the *National Food Survey*, an annual household survey for which we drew on the years, 1979, 1984, 1986 and 1989, and for which we calculated the food norms for various groups of foods and socioeconomic variables as discussed above. There are certain features of the Survey which need to be mentioned but which cannot be covered in detail here through lack of space. Specifically, the NFS has covered food purchased over a week for consumption within the home, not meals taken outside, and the vast variety of foods purchased have necessarily been aggregated into common categories of varying homogeneity. In our own work, we created our own food codes to cover finer divisions – beef as a single category instead of a range of beef products, for example. And we also created our own socio-economic variables out of the information available for the 7000 or so households surveyed.

The construction of our dramatrices was primarily undertaken around three different sets of foods. One was selected for consisting of dairy-type products (nine foods) – in part in order to investigate moves in diet such as those towards 'healthier', low fat milks and also towards low fat spreads and margarines and away from butter and cream. A second ranged across a variety of meat products (19 foods), again to investigate changes towards putative healthier eating, but also to examine the adoption of new products. The third range of 20 products was chosen specifically to investigate a number of foods which had, for differing reasons such as health or convenience, experienced quite rapid changes in consumption over the decade covered by the NFS Surveys used, as for the shift from white to brown bread or the drop in the direct purchase of sugar.

An extremely wide range of socioeconomic variables was also used to generate the food norms through sub-sampling. These included region, social class, income, household composition, with or without both men and women, and similarly for children of various ages, age of head of household (and retired or not), form of housing tenure, and ownership of freezer or not.

Table 6.1 shows a typical dramatrix for the meat items, although it represents an aggregation of the individual results for the four years studied (change over time could be examined by comparing the dramatrices for the four years). The entry in the row for lamb and in the column for age 25–34 years old for head of household, namely −15, shows that lamb is ranked 15 places lower than for the sample as a

Table 6.1 Aggregate dramatrix by age

Age	<25	25–34	35–44	45–54	55–64	65–74	>75
Beef	3	2	0	0	−1	−1	−1
Uncooked bacon	−4	−2	0	0	1	1	−1
Cooked bacon	−4	−1	1	0	1	−2	−1
Sausages	0	0	−2	−2	0	0	−1
Chicken	3	3	3	1	−1	−4	−4
Pork	−1	0	1	0	1	2	−2
Lamb	−28	−15	−8	0	0	6	9
Meat pies	6	1	3	−1	−3	−4	−6
Corned meat	−8	−5	0	1	5	−2	−4
Cooked meat	−14	−10	−10	0	1	4	4
Canned meat	13	11	1	−6	−10	−7	−5
Other frozen	22	11	6	−3	−4	−4	−4
Deli paté	5	21	15	3	−4	−3	0
Cold pies	−6	−6	−4	6	5	6	5
Liver	−11	−12	−9	2	12	15	16
Burgers	16	7	3	−4	−4	−3	−4
Ready meals	15	5	3	−3	−3	−6	−4
Cooked poultry	0	0	1	4	5	5	9
Turkey	1	1	0	1	1	2	0

NB: no separate category for frozen burgers in 1979
Source: calculated from National Food Surveys, as in Fine, Heasman and Wright 1996.

whole for this age group (or 15/4 places on average, taking account of the aggregation over the four years).

More generally, especially because age is a variable running from lower to higher, the rows of the dramatrix reveal relatively easily the impact of the variable on food norms as defined here in principle and interpreted in practice. For lamb, cooked meat and liver, for example, there is a heavy positive influence in ranking with age as the rows run from negative to positive values. On the other hand, exactly the opposite applies to canned meat, other frozen foods, burgers, ready meals and, setting aside the under 25s, deli paté. Similarly, by looking down the columns, it is possible to see which types of household are highly variable in the way they rank foods – if there are many large divergencies from zero in the column, as is especially so for the under-25s.

On the basis of such methods, whether with this group of foods or others, and with a range of different socioeconomic variables, literally hundreds of dramatrices were constructed and interpreted in order to tease out significant aspects of food norms. Before presenting some of the results, it is first worth reporting on the progress made in the understanding of food systems.

Food systems

The previous section has outlined our particular method for investigating empirically the presence and nature of food norms. There could be other understandings of norms, most obviously as average consumption rather than purchase or not by socioeconomic group. And there could be other statistical techniques used to identify and measure norms. For the moment, take the norms, however defined and measured, as given. How are we to explain them? An obvious approach is by appeal to the most immediate determinants or correlates of choice itself. Reference can be made to age, as in Table 6.1, or to prices, incomes and other such variables.

However, this is a relatively superficial stab at explanation however sophisticated it might prove in practice in terms of statistical techniques. It even borders on the tautologous, with the old or the wealthy, for example, consuming more or differently according to what the old and wealthy tend to consume, respectively. Apart from these factors, that economists would call demand-side, there are supply-side factors to consider which are crucial in determining what foods are available and how. A little thought while meandering around the supermarket, itself a profound influence on food choice, raises questions about how food has been transported, processed and grown – each aspect of which has experienced dramatic shifts of one sort or another, through industrialisation of agriculture and bio-technology. The issue is not whether demand- and supply-side factors should be taken into account in explaining food norms but how their interactions should be analysed.

The use of food systems is one way, although it is a notion that has been understood in a variety of ways. Perhaps the most common and simple is as a descriptive device – tracing, as it were, the passage of food from farm to plate. This has some purchase in organising empirical and historical material but, though rarely free of analytical content, this is only implicit in terms of the structures and factors considered to be of importance. As such, it offers very little by way of causal analysis, and much the same is true of relying on explanation in terms of shifting supply and demand. For this then begs the question of what has made these change in the way that they have.

More specifically, once it is accepted that food systems signify the presence of an integral structure, three questions present themselves. First, how are such structures reproduced and with what effects? Second, why and when do such structures change and in what way – at one level, there can be a restructuring of the chain of existing activities within a particular food system; more fundamentally, it would be possible for a food system to be restructured either to broaden or narrow its scope – do we have a single food system for vegetables, fruits and meats or does each of its products, at the other extreme, constitute its own food system, one for oranges or turkeys or whatever? Third, following on from these theoretical conundrums, how do we identify food systems empirically? What are the boundaries between one food system and another, with the possibility of interaction across them, as opposed to such interactions implying the formation of a single food system?

Clearly, such questions are germane to our analysis of consumption more generally, and they were debated as such between Fine (1993a) and Glennie and Thrift (1992, 1993). In the specific context of food, our work has drawn heavily on the field in which these issues have been most usefully debated – the sociology of agriculture, for a long-term overview of which see Buttel, Larson and Gillespie (1990). Until recently, even if with relatively minor differences, a common approach had been established with the following main features. First, emphasis has been placed on food systems as being made up of integral structures with, not surprisingly given the analytical origins involved, emphasis placed on the structural divide between agriculture and industry (or the rest of the commercial world more generally). Second, tensions have been placed on these structures by underlying forces that tend to undermine them, such as a technological treadmill in farming and the chronic problems of over-supply. Particular attention has been given to the industrialisation of agriculture which tends to shift the boundaries between it and industry in favour of the latter – as agricultural inputs (substitutionism) and agricultural processes (appropriationism) are taken over. Third, there is a crisis in, and shift or restructuring of, the food system once the technological or other imperatives are no longer accommodated within the existing structures of the food system (and for which the state is no longer able or willing to provide sufficient economic support). Fourth, agriculture has been globalised and rendered increasingly like the industrial mass production of uniform commodities, with the rise of a number of food complexes, such as grains, for example.

Our own approach offered some differences, some hotly contested, to this version of food-system analysis, as in the debate organised with Fine (1994a, 1994b) in *Review of International Political Economy*. First, raising that old chestnut of social theory – the relationship between structures, processes and agencies – we considered that structures within food systems were erroneously being given causal priority over the underlying pressures arising out of the pursuit of profitability through the accumulation of capital. In particular, such underlying tendencies were being interpreted simply as empirical trends that would eventually erode food system structures. Instead, we emphasised the priority of underlying, but contradictory tendencies – such as those of vertical integration and disintegration along the food chain according to whether competition takes the form of gains from economies of scale or of scope – with the added complication of the role played by the intervention of landed property where the agriculture/industry divide is concerned. It is through these that the structures of the food system are reproduced or transformed – possibly through a crisis.

Second, irrespective of the trend in the division of activity between agriculture and industry, it is necessary to recognise that it is the consequence of a complex outcome reflecting the pressures and potential for restructuring of the divide in either direction. Artificial fertiliser manufactured by the chemical industry, for example, might displace more 'natural' sources but would itself enhance the potential of agricultural production. Similarly, bio-technology has the same effect without simply shifting activity off the farm and into the laboratory. Moreover, similar considerations apply to the structural divides elsewhere along the food system.

Third, undue emphasis has been placed on the agriculture/industry divide without sufficiently examining how it is influenced by, and works in conjunction with, the other activities within the food system, such as food-processing and retailing, for example. One consequence of this has been the neglect of the organic nature of food systems other than at the agricultural end which perversely is then unduly exaggerated with leanings towards a form of naturalism in which capital is seen as being in confrontation with natural obstacles.

Fourth, particularly in the idea of global food complexes, the analysis has suffered from an overgeneralisation across foods from a few, admittedly important, foods. This has had the unfortunate but inevitable effect of revealing an ever-expanding portfolio of counter-examples, ultimately throwing the whole approach into disarray. With the rise of more varied and specialised food provision, and the deployment of concepts such as globalisation to express the local and differentiated response to the global, analysis of food systems has recently turned full circle – emphasising the heterogeneity and fluidity of food so that all structures are flexible and fleeting in response to the diversity and exotica of consumer tastes. As Goodman and Watts (1994) rightly observe, food studies in this regard has been subject to what they term mimesis – the presumption that agriculture mimics the development of industry – necessarily overlooking the unique features of food systems.

Finally, there have been historical anomalies in the food-system's literature. Not surprisingly in view of the previous points, the historical record has failed to conform to the theory that has been prepared for it. Different foods have not experienced the same rhythm and form of restructuring, and this is not simply a matter of timing but also of different food systems for the same commodity at the same time but in different countries. This is a consequence of the historically contingent, varied and complex ways in which underlying economic imperatives have interacted to create, for example, distinctly national food systems.

With these perspectives, our empirical research on food systems focused on sugar (and artificial sweeteners), on the meat system, and on the dairy system, specifically for the UK. However, these particular studies, partly in conjunction with our measurement of food norms, themselves furthered our theoretical work, especially concerning the definition of, and boundaries between, food systems. Broadly, three conclusions were reached. First, the formation of a food system is dependent on the strength and extent of the linkages across its various components other than at the level of consumption itself, for which the flexibility of material culture suffices, in principle, to render almost any two consumption goods as complements.

Two contrasting examples from food systems informed this stance. On the one hand, while sugar and artificial sweeteners both serve the same consumer demand of sweetening products whether directly or indirectly, there is practically no interaction between the two, and hence they are separate as food systems except in the competition for final markets (something which essentially characterises all commodities to a greater or lesser extent). On the other hand, the meat system is characterised by substantially divergent patterns of consumption, as we have already seen above for age, for example. Yet, away from consumption itself, there is an increasing integration in the functioning of the various means by which meat products are supplied, although this is by no means uniform given specialisation on farms, as opposed to the widening scope of input provision (feeds and pharmaceuticals), and meat-processing, packaging and retailing.

A second theoretical conclusion drawn out from our empirical work on specific food systems, especially from the meat example, is that the delineation of food systems is not always clear-cut and rigid. There is a continuing process of restructuring the elements within and across food systems. While it is important to identify the key aspects of change, and the reasons for them, they can evolve without dramatic restructuring from one well-defined system, or set of systems, to another. The issue is not so much whether the chicken is separate from the pork system or not, but how the two are being restructured individually and in relation to one another.

Third, and as a consequence of the previous points, while theoretically informed, the identification of different food systems is an empirical exercise, whose exact content cannot be laid out in advance by a formula whether mathematical or procedural. This is precisely because the formation of food systems is historically contingent, dependent on which structures are formed and how in response to underlying socioeconomic forces.

Selected results

In principle, our research was to have fallen into three components. The first is the empirical identification of food norms from the *National Food Survey*; the second the analysis of the corresponding food systems; and the third is to bring these two components together in order to explain socioeconomic patterns of food purchase. In practice, this is an extremely tall order, especially for the last two elements for which we had to be satisfied with merely attempting to identify the key aspects of the food systems and to sketch their potential connections with the measured food norms.

But first consider an insight that emerged during the course of our research, revealing the nature and significance of the difference in our approach to the understanding of food norms. As previously mentioned, it has been more usual, especially in the NFS's own Annual Reports, to define consumption norms in a different way, even if only implicitly. Attention is focused on the average quantities of a food purchased per household per week, possibly comparatively across sub-samples defined by various socioeconomic variables. Accordingly, our approach is different in examining whether foods are purchased or not rather than in averaging quantities over households, irrespective of whether they purchased or not. There is also a technical difference in the norms in so far as our definition is dependent on the purchase behaviour across a range of foods (relative ranking by frequency) although it could, like the implied NFS norms, be defined by reference to single foods by recording absolute frequencies of purchase alone (corresponding to absolute averages of quantities purchased).

It is crucial to recognise that there is a further issue involved, quite apart from whether a food is purchased or not and how much of the food is purchased on average. This is the frequency with which the food is purchased over time. The NFS surveys purchase behaviour over one week alone. Given the size of the sample, this is not liable unduly to affect estimation of the average quantities purchased. What we call the bulk purchase syndrome, in which household purchases are intended to last over more than one week (food durables, as it were), will lead to fewer households purchasing an exactly compensatingly larger quantity than if all purchases were required to be consumed within the purchase week. However, this implies that the identification of shifts in the average quantities purchased within a week, an increase say, does not distinguish between whether the same few households are purchasing more or more households are purchasing the same (or some combination of the two). In short, the two approaches can be interpreted as lying at two opposite extremes. The NFS proceeds as if all households within a sub-sample exhibit identical purchasing behaviour over time. Accordingly, all households are presumed to purchase all foods in the average quantities associated with their socioeconomic characteristics. The presence of non-purchase within a week is linked with the bulk purchase syndrome. Our procedure can be interpreted as assuming that there is no bulk purchase, so that within-week purchases alone reflect consumption over time (all food purchased within a week is consumed within the week) and the presence of households that never purchase particular foods.

Those associated with the NFS are fully aware of the assumptions they are making. But it is as if the presence of the bulk purchase syndrome serves as a rationale for setting aside the issue of the division between purchasers and non-purchasers. This has extremely important implications both for analytical purposes and for policy formulation. For the former, even estimates of average behaviour will be biased by the setting aside of the identification of the distinctions between purchasers and non-purchasers which is, in any case, an important analytical problem in its own right. For policy, given the goal of identifying the extent and the incidence of healthy and unhealthy diets and of targeting improvement, it is essential to distinguish between those who consume and those who do not, rather than averaging across them.

Obviously, our own approach can be legitimately criticised for setting aside the equally, if not more important, issue of the average quantities of foods that are purchased. However, our approach is open to the interpretation of posing, as a prior question, the different susceptibilities of different socioeconomic groups to purchase the various foods. This can be thought of as the first stage, of household purchase or not (together with frequency of purchase), in a two-stage process. Logically, the second stage follows in examining how much is purchased (given that it is not zero).

An example will illustrate the point. The proportion of households purchasing sausages has declined from 53.9 per cent to 34.8 per cent between 1979 and 1989 with a corresponding decline in ounces purchased per household per week from 3.29 to 2.53. As the fall in the former is greater than for the latter, it follows that those households that are purchasing sausages do so in ever larger quantities against the other two trends. According to the NFS approach as interpreted here, it would be presumed that all households are purchasing fewer sausages by buying them in larger quantities but much less frequently. This could even be explained by appeal to shifting notions of healthy eating as meat products, especially sausages, decline in popularity. However, it seems more plausible to suggest that bulk purchase is not involved but that the consumption of sausages is being concentrated and even increased in a particular section of the population whose behaviour is contrary to the more common trend. If so, the NFS approach can identify the socioeconomic characteristics of this deviant section, but it will tend to understate the extent of the problem by averaging across it as a whole. In this instance, given our knowledge of the increasing reliance on the one major shopping trip per week, it is reasonable to presume that sausages are not being purchased in bulk and consumed over a period longer than a week (unless being stored in a freezer). However, yet a further factor is the potential for a more or less regular cycle of consumption. Sausages may be purchased irregularly from week to week but still be consumed more or less instantly (and hence not form a bulk purchase).

In short, it can be argued that the issue of purchase or not, and how it is distributed across the population, is of importance even if requiring the complementary analysis of quantities consumed. The point is brought out very clearly by analogy with the case of smoking, although in more extreme form. In this instance, averages across smokers and non-smokers are of limited interest in the absence of an understanding of the incidence of who smokes. Interestingly, the NFS recognises the problem in a rather different context, taking care to undertake special analysis of the possibility of the concentrated consumption of those foods that are at greater risk of inducing food-poisoning.

Having obtained food norms as defined above, these could, although merely descriptive categories, be suggestive of proximate causes for their patterns – in other words, as found, the higher ranking of crisps, for example, in households containing children might be thought to be a sufficient explanation in itself. In what follows, however, we present a cursory overview of some of our food-norm results, together with an equally brief but more penetrating connection of the norms with the food systems involved.

For some dairy products, such as whole milk and butter, there are very sharp falls between 1979 and 1989 in the number of households purchasing them. This contrasts with the sharp increase for products such as skimmed milks and yoghurt (for which the young are particularly prominent). These changes appear to reflect a move towards healthier eating. The dramatrices for dairy products revealed a number of patterns, but the most consistent were those associated with the levels of food expenditure. Not surprisingly, the absolute frequency of purchase of any product tends to increase with food expenditure – more money is being spent, presumably across more items as well as more of the same items – although some 'inferior' foods might be expected to fall in frequency of purchase. These patterns of absolute frequency were particularly striking in the case of dairy products. However, while those who spend more might be reasonably expected to purchase more (and more of all) foods, there is no reason to believe that they should change their ranking of the foods.

But, for dairy products, there is a peculiar pattern for some of the foods. Those who spend more rank 'healthy' products, such as skimmed milks, less highly and an 'unhealthy product', such as cream, more highly. To the extent that other socioeconomic variables are associated with systematic patterns in the dramatrices, these are weaker than for food expenditure and appear to be correlates with it (such as class and income). In other words, high income or whatever might be weakly associated with these patterns in the dramatrices but this could be because of the association of high income with spending more. Whatever makes you spend more makes you spend in this particular way. Although yoghurt is an exception (with its association with the young and lower levels of food expenditure), what is striking about these results is the extent to which they contradict the absolute movements in frequencies over time. It implies that as more is spent, those who spend more do take on the 'new' products (since absolute frequencies are higher) but they are also relatively more likely to retain the 'old' products which is why their relative frequencies are higher. High spenders adopt the new patterns of consumption but shed the old products more slowly than they adopt the new. This might be explained by an association between spending more and the occasional but evenly spread ('bulk' or 'cyclical') purchase of such products but this hardly seems likely in the case of a staple such as skimmed milk, leaving aside purchase of UHT milk. It seems more likely to reflect common innovative behaviour across both 'healthy' and 'unhealthy' foods, and the lite/heavy syndrome in which consumption of something healthy justifies the consumption of something unhealthy – a sugarless diet coke allows a fatty hamburger, for example. In this light, the evolution of the UK dairy system was examined in terms of:

1 the tendency to overproduction as yields could be increased through artificial feeds and herd size
2 the division between liquid milk and processed products and the role of the Milk Marketing Board (MMB) in regulating (1) and intervening between farmers and manufacturers/retailers
3 the impact of stricter EC quotas, the rise of supermarket retailers and the erosion and ultimate abolition of the role of the MMB
4 the development of new products, and a variety of products, to serve the imperatives of healthy consumption (skimmed milks), supermarket retailing (one-stop purchasing with high expenditure), and the use and sale of the otherwise wasted butter fat in new products despite the decline in butter consumption.

Thus, the dramatic rise in the consumption of what are perceived to be healthy products, such as skimmed milks and yoghurt, is indicative of the success at one level of the healthy eating message, and it has been practically implemented by the increasing role of supermarkets in selling milk and new milk products at the expense of doorstep deliveries. But, by the same token, the very same changes in the dairy system (incorporating restructuring in the relations between farmers, marketing of liquid milk, processors, retailers and forms of household purchase) have promoted the sale of butter fat in new forms, thereby accommodating the particular organic properties of milk in terms of accommodating its perishability if not processed in the absence of rapid sale and consumption.

The dramatrices for meat products reveal a number of patterns. Perhaps the most important is that whether in the socioeconomic variables themselves or in those interpretations attached to particular meat products, there are not consistent variations. For example, the young have a particularly pronounced bias, conforming to the trend over the period from 1979 to 1989, against meat products which can be interpreted as incorporating the appeal of healthiness or vegetarianism. But for some products, attached to convenience and innovation, for example, they are also particularly favourably inclined. This leads us to the conclusion that, in demand, meat is a heterogeneous category and should be analysed as such.

A different factor in the meat norms concerned the greater overall purchases of meat products by those of lower income or class status, a reversal by 1989 of the previous association of meat purchases with higher status. This suggests that meat consumption, and possibly food more generally, has become a form of gratification for those who have more limited alternative outlets, whether these be through other forms of food provision, such as eating out, or through other aspects of personal or social life (holidaying, prestige car or house ownership). Paradoxically, as mentioned, in order to link these features of meat consumption to the food system, we emphasise the presence of a single meat system, rather than a series of individual meat systems for chicken, beef, etc., even though we have insisted on the heterogeneity of meat products. The meat system has the following features:

1 an increasing industrialisation of meat production favouring some products, such as chicken and pork, rather than others, such as lamb and beef. This reflects the cost-effectiveness and capacity in converting feed-stuff into meat
2 the development of meat products to utilise animals as fully and cheaply as possible and in conformity to the rise of standardised marketing through supermarkets at the expense of specialised butchers
3 increasing specialisation in farming with the corresponding scope of activity across meats shifting vertically up the system of provision.

Not surprisingly, like meat products, the dramatrices for the foods for which there have been major changes show that the food norms are varied across both socioeconomic variables and the significance attached to particular foods. Two themes were developed. The first was to explore the differences in patterns of consumption associated with class; the second was to examine the impact of the presence of children on food norms and how this differs in response to other socioeconomic variables. Thus, there are class, income and children effects, but they do not exist for all foods and they have complex interactions with one another and with the characteristics of the particular foods concerned. This means that the effects of class and other variables on food choice cannot simply be read off in terms of a direct reflection of their influence, as in a fish-and-chips and cloth-cap image, but nor does this imply the absence or insignificance of such effects. More specifically, without going into details, we were led to conclude that there may be a concentration of poor diets in households 'on the margins' – those on low income, with children, the unemployed – which may be overlooked in restricting analysis to average quantities consumed even within these categories at risk.

Other results and research priorities

Not surprisingly, in view of the broad scope of our approach, a number of different avenues for research were opened up, some of which we pursued and which we describe briefly below in order to illustrate the potential arising out of our work. In general, our focus has shifted away from the food norms and towards the nature and consequences of the food systems on which they depend. This is in part because an undue focus on food norms leads to the invalid proposition that food choice can be significantly changed by manipulating the immediate determinants of individual behaviour – make such and such a group at risk eat more healthily, for example, by targeted healthy eating campaigns. The desired outcome does not necessarily follow in the context of the functioning of food systems as a whole. While more effort could fruitfully go into refining the notion and measurement of food norms, this needs to be set against the task of examining how they are dependent on underlying socioeconomic factors.

First, in broaching the issue of consumption, food and gender, a review was made of the literature on eating disorders (anorexia and bulimia nervosa, and obesity) since these constitute medical conditions which represent an acute response to the socioeconomic pressures associated with modern food systems to which all consumers are subject to a greater or lesser extent with varying outcomes by foods (e.g. overindulgence or taboos) (Fine 1995a). It was found that the social science literature had neglected the extent to which these conditions were dependent on the simultaneous interaction of the compulsions to eat as well as to diet. Further, this was examined in terms of what had also been neglected, the economic factors underlying these compulsions – not just their culture and psychology – and, in particular, how the diet and food industries could coexist so symbiotically.

Second, while this chapter is based on a critical stance towards the choice *theory* associated with orthodox economics, there are also serious problems with its associated *empirical* work. In particular, NFS Reports have used standard demand analysis to assess the sources of change in the UK demand for foods over the past 50 years. The evolution of this demand analysis by the NFS can be shown to be seriously weakened by the standard assumption that demand depends on income and price effects derived from given preferences, with any unexplained residual being measured as a shift in preferences. This is most perverse especially as, for the vast majority of foods for most of the time, the residual is highly significant. In other words, the measurement of the impact of prices and income on food choice is being made on the basis of unchanging tastes even while showing just how important shifting tastes have been! In short, the demand for food cannot be legitimately studied in isolation from shifting preferences and shifting conditions of supply.

Third, drawing on previous work (Fine and Wright 1991), the understanding of the sources and impact of what is taken to be 'food knowledge' have been investigated, breaking with previous literature in a number of ways. There is a complex 'food information system' which is highly dependent òn the food system itself and interaction with it in generating choices; the model of more or less perfect trickledown of knowledge from the experts is totally inappropriate; and informational campaigns to promote healthier eating need to take account of the food system and can even be counter-productive if they do not. Once again, studying one aspect of food choice, the generation and use of knowledge about food, cannot be legitimately considered apart from other factors.

Fourth, as has been so forcibly brought to the attention of the British public in recent years by a sequence of food scandals, there is a lack of consistency between (healthy) food policy on the one hand and agricultural policy on the other. Nor does this simply raise the issue of making the two consistent with one another but of overcoming what has been an extremely dogged persistence of the hegemony of agricultural over food policy. Attempts to teach consumers to change their dietary patterns is doomed to failure if the food supply is not equally induced to conform to the desired changes. The food system has to be examined as a whole and cannot be manipulated by policy in one aspect without considering reactions and feedback effects from others.

Fifth, the last two issues open up the more general area of healthy eating and nutrition policy and regulation. Apparently good intentions and developments can prove counter-productive. Consider the example of so-called functional foods and beverages or nutraceuticals. Invented in Japan in the late 1980s, such foods and ingredients are being marketed as imparting specific health benefits in addition to their standard nutrient content: probiotic cultures in yoghurt, for example, claim to assist in regulating the human gut. This pushes food into the grey regulatory area between 'medicine/drug' and 'food' with regulatory agencies, the food industry and consumers squabbling over whether functional foods are marketing gimmicks or genuine break-throughs in contributing to improving public health.

The thrust behind the deregulation in food supply is the general belief that there is a need to free business from increasing administrative and legislative burdens to enable wealth creation.

However, in the case of food there is a strong counterfactual argument: that is, regulation in many instances is positively welcomed by the food industry itself. It is seen as setting standards, keeping 'cowboys' out of the food business and ensuring consumer confidence in terms of food safety. Research shows that many food businesses do not even know or bother to calculate the costs of compliance with food regulation, seeing such 'costs' as part of running a food business. The deregulation of the food industry is further complicated by technological and marketing developments moving faster than regulators can catch up. Powerful vested interests can also dominate the regulatory debate with other, often smaller producers, losing out in setting the regulatory agenda and seeing their interests adequately represented.

In short, we believe we have shown the importance of food norms and that the purchase/non-purchase decision has been unduly neglected. We also emphasise the need to eschew orthodox demand analysis based on price and income effects in response to fixed preferences, not to overgeneralise across foods which are of different composition and socioeconomic significance to consumers and attached to differentiated food systems, to assess the impact of factors such as smoking and drinking on diet (even if not covered here), and also to assess the impact of healthy eating campaigning in the light of the complex and varied factors underlying food choice and how these interact with differentiated food systems. For the latter, we are specifically concerned, in the case of dairy or meat products and sugar, for example, with how the differential impact of nutritional advice may predominantly redistribute food ingredients across the population, possibly in the form of new or different products. These are all issues worthy not only of further research but also as a means of providing entirely new policy perspectives and policies themselves.

Acknowledgements

Thanks are due to MAFF and the ESRC Data Archive for making data from the *National Food Survey* available, for the use and interpretation for which they bear no responsibility.

CHAPTER 7

How British retailers have shaped food choice

Neil Wrigley

Introduction

By the early 1990s, 'food choice' for the majority of British households was exercised within budget constraints in a food distribution system which, when viewed in international terms, had developed a series of quite distinct characteristics (Cotterill 1997). The nation's diet, in a very real sense, had been transformed in the 1980s by the emergence of a small group of retail corporations whose turnover, profitability, employment levels and sheer market power came to rival the largest industrial corporations in any sector of the UK economy. Those firms, operating in and actively shaping a regulatory environment supportive of their dominance of the food manufacturer–retailer interface, had assumed the role of 'channel captains' in the food system, in the process eliminating the wholesaler sector and shifting UK food distribution to a 'leading edge' position in world food system terms on dimensions ranging from inventory control to new food product development. A revolution in physical distribution, logistics and IT systems promoted by these firms had swept through UK food retailing. In turn this had facilitated the development of innovative own-label programmes, a unique chilled ready-meals market, and supply chain management techniques whose global reach incorporated previously exotic foods into the everyday diets of an increasingly wide spectrum of British households. Simultaneously, these firms had become locked into a highly capital-intensive form of competition with important conse-quences for the infrastructure of supply – the network of food retail outlets in Britain's towns and cities. British food retailers had been drawn into what, by international standards, were huge investment programmes in fixed assets – the £25m per site out-of-town super-stores, 'the cathedrals of Thatcher's Britain' (*The Times* 19 April 1997: 20). Directly consequent on that had come intense and innovative managerial concern with techniques aimed at controlling operating costs and reducing working capital.

What did all this mean for British consumers? In particular, how did it shape the manner in which consumers of the early 1990s exercised 'food choice' at the point and time of purchase? In addition, how did that differ from the experience of their counterparts in the UK a decade earlier or, in international perspective, the experience of, say, their US counterparts, at the same point in time, confronting the seemingly similar but subtly very different North American food-distribution system? Finally, why this focus on the early 1990s? Have there been facets of UK food distribution that have changed in the later 1990s to the extent that they have altered the nature of food choice?

This chapter explores these questions concentrating, in particular, on two issues. First, the way in which the major UK food retailers have shaped the range and type of food products offered to British consumers. Second, the way those retailers have altered the accessibility of different groups of consumers to food supply. Except tangentially, this chapter chooses to leave to Marsden and his research team (Chapter 9) issues relating to differential 'rights to consume' and the ways in which the major food retailers have attempted to construct and represent the 'consumer interest' in their dealings with government on matters of food quality and choice.

How retailers have shaped the range and type of food products offered

Any discussion of how British food retailers actively shaped the nature of the food products offered to consumers during the 1980s demands knowledge of two interrelated background issues. First, the way in which food manufacturer–retailer relations in the UK were transformed as power and profitability in the food system shifted in favour of corporate retail capital. Second, the way in which a revolution in physical distribution, logistics and IT systems swept through UK food retailing facilitating new forms of supply–chain management and shifting the major food retailers into a position of 'more and more actively mediating the producer–consumer relation' (Sayer and Walker 1992: 91). A considerable and distinctive body of research in the social sciences exists on these issues.

Food manufacturer–retailer relations: the shifting balance of power

Concentration of retail capital via merger and acquisition and organic growth provided one of the key trends of the 1980s in the UK food system. By 1990, just five food retailers – Sainsbury, Tesco, Argyll (Safeway), Asda, and Gateway (Somerfield) – controlled 60 per cent of the total UK 'grocery market' (Henderson Crosthwaite 1992) or 40 per cent of a more broadly defined total UK 'food market' which includes the sales of specialist food retailers (butchers, bakers, etc.), off-licences, chemists, confectioners, tobacconists and newsagents. The significantly increased market share of the major food retailers endowed them with potentially immense oligopsonistic buying power, and that power came to condition all aspects of food manufacturer–retailer relations. Social scientists of different disciplinary perpectives on economic theory have questioned both the retailer buying power and the changing characteristics of retailer–supplier relations which flowed from this shift towards a retailer-led food system.

Grant (1987) is typical of those who have considered in broad economic theory terms the nature of retailer buying power in the UK food system. His view of markets dominated by a limited number of large buyers (oligopsony) is that the principal effect of that buying power, exercised through bilateral bargaining between individual buyers and sellers, is to induce price-discrimination in favour of large buyers, typically through specially negotiated and arguably 'discriminatory' discounts. The key to understanding those discriminatory discounts in Grant's view is not the market-power of the buyers but that of the sellers. At very high levels of seller-concentration (particularly where excess production capacity is low and brand loyalty is strong) he suggests that oligopoly coordination (price/output coordination among the sellers) is likely to be effective. However, in the moderately concentrated oligopolies typical of UK food manufacturing (particularly if there is excess capacity), his view is that large retailers are likely to be able to use their buying power to induce a breakdown of oligopoly coordination, thus counteracting the market-power of the sellers and extracting concessions.

The consequences of increasing retailer buying power in the UK food system for the industrial structure of food manufacturing and retailing, the relative profitability of the sectors, and for the 'public interest' were subjects of intense debate during the 1980s (Wrigley 1992), generating two major Monopolies and Mergers Commission (MMC) and Office of Fair Trading (OFT) reviews of competitive conditions – Discounts to Retailers (MMC 1981) and Competition and Retailing (OFT 1985) – and 11 separate investigations between 1979 and 1991 of the use of vertical restraints in the UK food system. The early 1980s, in particular, was a period rife with acrimonious disputes between food manufacturers and the emerging retail corporations over issues such as retailer delisting of manufacturer brands, denial of selling space, withholding of supplies, and demands for the backdating of discounts (Davies, Gilligan and Sutton 1985). Nevertheless, despite evidence of increasing market dominance of the major food retailers and of a widening divergence between food manufacturers and the major retailers in terms of return on capital employed, the OFT's conclusion was that competition in food retailing remained robust and that the granting of 'discriminatory' discounts to the large food retailers had not been harmful to the public interest. The separate vertical restraint investigations of the MMC echoed those conclusions (McCorriston and Sheldon 1997).

The MMC and OFT investigations of competitive conditions in the industry provided, in effect, regulatory conditions supportive of the development of both a highly consolidated 'big capital' food retail sector and the retailer-led food system which had emerged in the UK by the early 1990s. Food manufacturers were increasingly obliged to learn to live with the realities of that retailer dominance and to seek stability and communication in their relationships with the major retailers, often within 'preferred supplier' type relationships (Crewe and Davenport 1992). In consequence, an important thrust of social science research in this area has focused on uncovering and understanding the nature of sourcing and supplier relations in an increasingly retailer-led system and the processes of supply-chain governance involved. In a series of studies, often supported by ESRC (Dawson and Shaw 1989; Knox and White 1991; Foord and Tillesley 1992; Foord, Bowlby and Tillesley 1992; Shaw, Dawson and Blair 1992; Hogarth-Scott and Parkinson 1993; Bowlby and Foord 1995) – and in recent PhD research (e.g. Doel 1995, 1996, 1998; Hughes 1996a, 1996b, 1996c, 1997, 1998; Duke 1996) the involvement of UK food retailers in food-product sourcing, innovation, design, development, quality monitoring, and so on has been explored and conceptualised. In particular, the rise and strategic significance of own-label/'retailer-brand' products has been considered and provides, as we will see below, a key element in the way UK food retailers shaped and altered the range and type of food products offered to British consumers.

The revolution in distribution and systems: delivering quality .

During the late 1970s and 1980s a significant frontier of cost-control and profitability in UK food retailing became focused on the areas of physical distribution, logistics and IT systems. In parallel with their increased buying power and growing dominance of the supplier interface, the major food retailers 'progressed from simply being the innocent recipients of manufacturer's transport and storage whims, to controlling and organising the supply chain, almost in its entirety' (Sparks 1994: 331).

In practice, this involved taking supply of stores out of the hands of the food manufacturers and developing centralised, quick response distribution systems (McKinnon 1989; Smith and Sparks 1993). Increasing amounts (up to 90 per cent) of a retailer's products were channelled via a network of dedicated, strategically positioned, multi-temperature, regional distribution centres (RDCs) through which deliveries to stores were consolidated and optimised. Both the RDCs and delivery to stores were frequently contracted out to specialist logistics companies (Fernie 1992). The development of dedicated RDCs and distribution systems within an increasingly concentrated food retail industry effectively eliminated the food wholesaler sector in the UK. In addition, by permitting shorter and more predictable delivery lead times (frequently below 24 hours), a significant reduction in the so-called 'conversion ratio' (the ratio of warehouse to sales space) within stores was facilitated. In turn, pressure was placed on food manufacturers to develop just-in-time, fixed-performance specification, production and factory-to-RDC systems to match. The result was a significant and progressive reduction in retailer inventory holdings, and the amount of capital tied up in those holdings, throughout the 1980s (Figure 7.1 shows the case of Tesco) as more and more of the costs (including 'uncertainty' costs) of inventory holdings were passed back to manufacturers/suppliers. By the early 1990s, 'nil' inventory levels for fast-moving, short shelf-life products had become increasingly common. In essence, stock only existed in-transit in the supply chain or on the shelves of the stores (Fernie 1994).

As the 1980s progressed, those centrally controlled distribution and stock-control systems provided fertile ground for the adoption of increasingly sophisticated computer-based IT systems. By the end of the decade fully integrated systems in which EPOS (electronic point of sale) scanning information was used to automate reordering and the linkage between within-store stock levels, the warehouse/distribution network, and central administrative functions had become the norm. Moreover, these systems were increasingly linked back via EDI (electronic data interchange) into the computer systems of manufacturers/suppliers, permitting 'paperless' supply chain control and sophisticated sales-based ordering and tracking. By the early 1990s, the EDI links of the major food retailers frequently covered more than 80 per cent of merchandise and lay at the heart of a 'demand pull' system of supply-chain management which included increasingly

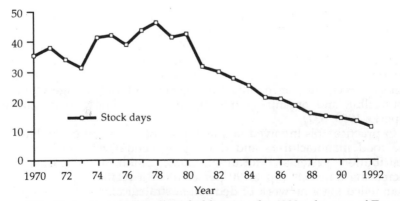

Figure 7.1 Reductions in inventory holdings in the 1980s: the case of Tesco. *Source*: redrawn from Smith and Sparks 1993.

refined waste/shrinkage control, activity-based costing, and space/ category management elements. It is widely accepted that, in terms of integrated logistics and supply chain management, the major UK food retailers were significantly ahead (perhaps as much as ten years) of their North American equivalents at this time, and also in advance of their major continental European rivals.

Implications for food choice: innovative retailer brands, chilled ready meals

What then were the implications for the food choices of British consumers of this increasingly retailer-led food system with its logistically refined 'demand pull' supply chain management? Two features among many which demand attention concern the rise and significance within UK food choice of retailer brands and the interrelated development of an innovative and, in many respects uniquely British, chilled ready meals market.

By the early 1990s retailer own-label products accounted overall for around 36 per cent of the 'packaged grocery' market in the UK (or approximately 48 per cent of sales when perishables are included), having risen in step with the increasing concentration of the food retail industry from 23 per cent at the beginning of the 1980s (Hughes 1994). The leading food retailers typically had higher own-label penetration levels than average (Sainsbury 55 per cent, Tesco 41 per cent) and, as a group, had increased those levels more rapidly (Table 7.1). In addition, the food sales of Marks and Spencer were 100 per cent own-label. In international perspective, these levels of own-label food sales were highly unusual. The equivalent overall market share figures in the USA, France and Germany in 1992 were just 14 per cent, 22 per cent and 24 per cent, with the top four food retailers in the USA having own-label penetration levels in the range 14 per cent to 21 per cent (J P Morgan Securities Inc 1995).

Table 7.1 Trends in own-label 'packaged grocery' market shares of the four leading UK food retailers

| | Market share (%) | | |
	1980	1992	1995
Sainsbury	54	55	56
Tesco	21	41	48
Safeway (Argyll)	28	35	44
Asda	5	32	41

Source: AGB Superpanel

117

Table 7.2 Trends in operating profit margins of the 'Big Three' UK food retailers' major operations 1985–92* (figures based on turnover exclusive of VAT)

Retailer	Operating profit margins (%)							
	1985	1986	1987	1988	1989	1990	1991	1992
Sainsbury	5.25	5.53	6.09	6.54	7.31	7.61	8.32	8.71
Tesco	2.72	3.10	4.10	5.21	5.86	6.18	6.62	7.09
Safeway (Argyll)	3.57	3.89	4.34	4.69	5.19	5.94	6.74	7.49

* Takes account of only major format/fascia of the company, not secondary formats/operations such. as Lo-Cost/Presto (Argyll/Safeway), Savacentre/Homebase/Shaw's (Sainsbury)
Source: Henderson Crosthwaite 1992

Why then did these unusual UK levels of own-label food sales emerge, and why are they important in the context of food choice?

The growth of own-label trading and the increased market dominance, profitability and supply-chain control of the major UK food retailers during the 1980s were intrinsically interlinked. Own-label products offered the major food retailers higher profit margins than comparable manufacturer brands and leveraged their heavy logistics investment more efficiently. They were thus an essential component powering the significant profit margin increases enjoyed by those firms during the period (Table 7.2). However, as Terry Leahy (1987), now Chief Executive of Tesco, outlined in the late 1980s, own-label also provided other significant advantages to the food retailers. The most obvious lay in market development, product control and product innovation. Retailers could use own-label to fill gaps left in the range of products offered by the manufacturers, in that way spurring broader market development. They could also develop own-label products quickly, under tighter control, and take more risks with product innovation. The result was that during the 1980s the major food retailers were increasingly drawn into making significant investments in product specification, development, packaging and quality testing, and the developmental role of the retailers' food technologists and home economists became ever more critical (Senker 1986; Doel 1995; Omar 1995; Hughes 1996a). New product innovation by the food retailers was aided by the consumer preference/sales information — item-by-item, store-by-store, region-by-region — which flooded out of their EPOS systems from the mid-1980s onwards. As a result, they could effectively take more risks than the food manufacturers, not only because they did not have to buy distribution and access to shelf space at the same marginal cost as the manufacturers, but also because their proprietary scanner data allowed them to position new products with greater precision at the leading edge of changing consumer tastes.

The consequence was that, as the 1980s progressed, the own-label products of the major UK food retailers were successively transformed away from the inferior quality, cheap, generic or sub-brand image which had been common in the 1960s and 1970s in the UK, and which continued to characterise own-label in many other countries (particularly the USA) throughout the 1980s and early 1990s (see Hughes 1996b). The image moved towards high-quality and innovation, placing UK food retailers, who were often adding over 1000 new own-label lines per year, at a leading edge position in world food system terms by the end of the decade. Own-label had effectively been repositioned as 'retailer brand' (de Chernatony 1989; Burt 1992; Sparks 1997) in which a link between the retailer's corporate identity and consumer trust in the firm's reputation creates a situation in which the retailer brand becomes the guarantee of quality and consistency. Innovation in retailer branding also became a key element in the enhancement of company image. Sparks (1997), for example, draws attention to Tesco's healthy eating initiative of the mid-1980s – an important element in the repositioning of Tesco's corporate image – and the way that was launched via extensive nutritional labelling on its retailer brands. Similarly, he notes how Argyll (Safeway) used the removal of contentious food additives from products in its retailer brand range to enhance its corporate image.

At the cutting edge of these developments was the emergence of the chilled ready meals sector – a market whose value in the UK was worth over £300m per annum by the early 1990s, but which barely existed in 1983, and which remained undeveloped in many other countries (particularly the USA) by the mid-1990s. This development, which differentially but significantly altered the food choices of certain socioeconomic groups of consumers in the UK, created the first major food market segment in the UK to be totally dominated by own-label. It was not only 'of immense symbolic significance . . . visibly epitomising the changing dynamics and shifting power balance within the food industry' (Doel 1996: 55), but also demanded entirely new modes of supply network initiation. Given that chilled ready meals were, in the mid-1980s, a completely new, retailer-initiated, product sector, complex both to manufacture and to distribute, there was simply no pre-existing brand manufacturer presence. That is to say, there was no manufacturer surplus capacity to appropriate as the basis of an own-label supply. As a result, the retailers – Marks and Spencer, the pioneer of the sector, closely followed by Sainsbury, Tesco and the other major firms – were forced to develop their own ready meals supply chains in the absence of organisational alternatives. The chains that developed had some distinct characteristics (Doel 1995, 1996). In particular, they were characterised by larger numbers of small and medium-sized specialised suppliers than was typical elsewhere in the industry and the early growth of those suppliers was frequently underpinned by retailer intervention/commitment. In return, the retailers' requirements were exacting. The supply chains that evolved were, in consequence, dynamically interactive, based around the imperatives of continuous new product development as the food retailers pursued product-centred competitive advantage. They were also characterised by stringent confidentiality and exclusivity contracts. The exacting requirements of chilled meals distribution also created and/or strengthened the trends towards contracted-out relationships between specialist logistics companies and the food retailers – for example, the growth of BOC Distribution Services was the direct result of Marks and Spencer's development of chilled food products.

Some wider implications

By the early 1990s, not only had UK own-label food products effectively been repositioned, as 'retailer brands', with all that implied for the consumer in terms of quality and consistency, but a significant proportion of those products were increasingly derived from a supply chain in which intensive new product development lay at the very core of the retailer–manufacturer relationship. Social scientists from several disciplines have sought to understand and conceptualise the nature of this new product development process, which is neither purely production-led or demand-led, and the supply-chain relationships on which it rests (Hughes 1998). Some, using the arguments of Granovetter (1985), have viewed the process as being deeply embedded in networks of personal relations – 'the ties that bind' – between individuals in the supply relationships. Others, while acknowledging that new product development is conducted through complex socially embedded organisational processes, have suggested that it is rather the product-centred competitive imperative of the retailers which structures the nature of the process. In this view, new product development is seen as having assumed a critical role in own-label supply governance in the UK (Doel 1995, 1998).

Irrespective of the theoretical interpretation which is placed on the process, however, the overall effect for British consumers by the early 1990s was marked. The range and type of food products offered by the small number of major retailers who increasingly dominated supply had some very different characteristics to that experienced in other countries or in the UK a decade earlier, as did the logistically refined 'demand pull' supply-chain management system which delivered these products to the stores and created, in practical terms, for those consumers their 'environment of choice'. Two facets of the food choice milieu faced by British consumers of the early 1990s are worth drawing out at this point.

First, as retailer brands increasingly squeezed out of the market the weaker manufacturer brands in each product field, British consumers faced far less brand proliferation on the shelves of food stores than their counterparts in North America or continental Europe. To some this might appear to be a restriction of food choice, but that is to confuse mere brand duplication with choice. For example, a US superstore of the early 1990s might easily have stocked between 20 000 and 30 000 SKUs (stock-keeping units – the most specific description possible for a single grocery item), double that of its UK equivalent. But did that imply a richer food choice for US consumers and/or enhanced consumer-welfare benefits? Many US analysts would suggest not, often lamenting the low-quality positioning and lack of innovation which characterised US own-label in the early 1990s, and suggesting that 'injecting a strong dose of British retailer-led vertical alliances with small and medium sized food manufacturers to produce top quality private label might be just what the public policy sector should order' (Cotterill 1997: 127).

Second, a majority of British consumers by the early 1990s exercised food choice in stores which, in international and temporal perspective, had very high levels of sales per square foot, very rapid stock turns (twice as fast as those in the USA), and low risks of 'stock-out' of any particular item (in comparison to the equivalent UK stores of the 1970s). The sophisticated logistics, IT systems, and broader supply-chain management which had created these conditions had developed inseparably from the growth of the often dynamically interactive, intensely innovatory, own-label supply networks of the 1980s. But as the major UK food retailers learned to manage those own-label supply chains 'in order to derive a fluid and differentiated portfolio of competitive advantages' (Doel 1998), they increasingly applied the same supply-chain management techniques to global produce markets (see Arce and Marsden 1993; Cook 1994). What this increasingly implied for British consumers by the early 1990s was the incorporation of previously exotic foods (from mange touts to mangos) into their everyday food choices, the erosion of seasonality of fresh produce lines (the year-round strawberry), and the increasingly sophisticated tailoring of certain food products and fresh produce to niche markets (Crang and Cook 1996). Often underplayed in the placing of these developments in international perspective is the differential extent of retailer control of food-purchase information. In the UK the major food retailers exercised tight control of, and exploited in increasingly sophisticated ways, the data outputs of their EPOS scanner systems for the mid-1980s onwards. In the USA, by contrast, it was the food manufacturers rather than the retailers that came to dominate the use of scanner data, with third-party information companies such as A C Neilson and IRI gathering, providing and analysing the information largely for food manufacturer-related purposes.

How retailers have altered the accessibility of different groups of consumers to food supply

Concentration of retail capital, shifting retailer–manufacturer power relations, the emergence of logistically refined 'demand pull' supply-chain management, and the dynamism and innovation which characterised the rise of UK retailer brands, although vital elements in their own right, represent only parts of a broader story of continuous reconstruction of the competitive spaces of the British food industry during the 1980s. An equally significant element, with very considerable consequences for the food choices of British consumers, was the transformation of the infrastructure of supply – the network of retail outlets through which food was delivered to those consumers. During the 1980s, that infrastructure was radically altered as the major food retailers were drawn into an increasingly capital-intensive form of competition and into what, by international standards, were huge investment programmes in fixed assets. Those programmes not only differentially altered the accessibility of consumers to food supply, but also linked back through the imperative created to 'work the fixed assets' into intense managerial concern with operating productivity and a strengthening of the many supply chain management innovations outlined above. What then·were the characteristics of the increasingly capital-intensive form of food retail competition in the 1980s, and what were the consequences for food choice?

Superstores and store wars

Larger stores, on highly accessible sites, with significant amounts of dedicated customer parking, simple/segregated delivery vehicle approaches, and negligible catchment-area competition from rival stores of the same vintage, rapidly became one of the critical 'drivers' of increased profitability of the major food retailers in the 1980s. Such superstores (see Table 7.3 for the case of Sainsbury stores) were able to operate at significantly lower wage costs and distribution costs as a percentage of sales, and were able to achieve substantially higher operating profit margins (Shaw, Nisbet and Dawson 1989; Richards and MacNeary 1991). The increasing profit margins came in part from the lower relative operating costs, and in part from higher sales densities (sales per sq ft). In turn, those higher densities reflected the ability to stock a wider product range (with more 'value added' items), plus a higher average 'customer spend' – a function of both consumer

Table 7.3 Sainsbury UK supermarkets: comparative wage costs, sales intensity and operating margins by store size group 1990

Store size group	Wage costs (as % of sales)	Sales/sq ft	Operating margins
<15 000 ft^2	124	95	66
15–25 000 ft^2	102	95	96
>25 000 ft^2	91	108	114
JS average	100	100	100

Index base 100 = company average of established supermarkets
Source: Richards and MacNeary 1991

122

preference for a food-shopping environment configured in such a way and the very real restriction of alternative competing food stores as a result of the local spatial monopolies conferred by UK land-use planning constraints on superstore development. As Moir (1990: 112) noted: 'ensconced and dominant in their own markets, the new large stores [of the 1980s] enjoy[ed] a degree of protection from all'.

By the early 1990s the average size of Tesco's food stores had risen to over 26 000 sq ft sales area from just 11 000 sq ft at the beginning of the 1980s, with the new Tesco stores being constructed averaging over 40 000 sq ft. Moreover, an increasingly large proportion of the food retailers' stores were of very recent vintage. Indeed, about a quarter of all Tesco and Sainsbury floorspace was in stores built within the previous three years alone (Guy 1994), and the major firms were generating a substantial proportion of their annual increases in sales from the new superstores opened in the previous 12 months. Essentially, what had occurred during the later 1980s was that strategic capital investment in new store expansion had become the all-consuming engine of corporate growth and of increasing concentration, and had become vital to the maintenance of the substantial annual increases in turnover and profit that the capital markets had come to enjoy (Wrigley 1991).

However, given an effective rationing of sites for large-scale development as a result of UK land-use planning constraints, even during the Thatcher–Ridley deregulatory free-market era of the mid-to-late 1980s, competition between the major food retailers for the most attractive development sites became intense. The late 1980s and early 1990s became, therefore, an era of 'store wars' in which an increasingly

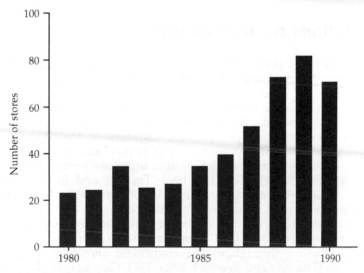

Figure 7.2 Food superstore openings in the UK, 1980–90.
Source: adapted from Guy 1994.

123

frantic store-building boom (Figure 7.2) forced up prices in a distorted land market, resulting in site costs alone rising to over £20m or between £2m and £3m per acre in several cases in south-east England. A form of collective corporate over-commitment to a single dominant strategy of accumulation – growth via out-of-town superstore development – occurred. On the one hand this raised barriers to market entry by other food retailers who could not match the huge sunk costs of the major firms, but on the other it substantially increases the potential vulnerability of those firms (Wrigley 1994).

During this period of the 'store wars', the British food retail industry became increasingly capital intensive. Huge investment in fixed assets, by international standards, created an imperative to work the assets hard in order to achieve RONA (return on net asset) levels which matched those in other countries (for example, in the USA equivalent stores could be built at less than one-third of the UK costs). The result was intense managerial concern with techniques aimed at controlling operating costs and reducing working capital. In other words, there was a direct feedback between the highly capital-intensive store-development programmes, and the leading-edge position which the major UK food retailers had evolved to in world food-system terms by the early 1990s in terms of innovatory retail brand development, logistics and inventory control, wider supply-chain management techniques, IT systems applications and exploitation of scanner data to enhance retailer profit. In a very real issue the major UK food retailers had been pushed still further into that highly active supply-chain management role by the demands of a form of competition which became increasingly focused on high fixed asset investment (Wrigley 1997a).

Implications for food choice

The overwhelming profitability advantages accruing to the major food retailers from the building of the superstores (see Table 7.3) were often best captured on green-field, edge-of-city sites able to meet all the criteria outlined above. As a result, the locus of food supply in British cities shifted outwards during the 1980s, and the accessibility of particular socioeconomic groups of consumers to that supply was radically and differentially altered. The nature and extent of those transformations generated a considerable literature (examples include Guy 1988; BDP Planning/OXIRM 1992; Thomas and Bromley 1993), plus one well-known case study (Guy 1996) of the local-scale impacts of the shifting food retail structure of a British city.

A general conclusion of this literature was that the development of the superstores 'resulted in a significant weakening of the [food]-shopping function throughout the traditional shopping centres' of British cities (Thomas and Bromley 1993: 131). Guy's (1996) case study of Cardiff during the 1980s and early 1990s – a city of 300 000 population, large enough to have experienced most of the developments typical of the period – suggests that this weakening occurred essentially as a result of a sharp decline in the number of small food stores in traditional local shopping centres or small store clusters in the city which accompanied the building of the superstores. Essentially, as a ring of seven edge-of-city superstores was gradually put into position in Cardiff during the 1980s, a wave of closures of smaller food stores in suburban and inner-city locations was induced. Although these two trends are clearly interrelated, it is more difficult to link them through a simple 'trading impact' diagnosis than might at first be imagined. Rather what appears to have happened is that the diversion of trade to the new superstores was mediated through, and accelerated in rather complex ways, trends which already existed (Guy 1996). Nevertheless, the results in terms of accessibility to food supply were clear cut.

As food retailing was unevenly stripped out of particular parts of British cities during the 1980s, or repositioned downward in range and quality terms relative to the expanded, often innovatory, offerings of the superstores, so the accessibility to food supply and the effective food choice of particular socioeconomic groups was differentially affected. The food-choice benefits of the edge-of-city supermarkets went, in practice, to the mobile, relatively more affluent, majority. As a result, the existence of 'disadvantaged consumers' – effectively constrained by mobility restrictions (e.g. dependence on public transport) to an increasingly eroded food retail environment – became a subject of debate and concern (Westlake 1993). In particular, the position of women food-shoppers, who as a group suffered relatively greater mobility disadvantages (Bowlby 1988), together with the elderly and disabled, attracted the attention of academics, consumer groups and the Royal Town Planning Institute (1988). However, so profound was the dynamic of retail change, and so subtle were the complex repositionings of food retail offerings through the portfolio of stores of the corporate retailers, that this literature often struggled to capture the food-choice implications of the increasingly capital-intensive British food retail industry. Nevertheless, these debates were contributory elements to increasing public disquiet about the adverse consequences of food superstore development – a disquiet which ultimately was to give rise to significantly tightened land-use planning regulation with respect to such development in the mid-1990s.

What has changed in the 1990s?

The capital-intensive, channel-captaincy mode of operation of the major UK food retailers, with its many consequences for the nature of food choice, was essentially forged during the retail revolution of the late 1970s and 1980s. By the early 1990s the conditions that had sustained the increasing market dominance and profitability of those firms was beginning to ebb away (Wrigley 1991). Two interrelated gaps in the barriers to market entry erected by the heavy capital investment in fixed assets of the major firms during the 1980s were suddenly exploited: first, a 'value platform' gap – a vulnerability to low-margin, low-capital-intensity, limited-line deep discount operators (Burt and Sparks 1994; Wrigley 1994); second, a locational gap – the potential loci of profit extraction represented by the urban 'High Streets' increasingly abandoned by the major food retailers as they had shifted out-of-town, together with smaller towns by-passed by the superstore building programmes of the late 1980s. The major food retailers also suddenly found themselves engulfed by the consequences of the more general UK property crisis, facing significant problems of property over-valuation, non-recoverable investment and capitalised interest, which came to a head in spectacular fashion during 1993/94 (Wrigley 1996, 1998a). Finally, those firms found themselves faced, after a period of growing public unease about the consequences of their dominance of the UK food system, with tightened regulation both in terms of land-use planning and competitive practices (Wrigley 1993, 1994). In effect, they were faced with the need to engage in the 'politics of market maintenance' in order to defend their competitive space (Marsden, Harrison and Flynn 1998).

It is not the intention of this chapter to explore this reconstruction of the competitive spaces of British food retailing during the 1990s, or the increased internationalisation of the leading firms which was one response. That task is addressed elsewhere by several authors (Wrigley 1994, 1997b, 1997c, 1998a, 1998b; Guy 1997; Langston, Clarke and Clarke 1997; Sparks 1996a, 1996b). It is sufficient simply to highlight some of the food-choice implications of that reconstruction. Three features are worthy of attention, each intrinsically related to the way in which the major food retailers have been forced, by changing competitive conditions and by the harsh consequences of their collective over-commitment to what increasingly amounted to a single dominant strategy of capital accumulation in the late 1980s, to seek new ways of maintaining and gaining profitable market share.

First, the discount reorientation of UK food retailing in the early 1990s – the market entry of the limited-line discounters from mainland Europe (Aldi, Netto, Lidl), and the amplification of their primary impact via the competitive response of the second-tier UK food retailers – spread price-competition ripple effects throughout the industry. Ultimately those effects engulfed the 'big three' firms and impacted on the profit-margin structures of the entire industry. Gross profit margins experienced a downward correction, and the upward trend of operating profit margins which had characterised the period from 1985 to 1992 (see Table 7.2) went into reverse. For the first time for many years, price competition became a significant feature of UK food retailing, forcing down during 1992–94 the prices of so-called 'core' food items in a rapid way throughout the country but particularly in some of the urban areas of the North and Midlands. In addition, the uni-dimensional increased quality movement of own-label products which had characterised the 1980s came to an end, as the major food retailers introduced price-fighter 'Value' and 'Economy' own-label ranges, alongside their standard retailer brand ranges, to match the discounter's tertiary brands on price.

Second, the coincidence of tightened land-use planning regulation – the revisions in 1993 and 1996 of Planning Policy Guidance (PPG) Note 6 *Town Centres and Retail Development* (DoE 1993, 1996), together with PPG13 *Transport* (DoE 1994) – and the need, following the property crisis of 1993/94, to re-evaluate over-commitment to a strategy of growth via out-of-town superstore development, has offered the potential to reassess old and/or previously marginal locations of food retail profit extraction (Wrigley 1998a). The major food retailers have returned, in a somewhat halting fashion, to High Street food retailing. This has occurred via new small (10 000 sq ft) Tesco 'Metro' stores plus the short-lived Sainsbury 'Central' stores experiment, via refurbishment of remaining High Street stores, and via contributions to the fledgling 'Town Centre Management' movement. More significantly, there has also been important reconsideration of locations (e.g. smaller towns) which during the height of the 'store wars' were regarded as having population catchments too small for profitable superstore development by the major food retailers. So-called 'Compact' or 'Country Town' stores – at 15–20 000 sq ft just half the size of the superstores of the late 1980s – have become a feature of the store-development programmes of the major food retailers. Together with the High Street 'Metro' stores, and the new stores of the limited-line discounters, the 'Compact'/ 'Country Town' stores are increasingly bringing the product range and quality of the corporate food retailers, and the associated food-choice possibilities, to groups of consumers previously disadvantaged in terms of their access to the more dynamic elements of UK food retailing.

Finally, changed competitive conditions have increasingly forced the major food retailers to seek new ways of gaining profitable market share based on the competitive advantages of their IT systems expertise. That expertise, and the EPOS scanner data which supported it, had for some time offered the food retailers the potential to respond in sophisticated ways to increasingly fragmented consumer markets. During the 1990s that expertise and potential has been built upon via customer loyalty/reward schemes, database marketing, new electronic channels to market, and the linked retailing of financial and other services.

The rhetoric which surrounds these developments would often suggest the primacy of new electronic 'channels to market'. The reality is somewhat different (Reynolds 1997). Although Tesco, for example, has run extensive trials in West London of the potential of electronic home-shopping, although several of the major firms have experimented with various forms of non-store routes to market, and although most UK food retailers have an Internet presence, the anticipated shift to such forms of food retailing is extremely low. Rather, it has been the growth of consumer loyalty/reward programmes, and the ability to tie into and retail potentially highly profitable financial services through such programmes, which has proved to be of greater significance. Despite the controversy which surrounds the cost/benefit ratio of such schemes to the retailer, in food-choice terms such programmes clearly present increased opportunities to the retailer to 'direct' choice in subtle ways. Particular segments of the customer base (e.g. the sub-group of Tesco loyalty scheme participants who are 'Baby Club' members) can be differentially targeted through 'reward' incentives with little of the resource wastage associated with old fashioned direct-marketing schemes. And, more generally, by using such schemes to add greater 'excitement' to a basic food retail format which in the USA would be termed EDLP (everyday low prices), differential consumption is clearly induced. In the longer-term, however, new electronic channels to market do pose some vitally important questions in terms of the retailers' role in shaping food choice. Not least among these is the possibility that such channels may allow manufacturers increasingly to by-pass retailers and trade directly with consumers. The extent to which that is likely, and its consequences for food choice, must surely depend upon how innovatory British retailers remain in their role as 'channel captains' in the food system.

CHAPTER 8

A sociological approach to food choice: the case of eating out

Alan Warde and Lydia Martens

Sociological approaches to consumer choice

Much of people's everyday behaviour is predictable to a degree of detail that cannot be attributed to their biological or psychological attributes. Such regularity is the consequence of what many sociologists would describe as the existence of normative order: a set of institutionalised guidelines about appropriate conduct which are generally held to be binding within particular social circles or contexts. This is a way of explaining processes entailed by human *inter*dependence, the necessity in complex and impersonal societies for coordinating personal interactions. Institutionalised norms regulate and steer personal conduct into acceptable, comprehensible and effective activities.

As a result of recognising these features of social life, sociology has generally been suspicious of the concept of choice, and has spent much of its history trying to identify the forces, mechanisms and institutional arrangements which restrict the practical range of options open to individuals. Because they live under the sway of collectively sanctioned beliefs, values and norms, the conduct of individuals belonging to the same social groups or categories tends to be similar. Durkheim's *Suicide*, first published in 1895, is a classic exposition of the connection between individual acts and social regulation. To commit suicide, he reasoned, is the ultimate individual act, a personal exercise of will that demonstrates control over our own destiny. It might be thought the extreme and limiting example of pure personal choice. Yet he shows that the incidence of suicide is patterned in such a way as to suggest that identifiable social forces, like religious affiliation and marital condition, underpin the propensity for suicide. It is less personal a decision than might be imagined; social circumstances as well as individual inclinations determine its incidence. We like to think there are strong parallels between suicide and consumption.

'Choices' are pre-programmed; people have dispositions that they

129

have learned from others in their social network, whether that be a peer group, an ethnic group, a social class, a local community or a nation. Such entities form the bases of cultures, and people sharing a culture will tend to behave in similar ways, governed by the orientations, preferences and sanctions authorised by it. Material constraints, moral codes, social pressure, aesthetic sensibilities and situational logics all steer consumer behaviour along predictable paths.

Shopping, for food as for anything else, entails decision-making. The reality of the choice involved in such decisions lies at the centre of sociological debates about consumption. Commonsense asserts that the consumer makes real choices; there are few formal sanctions requiring the purchasing of particular items, engagement in particular leisure pursuits, or eating particular kinds of food. This is the sense in which, as Bauman 1988 says, most people are less restricted in the field of consumption than in any other part of their lives. While he may be correct, we want to contest dominant perceptions of the extent and quality of such individual freedom.

Beyond the rhetoric of choice

Political rhetoric of the 1980s was dominated by an equation between private ownership, markets and freedom of choice. Choice became perhaps the most powerful talisman justifying state policy in a wide range of fields, including education, health care, housing, privatisation of state-owned utilities, the citizen's charter and so forth. In association, the consumer became a key figure to whom politicians and ideologues referred when proposing and legitimising policy. One misleading consequence of such discourse is exaggeration of the scope of the freedom implied by the concept of consumer choice.

Choice, according to our dictionary, conveys four different shades of meaning: (1) to select; (2) to pick in preference; (3) to consider fit, or suitable; and (4) to will or determine. The ideological escalation involved in the application of the term choice in the field of consumption arises, we believe, from conflating the first two meanings with the fourth. The fourth implies the existence of freedom for an individual to determine their own fate. The first two, by contrast, merely suggest picking among a given set of items. To connect closely shopping and existential freedom appears to misrepresent both: Sainsburys does not offer the ultimate form of personal autonomy. Potentially the distinctions made by the dictionary might be formalised and serve usefully to eliminate from social scientific language the term choice which currently conflates several different types of act.

To exercise will implies a degree of power or control, the capacity to make decisions which will result in desired outcomes irrespective of the countervailing wills of other people or institutions. Willing implies getting one's own way, deciding for oneself. Only an actor with infinite resources, no prejudices and a capacity to suppress social opposition could approximate to the level of control ascribed to the truly sovereign consumer. Much of sociological analysis has been devoted to showing that individuals often lack a capacity for determination irrespective of others. Many desired goals are impervious to the will of any single, even extremely powerful, individual. What can be achieved is institutionally highly circumscribed, even though in an individualistic culture many cherish the illusion that they have a significant impact on their environment. There are many conditions under which the individual will is ineffective even in the apparently discretionary field of consumption. Consider four concatenations of circumstances in which freedom and constraint are tempered by one another.

Suitability

People internalise notions of what is fitting in particular situations for people like themselves, such that no external intervention is required to induce acceptable behaviour. Even when it is possible to exercise will, people apparently invoke certain standards, judgements, rules or norms which govern both what they might desire and how they might go about fulfilling their desires. We cannot countenance being in a restaurant and demanding custard with roast beef or throwing food at a customer at another table. Such behaviour is considered unsuitable or unfitting. No one in our interviews reported having taken beef with custard, nor even having eaten gateau before soup. Despite apparent provocation, no one recorded having admonished a fellow diner. These are not practicable alternatives because there are a set of deeply structured internalised constraints which effectively prohibit people from such courses of action on pain of the embarrassment of being considered socially deplorable or grossly incompetent. The implied judgements about what is aesthetically or socially acceptable comprise perhaps the key sphere of sociological interest, but one which recent debates about consumption have tended to ignore or take for granted.

Picking in preference

To pick in preference implies a hierarchy of taste and the probability of picking one thing rather than another because it will give greater satisfaction. In economics it is assumed that consumers in the market place do exactly that: consumers have a fixed and transitive set of preferences in accordance with which, subject primarily to constraints of price and income, they will always pick that which is preferred. Economists do not pretend to know the origins of these preferences – some hope that sociologists will solve this problem for them – but rather take them as given. Picking in preference presumes that some fundamental decisions about suitability have already been taken; for example, we never consider picking among the dog foods at the supermarket because neither of us has a pet. Though it overlaps with the process of considering things suitable, picking in preference might be deemed analytically as a stage lower down the continuum of wilful choosing. There are, still, interesting social processes involved in the governance of picking in preference. We are subject to social steering mechanisms which guide us towards picking some things rather than others. Picking in preference indicates some active standard of aesthetic or practical judgement and such hierarchies often operate as a means of social communication. They disclose personal identity and social identification; green wellington boots are socially meaningful icons which suggest that their wearers identify with, or at least are not repelled by, a particular stereotype of a social group. Sociologists of consumption have always been interested in this kind of behaviour because it indicates social differentiation, social divisions and social exclusion. Sociology is particularly known for its discussions of practices of invidious social comparison, whereby superiority is symbolised through displays of goods and the enjoyment of services which confer social distinction.

Selection

We might define selection as a process whereby someone picks from a set of items considered, in a given context, as equivalent: to opt for salmon rather than trout from a menu, or to go to Pizza Hut rather than Pizzaland would be instances. While these are matters which may be of enormous importance to a market-research company they hold almost no interest for a sociologist. At the point at which a decision conveys no social meaning, as when one item can be readily substituted for the other without any consequence for the reputation of the person involved, then it has little relevance to a sociology of consumer choice. This is not to deny that there are important potential issues raised for understanding consumption more generally by the very notion of equivalence: one main line of criticism of mass consumer society has been that consumers are misled into believing that the sheer variety of items available for purchase guarantees free and meaning-ful personal choice. Wood (1994), for instance, suggests that commer-cial restaurants are, in large part, standardised and uniform, their differences more apparent than real; indeed it has been argued cogently that much contemporary advertising is the attempt to persuade people that they are picking in preference when really they are merely selecting from identical items. Selection, then, refers to the most limited degree of choice, the level before allocation, where we simply have to accept what we are given – Hobson's choice!

Allocation, or Hobson's choice

There are many circumstances, frequently pertaining even in the apparently discretionary field of consumption, in which the will of the individual is totally ineffective. Relationships involving coercion and manipulation by others is one example. Compulsive addiction is another. The greater authority or influence of other people in a collective decision-making situation is a third. Shortage of resources necessary to achieve the desired outcome, including money, information and time, is a fourth. Yet another is the absence of an accessible environment within which the outcome can be effected; for example eating a Japanese meal in Lancaster is impossible because no Japanese restaurants exist. The individual has no practicable opportunity to exercise discretion. Such circumstances imply the absence, for all practical purposes, of any form of choice; they constitute the denial of the opportunity to enter the field in which will might be exercised. These disempowering circumstances are found in many fields of social activity and often operate prior to any consideration of consumer decision-making. Choice is pre-empted.

These gradations of the process referred to as choice raise potentially different questions for an understanding of eating habits. Sociology has a legitimate interest in them all and sociologists of consumption will often weave competing accounts of these various stages. Bourdieu, for instance, the most influential modern sociologist of consumption, argues that styles of consumption are means not just of using up resources, but of acquiring new forms of economic and social 'capital', because the display of goods is part of a system of reputation, wherein judgements about suitability, framed as definitions of good taste, result in members of different social classes systematically picking some items in preference to others. Some styles are socially more prestigious than others. But also among his axioms is the claim that different classes pick different items because, having developed a set of dispositions which are deeply entrenched in their consciousness, they have learned those preferences. His work, especially *Distinction* (1984), is the starting point for many debates. Some argue that judgements of suitability have now become so unpredictable and unpatterned as to suggest that group-based judgement has fragmented and consumption been disconnected from social identification. Other commentators see the activity of picking in preference as no longer seriously compromised by the unequal distribution of resources and thus a field for the playful expression of self-identity. Yet others, postulating the existence of a mass culture, deem consumer behaviour nothing but producer manipulation and trivial consumer selection. The area of competing theories of consumption is a highly contentious area and one where there are as yet few reliable means for adjudicating empirically between them. This is partly because of the difficulty of devising satisfactory methods for estimating patterns of consumption and interpreting their associated meanings.

Operationalising constraints on choice

Sociologists infer the existence of social steering and institutional constraint from regularities of observable behaviour and from reports by individual subjects which reveal shared understandings. When it is discovered that people with low incomes eat out less frequently than the more affluent it is deduced that money is an unequally distributed resource the shortage of which restricts eating out; when many people tell us that for them eating out primarily means taking a substantial and organised meal with others on a special occasion we can infer that it is recognised as a particular category of event with its own distinguishing features and therefore governed by shared norms. In the first case the sociologist uses the probability of certain outcomes as evidence of constraint or structure; in the second it is the appreciation of jointly held understandings about appropriate conduct in particular contexts that indicates the existence of prior collective learning processes.

Sociologists, therefore, employ a wide range of techniques for collecting evidence of the social constraints which operate on individuals. One of these is to examine statistical patterns of association between behaviours and collective affiliation or belonging. The point here is not to predict accurately the behaviour of particular individuals, which is quite simply impossible, but to estimate the probabilities of behaviour. Another is to try to understand, through interviews, what people are thinking, how they see themselves when in situations of making decisions about what to consume. The latter will hopefully produce a set of specifiable operational rules, or criteria of judgement, used by lay people when put in a situation where preference has to be exercised. A third is to examine collective representations of the items to be consumed: the examination of images, advertisements, popular information sources like newspapers and TV, visual and literary associations between food and social contexts, gives an analytic handle on processes of communication in the context of which people form, reproduce and alter their judgements about desirable comestibles.

Our study attempted both to identify statistical patterns and to explore the collective meanings associated with one aspect of the nation's diet: eating out. Initially it involved interviews with 33 principal food providers in households in diverse circumstances. All the interviews were in Preston and the surrounding area, in the autumn of 1994, and each lasted between one and two hours. All interviewees were asked a number of questions relating to aspects of eating at home and eating out. The interviews were of a semi-structured type and discussion was wide-ranging around the key topics. Subsequently, 1001 people were interviewed in three English cities: London, Bristol and Preston. A quota sample matched respondents to the overall population of diverse local wards by age, sex, class and ethnic group. The survey was undertaken in April 1995 and questions were asked about the frequency of eating out, types of outlet visited, attitudes to eating out and the nature of the most recent meal eaten away from home. The answers to these have been analysed to explore social variations in eating out by class, income, age, gender, education, place of residence, and so forth. We use the term 'interviewee' to refer to the people involved at the qualitative stage, and the term 'respondent' to apply to those contacted by the survey.

There was almost no reliable empirical sociological research on eating out at the point when this study was commissioned. Subsequently the

National Food Survey (Ministry of Agriculture, Fisheries and Food 1995) published the first detailed statistical analysis of eating out in Britain, though driven by a primary concern with the nutritional aspects of its expanding contribution to the national diet. Eating out constitutes an interesting case for the exploration of food choice precisely because it is apparently discretionary spending, usually interpreted as a form of entertainment on special social occasions. It might appear to be the aspect of eating which is least determined by external pressure and the decisions of others; it is often contrasted with the routines of the household where members eat what is prepared as part of the necessary basis for physical survival. Yet close examination of the practice of eating out reveals many ways in which behaviour is materially constrained, normatively regulated and socially structured.

In this chapter we seek simply to give some illustration of how the capacity for an individual personally to will or determine the form and content of a meal away from home is restricted. We use primarily data drawn from the qualitative interviews, which indicate the naturalness with which people accommodate to constraint without even necessarily perceiving it as such. We supplement quotations with some statistical evidence. It is not feasible to present evidence which maps directly on to the abstract categories of types of constraint identified above. To do so would result in the reporting of a series of unconnected, uncontextualised and therefore apparently trivial examples. Instead we examine some circumstances and some mechanisms which serve to restrict individual discretion in the activity of eating out.

Logics of restricted choice

In this section we consider four ways in which choice is effectively limited. First, we examine briefly the impact of limited resources on the capacity and likelihood of any individual to eat out. Second, we examine some social processes which restrict any individual's control over decisions about particular eating out episodes. Third, we investigate the ways in which judgements about suitability and preference operate to eliminate options. Finally, we isolate some instances of a process that might be called 'situational entailment', where every 'decision' taken narrows the range of subsequent options.

Limited resources

It will come as little surprise that shortage of money restricts people's likelihood of eating out; any economist would predict precisely that. However, although income was often a factor isolated in regression equations, attempting to predict the frequency of eating out, or the likelihood of eating in particular types of restaurant, it was never the only, and rarely the most powerful force operating. Money, as our interviews indicated, is one constraint interwoven with others, like time, social obligation and social opportunity. Asking people whether they would like to eat out more often than they did currently proved a useful device for getting people to discuss the constraints on them.

About half of our respondents said they would like to eat out more often than they did at the time of interview. They identified a number of constraints among which money was certainly one, typical responses including, 'Yes I would love to be able to eat out more often. It's more a case of not being able to afford it than anything else' (Steve), and 'Yes. Yeah . . . It's economics . . . more than anything else I would say' (Liz).

But money is just one, if important, resource. Among those who felt they could afford to eat out more often, other constraining factors were identified which amounted to shortage of resources. Time was often scarce. Work schedules and alternative leisure activities, of their own or of other household members, competed for time. Another restricted social resource is the availability of potential companions. Some interviewees mentioned this as a problem and another reluctantly concluded that current disharmony in her marital relationship meant that her outings were restricted. Company is a critical social resource precisely because most people consider eating out alone to be undesirable.

Another limited asset is the availability of what Bourdieu (e.g. 1984) calls 'cultural capital' – a stock of knowledge and social facility regarding meaningful social items. We asked interviewees about what might be described as their 'fantasy meal'. Thus we asked Smina, 'If you were taken out for a meal and your mother was looking after your children, and you could choose where to go and money was no object, where would you go?' Her initial response was to identify an Indian restaurant in Manchester in which she had had a meal very recently and which she had been to on several occasions previously and described as friendly, relaxed and familiar: 'I like the service over there . . . Atmosphere's very nice, relaxing, it's quite nice.' Then she reconsidered and reflected that she might like to go to 'a posh restaurant, when we were in London: is it the Hilton or something?' She continued, 'I could do if I win the lottery. Somewhere really posh, really expensive in London, yeah.' When then asked 'You think you would be able to enjoy yourself there?', Smina replied, 'Oh, no, I don't think you would, you'd have to be really upper class then wouldn't you? You'd have to be a proper snob.' Then, in the process of interrogating the interviewer about how she would feel about the Hilton, Smina concluded that 'It would be an experience to see how, it's like, how the other people live.'

Limited control: decision processes, allocation and domination

Other people, and other institutional demands, propel the individual into activities that they might otherwise either avoid or accomplish by some alternative means. In fact, although eating out is popularly considered a leisure activity, a good deal of eating away from home is necessary rather than optional. Because it is uncomfortable to delay eating for any substantial length of time, people often deem it necessary to eat away from home. This applies to people living in institutions, to people in employment who might eat during a break at work, to those involved in extensive travel (the lorry driver, the travelling salesman), to people undertaking informal work activities (for instance, shopping) or engaged in other leisure activities (e.g. visiting the cinema) which make it impossible to fit in with domestic meal-preparation cycles.

Discussions with our interviewees about the eating out behaviour of other household members gave some graphic indications of how the arrangements of other people affected their own behaviour. One husband was reported as having to eat in restaurants regularly for business purposes and hence preferred not to as leisure. The consequence was that his wife, though she said he would take her out to eat if she asked, was effectively and somewhat ruefully deprived of opportunities that she would have appreciated. Another husband did a lot of overtime during the week and his wife observed: 'Often on a Sunday Mark doesn't want to do anything because it's his one full day off from work. He's happy to plod around the house all day, whereas I'd rather go out and have dinner somewhere or go out for the day therefore you are eating out' (Anne).

Not only do the occupational obligations of partners affect recreational activity and the possibility of going out to eat, but so do their tastes. When asked about the behaviour of their children, particularly grown-up children, differences in taste were often acknowledged. But this was not so with partners. Except for occasional reference to partners as more or less adventurous or as having smaller or larger appetites, it was always implied that tastes were shared. This might in part be explained by the fact that eating out is an activity that those with a partner usually do together. Indeed, of 59 meals described to us, a partner was present on 41 occasions. Thus choice of venue will usually be a practical compromise, since generally both will attend together. It is not difficult to imagine that people come to assume that they prefer the types of restaurants they use regularly, which are the same ones that their partners frequent. Effectively some form of negotiated preference pertains which, by habit, restricts options and confirms people in their view that someone else's taste is also their own.

The same process of the outcome of social negotiation becoming routinised was apparent in the behaviour of Lisa whose only current involvement in eating out was with the same very large group of people all of whom went out together about every six weeks:

> We eat out as a social gathering. I mean we might not see our friends for six weeks but we'll be going out with them for a meal and that's, we all get together for this meal . . . we always make a point to have a meal, to go out with a gang of us, you know. I mean there can be anything up to 18 or 19 of us going out for a meal, and we always try and make a point of having one every six or seven weeks.

Again, other people effectively remove the possibility of personal initiative and personal control, a side effect of the size of the group being that the choice of venue was restricted to one where everyone's food tastes could be accommodated.

The extent to which people were often not in control was underscored in the survey results. Many people claimed to have had no say in whether or not to eat out. Only 45 per cent of respondents claimed to have been involved in the decision about whether to eat out on the last occasion that they had taken a main meal away from home. Moreover, we need not be consulted about where to eat: the question, 'Did you have any say in the decision to eat there?', elicited a negative reply in 20 per cent of instances.

It might be fanciful to consider inequalities of power and to bemoan a lack of choice over whether to eat out given that it is, overwhelmingly, a pleasurable and much welcomed activity (see Martens and Warde 1995). However, it might be inferred from the analysis of the responses in the survey to the question of whether people would like to eat out more often that there are indeed some systematic divisions in control over such matters. One of the survey questions was 'Would you like to eat out more often?' and respondents were offered one of five responses ranging from strong agreement to strongly disagreeing (see Figure 8.1). Multiple linear regression analysis on the answers scored on a scale

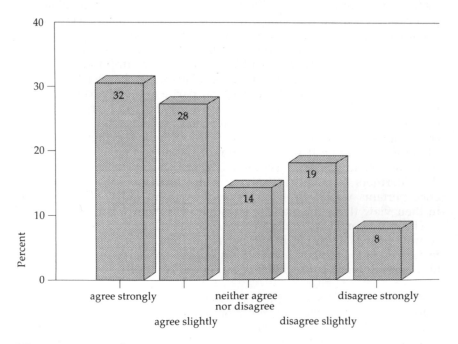

Like to eat out more often

Figure 8.1 Would you like to eat out more often than you do now? (percentages)

138

Regression equation

wants to eat out more = 2.64 (constant) + .04 years of age** + .23 (female)**
[.17]   [.00]   [.07]

− .39 (divorced or separated)** − .01 thousands of pounds*
(household income)
[. 12]   [. 00]

+ .23 (degree level qualification) − .22 (non-White)
[. 10]   [.10]

Adjusted R square = .20

Standard error pf parameters estimates in [ ] brackets

Significance t <.001 = **, t<.01 = *, t , .05 = others

Figure 8.2 Sociodemographic factors affecting the desire to eat out more often.

one to five, using standard sociodemographic independent variables, explained a level of variance (adjusted R-squared of 20 per cent) respectable for attitude questions.[1] The regression model is presented in Figure 8.2 with the variables listed in order of their significance (as measured by a t-test).

Once other factors were controlled simultaneously, older people want to eat out more.[2] Women were much more likely to desire more opportunities to eat out. Those separated or divorced were less likely than couples to want to eat out more. Personal income was not significant, but it was those with lower household incomes who seek more opportunities. People with a degree or equivalent educational qualifications also wanted to eat out more, despite their already registering a disproportionately high frequency of eating out. Finally, people who classified themselves as White would like to eat out more. The computation suggests that gender, age and marital status were of greater significance than current income. The significance of gender implies that at least one group in the population, women, may be somewhat aggrieved about their inability to control decisions about whether to eat out. The most prominent, and easily understandable, reasons exposed by our qualitative interviews were that most women appreciated eating out as a relief from personal domestic labour and considered being served by someone else as a luxury,

Limited imagination: suitability and preference

Once a decision to eat out has been made, and resources have been allocated, there is a potentially extensive range of possible places to go and types of food to eat. If, as seems likely, the most dramatic change in the catering industry in the past 30 years is the increased number and variety of outlets, then the options are considerable. Arguably, immense variety is the most seductive feature of contemporary consumer culture and one which has been said to cause indecision and anxiety (see Warde 1997). However, systems of judgements about quality and acceptability, which are in part modes of personal and social classification, are employed to guide decisions. The values invoked varied among our interviewees and the nature of that variation is worth remarking on, not least because it challenges the idea that there is some dominant understanding about the quality and desirability of different venues.

Some people hold strong opinions about hierarchies of venue, as was revealed by Jane. Jane was a full-time housewife and mother of two teenage children. Her husband was the only breadwinner and worked as a marketing manager. Jane's household had known more affluent times, and money was a constraint at the moment of interview. Although the household income was one of the highest among our interviewees, it supported two teenage children, as well as a large detached house, and Jane commented that the frequency with which they ate out at the time of interview was lower than it had been in the past. When answering the question whether she would like to eat out more often, Jane, unlike some of the other respondents, did not lack imagination.

Interviewer: And what sort of places would you like to eat out more?
Jane: Money no object?
Interviewer: Well, yes.
Jane: Well, actually, I would like to go to top-class restaurants with the top-class chefs like Raymond Blanc's place or up in the Lake District, what is it called – Miller Howe. I'd like to go to those types of places. Oh, and also round here I've been to Heathcotes' you know Paul Heathcotes' restaurant. I'd like to go there again. And then I would speak to friends who've got plenty of money and find out where they've had a nice meal. So those type of places really nice, top-class restaurants where they make food, cook food that I wouldn't make at home. The last place I would want to go would be a Beefeater restaurant. I just wouldn't, even with plenty of money, I would go and eat, I'd rather eat at home, you know.

Certainly Jane, who went on to elaborate the grounds of her dislike of places like the Beefeater chain, eliminated 'cheaper-type' eating places from consideration. Trisha, on the contrary, did not discount eating places on such a basis, contending that 'I think you can eat out quite inexpensively, if you want to.'

Most people held a view that some places were better than others, and most, like Jane, went to places that they ranked most highly. The notion arose several times that there was a threshold, places beneath which would be avoided, the criterion usually being the ability to prepare better, as well as more cheaply, the same food at home. (In a sociology of consumption the insight obtained from studying aversions may often be greater than from asking people what they like.)

Other interviewees expressed a more flexible attitude to variety, claiming either that they liked to try as many places as possible or that it depended on the occasion which place would be appropriate. Trisha, in her twenties, living in a couple, without children and in paid employment, exemplified the first case by her remarkably open experimental approach to different kinds of foods:

> Yeah, well, I mean I hadn't tried Indian food till about two years ago and I didn't think that I would like it and I've never been offered it at home but when I tried it I thought it was really nice and you know there's so many varieties that you can eat so you should just try different things, even if you don't like them at least you know for future. So we do tend to, especially when we go out, we don't choose the same thing on the menu. You know, every time we go out we tend to like go somewhere different and try a different meal and things like that. We get a bit [of] variety.

In this instance the challenge of variety is met by renunciation of the notion of transitivity of preference; the interviewee is, in our vocabulary above, selecting among equivalents. In effect, she maintains that any place is suitable. This could be interpreted as a particular sort of social statement, an attitude identified as typical of postmodern culture, rejecting hierarchies of taste, asserting the value of new experience and, above all, taking breadth of experience as a dominant objective. The notion that any place is suitable is the limiting case where the dominant sociological perspective outlined above becomes inapplicable. One of the most discriminating and adventurous of our interviewees (Steve, graduate, engineer, twenties, middle-class background) showed an associated, but more qualified, fascination with variety. When asked about his 'fantasy' meal he replied:

> Thing is, you see, if I had a choice of somebody taking me out for a fabulous expensive meal I'd probably want to go out for about six meals, 'cos you can try lots of different places and lots of different meals. 'Cos when you go out to eat you're, I mean however hard you try you can only eat about one main course really, so I think I'd like to have about six meals and I'd get to try like five more things, but, yeah. I like knowing about different types of food you see, so, if I had the chance I'd like to go out for a few, instead of just the one, but if I could only have one I'd go somewhere really special, a gastronomic delight.

Other interviewees proffered the principle of suitability as a fit between occasion and venue. This is perhaps the most sophisticated understanding of the social role of eating out, indicating that different venues are appropriate to different kinds of event. It tended to be held by the most experienced respondents. The effect of trying everything once is probably that some options are eliminated because they are not personally very satisfying, so reducing again the number of remaining practical alternatives.

141

While some were devoted to the pursuit of variety, other inter-viewees were not. Interviewees fell quite evenly along a continuum between the conservative and the adventurous. A significant proportion sought familiar foods, and said that they sought to eat foods which they knew they would like. So Debby, a woman in her twenties, à propos of having tasted a companion's swordfish, which she pronounced 'quite nice', said, 'I won't order anything I don't know. If I don't know what it tastes like I won't order. I'm very, you know, stick to what I know.' Again, Smina, also in her twenties, indicated similar reluctance to try new foods:

> Interviewer: Would you say that you like to try out new things when you go out for something to eat?
> Smina: No, not a lot. We normally get the same things that we like. But no we never try new things unless we take somebody along with us, and then we order different dishes and try different ones. If it is just me and my husband we normally get the same thing.

In practice, many people limit their options by repeatedly going to the same place. It would appear from our survey data that people insulate themselves from potential disappointment with new experiences by revisiting the same restaurants. In response to questions about the last eating out experience, 62 per cent said they had been to that same venue before, among whom over 99 per cent reported having enjoyed themselves overall. Moreover, 84 per cent of respondents said they would be likely to return again to the venue they had last visited, which partly reflects the very high level of satisfaction expressed throughout our study with eating out. On the basis of a previous similar experience, people presuppose the suitability of their excursion, picking in preference what they are confident they will enjoy.

A final step in the demonstration that a social process of collective judgement operates would be to indicate the social patterning of preferences. This is complex and a major aspect of the research findings for which there is not space in this chapter. Suffice it to say that when we asked respondents whether they had eaten in various different kinds of restaurant during the previous year, answers were frequently related to educational level, occupational class, ethnic group member-ship and age cohort, as well as income and household structure (Warde 1996b; Warde, Martens and Olsen 1997). There is a socially determined distribution of taste which implies a differentiated, but collective, framework with which social groups determine the suitability of alternatives.

Limited manoeuvres: situational entailment

The final form of constraint to be discussed is that which the restaurant itself imposes. Although there is a danger, exemplified by Finkelstein 1989, of exaggerating the extent to which the behaviour of customers is manipulated or directed by the owners, staff, design and organisation of restaurants, it is nevertheless true that the environment of the establishment imposes restrictions on behaviour. Once in a restaurant customers are obliged to conform to certain conventions, both of the particular establishment and of eating in public places in a competent fashion. The dramatic performance of eating out is complicated, as detailed ethnographic scrutiny reveals. Here we comment on just two examples.

Some schools of sociological thought emphasise the importance of situations in determining how people will behave. The competent person can identify the behaviour, opinion and mood expected in different circumstances and much of the time will feel constrained to act accordingly. The imperative of conviviality when eating out is particularly strong and probably explains in part the degree of pleasure expressed by our respondents (Martens and Warde 1995). Many of our interviewees gave details of the way in which they modified their behaviour or suppressed opinions with a view to maintaining an appropriate mood around the table. This resulted in some reduction of the potential level of complaints to the restaurant, for instance. This we interpret as both evidence of social competence and also of the definition of the situation of eating out wherein all participants must be happy and contented (Warde 1996a). Eating out properly requires drawing on a certain repertoire of behaviours, and failure to act appropriately leads to embarrassment, unpleasantness or disappointment.

A second, more obvious sense of situational entailment usually operates because prior decisions restrict subsequent ones. This happens in many ways. Take for example the order in which foods should be eaten. Taking soup usually eliminates taking a starter, and either may reduce the likelihood of eating a dessert; conventionally, choosing fish as a first course will eliminate it from choice for a main course. Or consider what food is devoured. Having decided to eat out often results in relaxing disciplinary rules: our respondents reported themselves likely to eat more than normal and to pay less attention to health when away from home.

A further interesting example of situational entailment is the degree to which the choice of restaurant entails a likelihood of eating particular foods. In most cases customers have to pick from a menu, which itself serves to reduce millions of possible combinations of recognisable dishes to a few on offer. Often the menu is specialised on the basis of a particular cuisine. Consequently, having decided to eat in a Chinese restaurant it is very unlikely that we will eat pizza, and highly likely that dishes selected will come from Chinese culinary tradition.

It is inevitably somewhat arbitrary to allocate dishes to different culinary traditions: the issue of authenticity – whether a given dish is an Italian pasta, whether *coq au vin* is done in such a way that it might pass as French – is one which connoisseurs persist in discussing. Nevertheless we collected some information which suggests that there is an increasing general recognition of culinary tradition. We used a rough-and-ready coding scheme to categorise the cuisine from which were derived the meals described as having been eaten by our respondents on the occasion of their last meal out. Of 584 respondents who had eaten last in a commercial establishment, 41 per cent ate a main dish with an identifiable foreign attribution. We also presented them with a list of some 20 types of commercial venue, including 'pub bar', 'fast food restaurant', specialist pizza house', 'Chinese/Thai restaurant', 'Indian restaurant', etc., from which they identified the site of their last excursion. This allows some indicative conclusions on operative rules about which dishes are deemed suitable when dining in different venues.

Of the 39 meals that had been eaten in an Indian restaurant on the last occasion, 35 were coded as being of Indian derivation. Of 32 people reporting having eaten their last meal in a Chinese or Thai restaurant, 26 main courses were identified as Chinese, the remainder being classified as Indian, Mexican and Japanese, with three unattributable. These data indicate that Britons when in 'ethnic' restaurants eat primarily ethnically appropriate dishes and that the practice of 30 years ago, whereby Indian and Chinese restaurants routinely advertised and sold conventional British dishes is declining, signifying a greater specialisation of cuisine.

Conclusion

This chapter has defined the character of the dominant sociological perspective and illustrated its application to the practice of eating out. While popular impressions of eating out are couched in terms of consumer choice, freedom is circumscribed. The term 'choice' inflates the importance of individual decisions and conflates qualitatively different aspects and levels of discretion. We have considered only a limited range of restrictions on personal choice, but sufficient to identify a series of processes, with wide applicability, which serve to contain freedom, understood as determination or will. The availability of resources, systemic inequalities of power in decision-making, shared cultural and aesthetic judgement, and 'situational entailment', all constrain the individual. Sociology is particularly adept at isolating and describing these, the component parts of the social logic of restricted choice.

Notes

1 We are grateful to Wendy Olsen for this computation.
2 This is the inverse effect compared to using simple bivariate analysis.

Part Two

Social Sciences and Food Choice

Analysing Sociopolitical Processes and Cultural Constructions

Overview to Part Two

Rounding off Part One, Alan Warde and Lydia Martens' chapter showed that even where a high degree of individual discretion might be assumed, choice turns out not to be a matter of each individual determining, solo, what they will eat: collective judgements and collaborative decisions are integral to the flow of social processes involved. Mention of social processes serves as a reminder that the basis for grouping chapters into Parts One and Two can only be approximate and is intended only as a convenience. There are at least two grounds (attention to social processes and the use of qualitative data-collection techniques) on which Warde and Martens' chapter is a possible candidate for Part Two, thus providing a bridge from Part One.

None the less, the reader will no doubt spot the logic lying beneath the division when moving between them. Chapters 9 to 16 include work for which relying on axioms or concentrating on measurement is beside their current purpose. Here, broadly speaking, attempting to grasp and duly detail quite what is happening is as important, if not more so, than investigating how big or how frequently it happens, measuring or counting it. The overview provided above indicates that Part One began with demand (in the form of dietary change in individuals), went on to range right across to the supply side, before doubling back to the conspicuous consumption of eating out.

Part Two begins by coupling consumption rights and the manner in which those engaged in supply create the circumstances and shape the opportunities in which food selections are made. In Chapter 9, Andrew Flynn and his colleagues draw on work developed in relation to property rights. This allows characterising consumption rights in terms of the mutual duties (of providers) and rights (of consumers) in the social relationship between the two in respect of food standards, hygiene and safety. In turn, this allows Flynn *et al.* to distinguish between two valued principles: the freedom to consume and the freedom from adverse effects of so doing. They do so, however, noting that the former has tended to expression as an individualised freedom or right and the latter as a collective matter. Although at times these two seem to be competing, they are shown to be operating side-by-side, not necessarily mutually exclusively. By separating the various elements, Flynn *et al.* make more readily visible the underlying forces that during the 1980s and 1990s resulted in a division. On the one hand the public sector retains a role as guarantor of food standards but the rights concerning freedoms to consume are devolved to the private sector (the retailers).

Chapter 10 widens the viewpoint still further. In it, Pat Caplan and her colleagues provide a broad, social anthropological angle on the cultural contexts of food. They introduce several sociocultural variations, especially gender, age, class/socioeconomic background and ethnicity. Based on a two-phase project portraying contrasts between two regions, they detail elements of these variations in relation to the nation's eating. Able to compare a south London borough with a small town in west Wales, they provide some novel insights into different nuances of 'ethnicity' as it concerns food and eating.

Younger, Black, British-born, London residents told the researchers they may not regularly eat according to the culinary traditions of the Caribbean, and may not even much enjoy the cuisine. But they still said they tended to join middle-aged and older residents for such meals at weekends at family reunions. For some, doing so is important to their identity as a Black person. On the other hand, Welsh cuisine appears in two rather separate guises. One echoes the self-conscious allegiance to, and perpetuation of identity of Londoners who describe themselves as Afro-Caribbean. In Wales, however, it is identity as Cymry Cymraeg, i.e. Welsh, born and bred as well as Welsh-speaking. The other is cast in a different light and looks to be closely connected to tourism, the leisure industry and a recently cultivated interest in 'heritage' (Murcott 1996) – the 'Welsh' cooking of commercialised spheres of restaurants, cafés and recipe books.

Caplan *et al.*'s chapter paves the way for the others in this section. In one way or another, the remainder concentrate on social processes and relationships in daily life, or on the social organisation of ordinary routines and the place of food and eating within them. Chapters 11 and 12 both deal with the household. Spenser Henson and his collaborators set out to discover what happens, if anything, when someone at home decides to change their diet. Never mind whether it is on medical advice, to lose weight or to cut out eating meat, it is the alteration by just one person that is of interest: does it affect the others and, if so, how? Chapter 11 shows that so far, the evidence suggests that the whole household adapts really very smoothly to such a change and that despite a good deal of extra effort on the part of the 'home manager' (much more usually a woman than a man), the rest of the household is well protected from unduly disrupting consequences.

As a type of living arrangement sometimes even defined primarily in terms of sharing a table and keeping a common larder, households are not necessarily composed of families (Murcott 1986). But like Henson *et al.* Debbie Kemmer and colleagues elected to concentrate on this type. Their interest, however, is on the stage when a household is newly formed by a (heterosexual) couple's deciding to live together or to get married. Like Lowe, Dowey and Horne, their interest is very directly applied to the public health call for changes in the nation's eating habits. Also like Lowe *et al.* they sought to develop a basic scientific study that would address this interest. Where Lowe *et al.* adopted an experimental approach to investigation about what shaped dietary change, they pursued investigation of what happens in any case. A virtually uncharted field, the formation of a new household seems promising as one set of circumstances in which dietary change is likely to occur naturally, in the ordinary run of social events. Chapter 12 is based on their project that studied couples before and after moving in together, and confirms that they do indeed report a change in their food habits and eating arrangements. More specifically, the changes involved a high valuation placed on a regular evening meal taken together and shopping that is more likely to be planned in advance. Thus the way is paved for looking more closely for processual elements in the social relationship of the couple which will shed light on the way these changes are achieved.

Chapter 13 moves from the site and social organisation of the household to that of the school. The connection between the home and school, however, remains in focus. For if nothing else, a long-standing policy debate about school meals revolves around the balance between the private responsibilities of the family and the public obligations of the state. Robert Burgess and Marlene Morrison's chapter provides evidence of the practical and cultural influences from home that travel into school via pocket money or the contents of a lunch box. But it also provides evidence of the effect of social processes and organisational features peculiar to the school on opportunities for learning and teaching about foods. School timetables, for instance, incline towards a 'conveyor belt' system in the dinner hour. As a result, concentrating on ensuring a child eats enough can supplant attempts at an educative concern with nutritional balance. What on the face of it seems an ideal occasion to reinforce classroom teaching about the composition of foods and dietary advice is liable to be overwhelmed in due attention to the smooth running of the school day.

Burgess and Morrisons' project, like other studies in 'The Nation's Diet' serves one of the Programme's purposes of bringing work and expertise developed in other substantive fields in the social sciences to bear on questions of food choice. Among other studies similar in this respect (for example those reported in Chapters 6, 9 and 15) is the project on which Chapter 14 is based. Here Sally Macintyre and colleagues introduce parts of a study that seeks to unravel the influences associated with the mass-media coverage of concerns linking food, health and safety. Coverage results in dramatically different effects on the nation's diet – measured at least by the public's food-shopping habits. On one hand, health-promotion advice especially about fat intake and coronary heart disease seems to be by-passed. On the other, reports about the safety (or otherwise) of food have a marked and almost immediate effect. Their chapter presents new evidence detailing the manner in which the newspaper-reading/TV-watching public is heterogeneous and discriminating. The combined implications are that socioeconomic variables are clearly associated with people's receptions of media coverage and that they actively interpret, and can be sceptical about, what they read/watch.

Being active rather than passive, thoughtful rather than merely reactive or habitual, are significant aspects of decision-making about infant-feeding addressed in Chapter 15. Elizabeth Murphy and her colleagues present some of the work from their project that, at the time of writing, is still part-way through its funding period. Designed longitudinally, they prepared to follow first-time mothers from late pregnancy until the child's second birthday. During this crucial early period of life, deciding and then planning what and how to feed, putting it all into practice and checking on how it is going, is complex and detailed. Its study requires it be matched with methods to collect suitably detailed data and correspondingly suitably detailed analytic modes for their interpretation. Chapter 15 documents the intricacies, showing that what some might be tempted to see as wayward failures to abide by antenatal decisions are to be understood as the outcome of fine-grained rethinking following the birth, in the face not just of complexities in events and social relationships, but of circumstances that could not have been anticipated.

Reserved for last in Part Two is work which returns to take account of both supply and demand. This twin focus is integral to the point of departure for a project investigating a practical problem of health variations across differing ethnic minorities resident in Britain. In Chapter 16, Rory Williams and his collaborators provide a sociological thread through a labyrinth of possible interrelations between body size and shape; origins in peasant-based economies on different continents; changes in fortune on migration; the same style of allegiance to so-called 'traditional' cuisines that Caplan et al.'s Chapter 10 reports; generational changes in opportunity or outlook; and cultural conventions governing the micro-politics of social relationships in the food-sharing group. This exceedingly complicated web of factors represents the background to the study mounted by Williams et al. of South Asian and Italian women (plus controls) in Glasgow. They assessed diet and levels of exercise, and compared the effects of several major dimensions, including religion, gender, the importance of meals and of hospitality, and the experience if any of racist hostility.

Implicated in these particular ethnic comparisons is one of the sharpest contrasts in the nation's diet. On one hand, both South Asian and Italian cuisines centre on the low fat/high carbohydrate diet now advised to promote good health; on the other the Scots are found to have an even poorer diet than the English/Welsh (Scottish Office 1994). A good many of the dimensions involved in the study continue to be disentangled. But thus far, the chapter reports that images of body size linked to good health and good diet, conventions which emphasise the importance of traditional dishes prepared at home, outlooks that have comparatively little space for the idea of exercise as leisure, are among the cultural values found to shape, and in part, serve as constraints to the food choices reported in the two Glaswegian minorities. Mindful that culture is not usefully thought of as some unyielding straightjacket for meaningful human action, Williams *et al.* suggest realising that members of ethnic minorities are blending individual choice with collective choice about eating to maintain culturally inherited cuisines. They end by recommending that anyone interested in supporting the maintenance or even recovery of these well-advised cuisines be alert to the sociological niceties involved.

CHAPTER 9

Regulation, rights and the structuring of food choices

Andrew Flynn, Michelle Harrison and Terry Marsden

Introduction – structuring choices

Most of Britain's food is purchased from the shelves of the multiple retail outlets. A key question concerning food choice lies in why some products and not others will reach those retailers' shelves. Supermarkets are not simply 'empty vessels' passively responding to the demands of consumers. To sustain their markets retailers, along with producers, manufacturers and processors, and distributors are involved in *creating* food choices for consumers. The corporate retailers also operate in a complex regulatory framework governed by national and increasingly European requirements. By establishing what is and is not permitted in terms of hygiene, content and production, state regulation also helps to set the boundaries which structure food choices.

That structuring of food choices is intimately linked to prevailing notions of *consumption rights*. By drawing on the seminal work of Daniel Bromley (1991) in relation to property rights it is possible to characterise consumption rights as social relations. That is relations between rights holders (in this case consumers) and duty bearers (here farmers, food manufacturers and retailers) in relation to food hygiene, safety and standards. It has traditionally been the role of the state to protect the benefits that consumers derive from these rights. Importantly, though, the state may perform its role in different ways, for example, as a result of regulatory reform. Since it is a social relationship that defines consumption rights, they are, as we shall see, subject to contestation.

In this chapter we examine how some of the core themes within food-consumption rights have changed and link those to the economic restructuring of the food system and the regulatory framework. Our argument is that as economic power has shifted from farmers to food manufacturers and increasingly to retailers, along with changes governing the regulation of food standards, the rights which consumers can expect in relation to food will also alter. As food rights are modified, so too are food choices. Our perspective on food choice does not, therefore, extend to *how* consumers make decisions on what products to buy from shop shelves or *why* they make those choices. Below we briefly explain our project's approach to food choice.

Constructing the consumer interest: retailing, regulation and food quality

We are concerned to bring together for the purposes of analysis of food regulation and quality three different sets of interests: retailers, the state and consumers. In recent years relationships between the three have become significantly more volatile. Four factors in particular have been at work. First, there has been intense competitive pressure within the retail sector, accentuated by the entry into the market of some foreign-owned discount retailers. Food retailers in the 1990s are increasingly having to participate in the politics of market maintenance in which they engage in much more diversified sets of economic and political relationships with local, national and European governments. Second, the growing intensity of competition has been complemented by a decline in regulatory stability. On the one side there has been concern that consumers pay excessively high costs for foodstuffs and on the other side that Britain's trade gap in food and drink is unduly large. Themes one and two raise questions surrounding the relationships between public policy and the private sector in the sourcing and provision of food, and the degree to which 'national' and private interests dovetail with those of the consumer. Third, has been the rise to prominence within food regulation of hygiene issues. Here, the multiple retail outlets, by dint of their dominance, are becoming increasingly important agents. A key area for us has concerned the extent to which the key retailers do regulate food-quality standards within their supply chains and whether they take a different approach to regulation to that which previously prevailed. Fourth, as part and parcel of its new regulatory responsibilities the retail sector must be able to represent itself effectively to different tiers of government. We have been analysing whether this has happened and if the major retailers are also to 'speak for' the consumer.

In order to explore the combination of public and private relations and how they may sustain the consumer interest demanded a methodology that placed at its centre the interactions between policy and regulation, the activities of the retailers and consumer groups. This has involved research at three different levels. First, there has been the study of key private and public sector organisations. Over 50 key person interviews have been undertaken with representatives of retailers and their trade associations; officials in local and national government as well as at the European level; and with consumer groups. There have also been two pieces of extended fieldwork; one an inner-London borough and the other a county in south-west England. Second, we have explored the role of professional groups engaged in the process of food-quality regulation. Throughout we have guaranteed anonymity to our informants and the field locations because of the sensitivity of the issues we are addressing. We have made extensive use of our interview sources in this chapter because they provide an unrivalled insight into the perceptions and practices of key actors in relation to food regulation. Third, we have examined 'landmark' legislation and policy developments in order to assess how the public interest is being reformulated.

Based on the perspective of our project we would wish to argue that ideas of choice are not to be understood simply as expressions of individual preference. Food choice does not just concern 'consumer choice'. Significant choices are made by the public and private *providers* of food. Providers of food here means the manufacturers and retailers of food and the regulatory activities that they and the public sector (for our purposes this has largely been Environmental Health Officers) undertake. Public and private sectors construct choices and then influence the choices of others. Currently, key providers of food choices are the retailers and the state. Far weaker, as we illustrate, are consumer groups.

Chapter structure

In order to explore further the links between food retailing, regulation and choice we aim here to reflect on the analysis and framework that we have developed, to bring key insights to bear on food choice. The chapter is divided into two sections. It begins by charting the relationships between the restructuring of the food system and shifting food regulatory strategies. The Conservative government from 1979 to 1997 made much of the need for deregulation, or more accurately 'good' regulation, and creating 'quality' choices and opportunities. The overall result has been a change in the nature of consumption rights (i.e. the structuring of consumer choices). To appreciate the extent to which consumption rights have changed it is necessary to examine the roles played by key elements within the food system. To understand the shaping of these consumption rights it is necessary to adopt an historical perspective. Moreover, viewing events through a longer time frame vividly indicates the extent to which there have been substantial shifts in the nature of consumption rights.

The second section of the chapter draws specifically on our recent research of the major food retailers, food regulators, civil servants and consumer groups. It details the transformation of consumption rights and examines how in the late 1990s notions of rights are played out in practice. What emerges is the way in which changes in economic power within the food system, regulatory practices and rights to consume are inextricably bound together. As consumption rights change over time, so this, in turn, structures food choices. Below we outline some of the changes in these rights since 1945.

Food regulation and the restructuring of the food system

In the postwar period we have witnessed a relative decline in the significance of food rights linked to supply and the rise of rather different rights linked to consumption. In order to examine the manner in which these rights have changed and their implications for food choice, this section is organised around the following themes: producer-led choice; the ties between economic interests and the Ministry of Agriculture, Fisheries and Food; consumer groups and the Ministry; and the administrative structure for the regulation of food within central government. These themes emphasise the role of key actors, such as farmers and retailers. They draw out the links between them and patterns of regulation, and show the pattern of evolution of *food consumption rights*.

Producer-led choice

The early postwar years were characterised by a producer-led domination of food choices. Its essential features were pervasive and have only recently been usurped as the major food retailers began to imprint their own characteristics on the regulatory process. Perhaps two factors more than any other were responsible for the initial producer domination of postwar food choice. One was the political strategy of the National Farmers' Union (NFU) and the other the government's response to food shortages. The following discussion draws on several sources, including the work of Self and Storing (1962); Wilson (1977); Grant (1983); Cox, Lowe and Winter (1986); and Foreman (1989).

Compared to other elements within the food system, farmers are distinguished by their sheer number – though that has fallen markedly – and thus the minute market influence of any individual farmer. Faced with ever more concentrated operations upstream and downstream – that is, those who provide them with inputs such as fertilisers and purchase their products like food manufacturers – who could use their market position to squeeze the profit margins of farmers, the latter have been successful at organising themselves to protect and promote their interests through political means. The NFU had an enviable reputation for its expertise and skilful lobbying and long enjoyed close contacts with the Ministry of Agriculture, Fisheries and Food (MAFF). Indeed, the closeness of the links with

MAFF have been a source of comment and, perhaps, these contacts go much deeper than those of any other interest group and government department. The NFU has supported successive postwar government's policy of making farming more productive through increasing intensification as, it was believed, this would ensure the long-term prosperity of farming.

The political strategy of the NFU dovetailed neatly with the concern of the postwar Labour government (Williams 1965) and its Conservative successors to increase food supplies. The war years and early years of peace were marked by considerable government intervention in the management of food. At a time of genuine food scarcity, which worsened with the ending of hostilities, the government had to play a role in ensuring food reached a largely urban population. Obviously a key means was through the stimulation and control of domestic agriculture. Farmers received guaranteed prices for the major agricultural products and sold to an assured market. In short, farmers were directed as to what to grow and the government engaged in bulk purchase.

The close links between farmers and government were crystallised in the 1947 Agriculture Act. This provided for a privileged position for the National Farmers' Union, as *the* representative of farmers to engage in annual negotiations with the government through an annual review of the general economic conditions facing agriculture in the year ahead and to set prices for products accordingly. Other interests, such as consumers, were marginalised. With the easing of food scarcity concerns in the 1950s and the election in 1951 of a Conservative government that was committed to relaxing controls on food, a more liberal pricing and distribution system emerged, although rationing on such staples as butter, margarine and meat lasted until 1954 (Foreman 1989: 56). Nevertheless, the NFU retained its pre-eminent position and, along with the then Ministry of Agriculture, set the tone for much of the postwar agricultural and, by default, food policy. In terms of choice, the overriding emphasis was ensuring adequate supplies of affordable, safe food for a largely urban population. In terms of food rights, it can be expressed as government action to provide collective food security: that is, *freedom from want*. The role of regulation here may be characterised as public interest regulation in which government takes a leading, strategic and directive role. It is to be contrasted with that of private interest regulation which characterises corporate food regulation in the late 1990s, discussed below (see also Harrison, Flynn and Marsden 1977). In short, *choice was in large part determined by the state-induced construction of supply*: the interactions between what farmers produced and what government wanted them to produce. Indeed, the rights emerged from the common interest (i.e. expectation) at the time in the need to safeguard food supplies, requiring positive state action (i.e. duties on the government) in the agricultural policy sphere.

Economic interests and MAFF

Through a combination of factors, farmers since the 1970s have generally found themselves in a difficult position. They have been squeezed between their suppliers and food manufacturers and retailers who increasingly dictate how products must be farmed by setting stringent quality standards. The favourable political framework within which farmers have been accustomed to operate has also come under closer scrutiny. Farming practices have been questioned for their effects on animal welfare and the environment and the costs of supporting farming is no longer unquestioned (see, for example, Cottrell 1987; National Consumer Council 1988; Body 1991; Clark and Lowe 1992; Clunies-Ross and Hildyard 1992). Almost inevitably the close links between the NFU and MAFF have come under critical scrutiny, not least from some Conservative MPs who may traditionally have been regarded as natural allies (see, for example, Body 1982, 1984, 1987). Thus, economically and politically farmers have increasingly found themselves in a defensive position.

The protracted relative economic and political decline of farming has been accentuated by the dramatic rise to prominence of first food manufacturers (Flynn, Marsden and Ward 1991) and more recently retailers (Wrigley 1991, 1992, 1994). These have proved to be the two most buoyant sectors within the food system, and are dominated by a small number of large firms. Key food manufacturers include AB Foods, Booker, Allied Lyons, Grand Metropolitan and Unigate, while the most important food retailers are Sainsbury, Tesco and Safeway, followed by Asda and Somerfield. Throughout the 1980s and into the 1990s the major retailers underwent considerable expansion such that today they have captured about two-thirds of food retail sales. In contrast the smaller independent retailers account for an ever declining proportion of sales. It is the major multiples which increasingly determine the shape of the British food sector and are able to influence the food choices on offer. Together retailers and manufacturers have been the sources of considerable innovation across a range of areas from new products, to the distribution and storage of those products.

Within the food system it is the manufacturers and increasingly the major retailers who will be exercising influence (Flynn and Marsden 1992; Marsden and Wrigley 1995). Such influence carries with it a regulatory dimension. Retailers, in particular, have found themselves both drawn into and actively seeking a regulatory role. For example, during the late 1980s to 1990s it was by no means apparent that key retailers would move into the dominant position within the food system they enjoy today. Retailers faced intense internal competition and growing criticisms of their sourcing strategies and as a result had to grapple with the challenge of market maintenance (Marsden, Harrison and Flynn 1997). This involved them in a more diversified set of relationships with the state at both the national and European level. Perhaps fortuitously, at the same time, MAFF, which has considerable regulatory responsibility throughout the food chain, had been seeking to share some of its regulatory burden, often under the mantle of deregulation (see below). That such a coincidence of regulatory interests could be realised owed much to MAFF's knowledge of, and involvement with, the industry built up over long years of its support. As one industry interviewee put it: 'The food industry has always had a good working relationship with MAFF because MAFF needs such a relationship. You see MAFF is sponsoring the food industry.' Today MAFF has much closer contacts with the food sector which it is keener to foster (interview with MAFF official) than, say, the Board of Trade with the energy industry. It is significant that the DTI publicly distanced itself much more from its sponsorship of industry role than MAFF (see Cmnd 278). Contacts between retailers and government will occur on a regular basis and at a variety of levels from the highest circles of policy-making to local level policy implementation.

Consumer groups and MAFF

The position of the supermarkets in relation to government is in marked contrast to that of consumer groups and consumers. It is worthwhile briefly contrasting their experiences with those of key producer interests in the aftermath of the Second World War. While the NFU was embraced by government and its privileged position with the then Ministry of Agriculture protected, consumers had their interests looked after by the Ministry of Food. As long as food shortages and rationing remained, there was a role for the Ministry of Food, which had been formed in 1939 (it had previously been disbanded in 1921 following the easing of food supplies after the First World War). Once those conditions changed, the rationale for a separate Ministry was lost.

In October 1954 it was announced that the Ministry of Food would merge, but very much as junior partner, with the Ministry of Agriculture. The proposed reform provoked considerable controversy, with significant implications for the subsequent construction of food choice. One junior Minister of Food, Dr Charles Hill, was moved to argue that 'in essence it [the Ministry of Food] had been a consumer's organisation and I doubted whether the consumer's interests could be fully protected if what remained of the Ministry of Food passed to the Ministry of Agriculture' (quoted in Foreman 1989: 57). Similarly critical comments were made in *The Times*:

'The worst of the possible alternatives has been chosen. If there could not be a separate Minister of Food, his remaining responsibilities should have gone anywhere rather than the Minister of Agriculture. It is asking too much of any Minister to be able to hold the balance fairly between the interests of the consumer and the powerful agricultural interest' (quoted in Foreman 1989: 57).

Concerns about consumer representation within MAFF never entirely disappeared (Smith 1990) but were muted while food itself remained a politically quiescent issue. Once that changed in the 1980s and 1990s MAFF found itself encountering real difficulties fending off charges that it put producers before consumers. In the early 1990s, in response to criticism of its aloofness from consumers, MAFF formed a Consumer Panel. Various consumer groups have members on this committee and they have welcomed the opportunity this has opened up for them to represent consumer views to government. As one interviewee put it: 'I think . . . our influence has grown . . . [This is] [p]artly through the setting up of the consumer panel, partly because we have quite a lot of people now on MAFF committees.'

Cultivating links with MAFF depends on groups observing codes of behaviour and practice. Consumer groups must show to government that they are responsible, credible and sources of useful information. Indeed, as one consumer group interviewee argued 'we have built up the relationship with government departments . . . built up the trust of government in that all our work is usually based on sound research'. Another interviewee, however, hinted that at the time links between MAFF and consumer groups were not that strong: 'in common with the other consumer organisations we were extremely sceptical when [the consumer panel] . . . was set up. But I think they've [MAFF] largely won us over, in that it isn't a hollow PR exercise, and they have moved quite considerably on a lot of things that the consumer panel has been pressing for.' While the influence of consumer groups within MAFF may have grown, it is from a low base. Moreover, it is largely confined by MAFF, to the less central (i.e. non-economic) areas of its work. There is, for example, little evidence to show that consumer groups have anything but limited or sporadic influence on *agricultural policy*. In any case, consumer groups find their ability to make inputs into the policy process constrained by limited resources. For example, in the summer of 1996 it was announced that the National Consumer Council faced swingeing cuts in funding from government and was to make one-third of its staff redundant.

Central government and the regulation of food

By changing the regulatory and policy styles of government, merging the Ministries of Food and Agriculture changed the way food choices were structured. As the Ministry of Agriculture, the department's preferred administrative style was to incorporate favoured (i.e. economic) interests into the decision-making structure in an attempt to ensure that the two moved together. When the need to ensure food supplies was a national priority the incorporation of farmers, presumably, made much sense. The merger with the Ministry of Food did not change the department's operating style. Thus, as part of the merger the Ministry of Agriculture took over the Ministry of Food's responsibility for food standards. For example, the latter had set up a Food Standards Committee in 1947, to be followed in 1964 by a Food Additives and Contaminants Committee (Foreman 1989: 56). These Committees exist to help protect the consumer; they also assist in the coordination of government and industry activities (National Consumer Council 1988). They were replaced in 1983 by the Food Advisory Committee but like its predecessors it has been increasingly criticised for its lack of independence, unrepresentative membership and secrecy of proceedings. When, for the first time in 1993, the financial links between members of the Food Advisory Committee and food companies were published, 'Twelve out of 17 members . . . declared some cash reward' and that may have been an underreporting (*Guardian* 12 May 1993).

Today the deliberations of food-related committees and their recommendations are significant for food choice because they are able to propose modifications to the boundaries of existing regulations. As the food companies and retailers search for new products and processes there is frequently a need for new regulations or the amendment of existing regulations. A good example of the types of changes that may be made are reflected in MAFF's attitude to food regulations which have 'tended to move away from imposing compositional standards on food . . . to provide more effective ingredient and nutritional labelling' (Foreman 1989: 118). The extra flexibility this modified stance has given food manufacturers is reflected, for example, in low fat products which were previously outlawed by specifications on minimum fat content.

The case of food composition provides a good example of how rights related to food choice have been reformulated. The move towards more 'effective labelling' is one based on the assumption that the *informed individual* is best placed to make decisions on consumption. In other words, the consumer is being given the right, the *freedom* to consume. Such a notion of rights is quite different from that which prevailed at the end of the Second World War. Then there was a sense of a collective consumer interest whose choice was largely determined by government. The role of governments was to ensure *freedom from* want through the provision of affordable and safe food. Now it is the corporate retailers who play a central role in promoting to individualised consumers their vision of quality and diversity of consumption. This is one of variety and a hierarchy of standards. Different retailers seek to imbue their products with notions of quality and to do this they must be able to exercise considerable influence over the supply of products. This may be termed *private interest regulation* (Harrison, Flynn and Marsden 1997), because retailers are creating their own standards and operating food-safety systems which go beyond that required by more traditional forms of public regulation. Below we explore how contemporary food rights are being played out by the retailers and other key actors, notably consumer groups and government.

Food choice and rights to consume

As we have argued above, the food regulatory framework is a dynamic one and plays a key part in structuring the choices that consumers make. The key constituent elements within the framework are economic interests, although government remains the ultimate arbiter of rules. Government's role is not static, and, increasingly in conjunction with private interests, is modifying consumer rights, particularly around contestations concerning quality parameters. This restructuring of rights, which we explore in terms of food choice, is determined at the national level but mainly played out at the local level in the food-enforcement practices of Environmental Health Officers and Trading Standards Officers.

Ministerial thinking on the market and regulation has resulted in a reconstruction of MAFF's traditional public interest form of regulation which prevailed until at least the late 1970s, and is deepening its relationship with the multiple food retailers. As one official remarked in the mid 1990s:

the government's position is that the market is, broadly speaking, the best determinant of what happens in industry and business. Ministers see us at MAFF as a group of people who are able, through *releasing powers of regulation*, as being able to facilitate the success of business. The attempt has been made to reduce all regulations to an absolute minimum ... The point is that present ministers neither believe in regulation nor in spending money. [But] they [do] believe in encouragement, facilitation, knowing a lot about business ... that's the sponsorship role, in a sense.

Releasing powers of regulation has not meant that the traditional public sector role of protecting the consumer *from* health risks associated with food have been subverted. Rather what has happened is that different sets of rights, intimately linked to private sector provision, have been fostered. Consumers are empowered, are free *to* make the choices as they see fit. These are competing notions of rights, and are associated with different regulatory arrangements. The public or the private sector may take the lead as appropriate, but in practice they are to be found alongside one another. The resulting tensions within the regulatory framework have been particularly acute at the local level of implementation. What we are witnessing, therefore, is the government essentially trying to act as backstop, to ensure basic standards of food safety. Over and above this the multiple retail outlets are creating additional *rights based on their different guarantees of food quality* which are available to their customers. This requires that these firms police and regulate their own food chains.

For the major food retailers quality is linked to competition among themselves. As a leading figure in one of the major food retailers put it: 'For our customers, we're in the business of offering quality.' He continued:

> Well, we're all competing for the same share of the purse. There is only a finite number of calories that people can eat in a day. Our job is to make sure that it is our calorie that they are buying and not someone else's. So, we only make our profits by satisfying our customers, and we have to discover what it is that satisfies them. . . . They're saying that there is a particular level of quality that they want, and we have researched this exhaustively, and every product that we produce goes through customer research to find out whether it is of the right quality.

To be sure of the quality of a product means that the company has confidence in the ability of food manufacturers to deliver appropriate standards. The interviewee went on to outline the procedures involved:

> The work that we do with the manufacturers – we do not make any products ourselves, but prior to anybody making any food for us, they have to satisfy one of our food technologists that they have complied with the criteria that they have set out in their quality management system manual which involves an audit . . . We devise this, in consultation with the suppliers who are involved. Sometimes suppliers say, well that is very interesting but we can't do this and we can't do that, so this consultation process is important. There is a lot of prior consultation. At the end of the day, there is a set of criteria, a set of standards, that we have set out for any manufacturer, and if they can't adhere to those standards in the audit, then they are not in the frame. This has to be sorted out before we start on the negotiations involved in buying stuff. Any buyer in this building knows that he/she does not go to any factory unless they have been formally approved. We will definitely not accept any food from unapproved sources anywhere by anybody.
>
> So once the supplier is approved we start to talk about the product that is to be developed. In that development process, there will be customer research . . . through our stores. We have market research agents in our stores asking customers to taste food in kitchens blind, to satisfy quality criteria, so that when we have a satisfactory customer report then we can market the product. So the technologists are really the key people who work in partnership with the producers to design, develop and procure the products. So the quality management process is governed by technologists effectively. They are backed up by laboratories here. We have got consumer kitchens here. We have got sensory panels, fragrance panels, wearer trials of clothing, packaging laboratories – and the whole thing that backs it up by saying there is a need for subjective information to meet our objectives. But what the analysts do is to check the competence of our suppliers. This is not endpoint testing. We are relying on the laboratories, to give the factories the information they need.

The competitive nature of food retailing means that products supplied by manufacturers cannot be stored to wait for tests to be made on them because this would be an inefficiency in the supply chain. Instead, as a senior retailer explained, what they will say to the manufactures is that:

> our truck is at the end of your production line waiting for that food. It will be in our depots tonight, our stores tomorrow, and sold the day after. So you had better start sorting out your quality management because what I want from you is confidence that what comes off your production line is OK without endpoint testing. There is no time in the world to interrupt the supply chain with endpoint testing. There is no time; you've got to get the job done on the production line. So we went round and said that we wanted the manufacturers to adopt hazard analysis, critical control point techniques, to apply those principles to food processing, so that what comes off the production line does not need endpoint testing to say it is OK to leave the factory.

The food retailers' ability to regulate the flow and quality of food is thus quite different from that of government, which relies heavily on local government officials. Nevertheless, the supermarkets' regulatory activities in this sphere, what we have termed private interest regulation, does derive some of its legitimacy from the government's own regulatory approach. Thus, the Food Safety Act 1990 and the requirement of 'due diligence' put the onus on food-retail outlets to be able to show, should there be a problem with food, in a court of law that quality and safety had been managed. For the major retailers it simply legitimated what they were already carrying out as good practice. There is also a difference in emphasis between private and public interest regulation which we can observe. The public interest is largely concerned with baseline measures. For the private sector, there is an additional element in which quality too has a value from which profit and competitive advantage can be extracted.

The results of the supermarkets' strategies are significant for the choices that consumers make. As a retailing interviewee put it:

> We don't have any control over brands. What Mr Mars does, or what Mr Kellogg does, is up to them. But 50 per cent of food in Britain is bought under own-label, and we have total control over our own-label – in terms of source manufacture, specification, composition, nutrition, packaging right through to the whole thing. It's totally under our control.

Other major food retailers adopt similar procedures to ensure the quality of the food they sell. But as we illustrate below, the different tiers of food retailing have slightly different ideas of quality and the choices they can offer their customers. Thus a very senior figure in one of the second tier of national retailers (Somerfield would be an example) argued:

> every single supermarket chain will establish its own [quality] benchmark, and that will vary. You will get a different benchmark talking to say, Kwiksave than you would talking to us. I mean our benchmark is saying that, on our own-label, we have to have a product that is among the top three in its field. In terms of product development, we tend to be a follower rather than a leader, given the nature of our business. We don't, for instance, go out and develop new areas of eating, we are happy to let Marks and Sparks and Sainsburys go and do that for us. When they develop something that is a winner, then we will piggyback on it. And, therefore, where there are existing products in a particular market, we will continue to make our own. We will say that we want to be at least as good as the best three. So, our buyers will get samples, and food developers will test them, and they will dissect them and they will create a specimen. Sometimes, we will go to the same supplier, and what we aim to do is to get the product that effectively eats and tastes like the best of them. The message that we give to our suppliers is that we are not interested in you adding cost into a product unless it delivers the eating, taste, and utility criteria.

The point that this retailer was keen to make was that price and quality go together:

> You can't persuade the consumer to eat cheap rubbish. But we will seek to make a price point. So . . . take ready meals, which is a classic example, we originally developed products which were selling at £1.40 or £1.50 for a lasagne, and this didn't sell. So we now make to a 99p price point, a slightly smaller meal, and slightly less packaging, but of perfectly good eating quality. These sell at an enormous rate. So . . . you've always got a price point, as opposed to price, in mind.

In short, quality is constructed by retailers and manufacturers. As such there will be variations in the quality of products between different food-retail outlets.

The elusive nature of food quality is well recognised by consumer groups. Rather than comment on quality directly, consumer groups will address other criteria (often as surrogates of quality) such as safety, price and choice. Where consumer groups would want to go further than, say, retailers is to link choice with knowledge: the informed consumer. As one consumer group official put it: 'We're not there to dictate what consumers should or shouldn't do, should or shouldn't have, but we do believe people should have the information they need to make up their own mind.'

Similarly, within government, the idea of choice is important. Once safety criteria have been satisfied, consumers should have the freedom to make decisions about what they want to buy. For MAFF this involves first, making sure that food purchases 'are not going to make consumers ill or kill them'. And second, that 'the consumer is not deceived' (interview with official). MAFF is here performing a

164

balancing act between its traditional role of protecting the consumer from dangers with products and a newer role of enabling consumers to make choices. The balance then shifts between government and private sector as to who has responsibility and rights for ensuring food safety. As one senior MAFF official explained:

> we therefore set a legal framework *putting the onus on* the trader, the producer, the distributor, the retailer, the manufacturer, whoever to do certain things so as to make sure that the consumer can make the purchase with confidence that the information given to the consumer at the time of purchase is correct. And that the food is safe. So that's the essential purpose that we're here for.

The shifting balance of rights and responsibilities for food safety means that government is also increasingly engaged in sharing its authority. The implications for the construction of food choice and the relative power of the key actors in that construction are thus undergoing some changes. The case of food irradiation provides an interesting example of the way in which government and supermarkets help to construct consumer food choices. One MAFF official explained the situation as follows:

> We as a department are very, very nervous about legislating to make food irradiation legal. But there were simply no scientific grounds on which you could continue not to permit this process. There were quite a lot of emotional grounds on which not to permit it. But ministers eventually decided that this was no basis on which to restrict consumer choice. [T]he process of irradiation [did not create additional risks], and could arguably be said to have real benefits because all the microbiological risks associated with that food product were eliminated in the process. So the scientific arguments were that this process should be approved immediately. But the fact of the matter is it is simply not being used in this country because the retailers have said that they are not going to handle it. Consumers will take fright you see.

As a result, on this view, choice is diminished. Curiously, in this case, the traditional roles of public and private actors have been overturned. The government argues that consumers should have the freedom to consume irradiated food if they wish, while the supermarkets, conscious of their growing responsibilities to protect the consumer interest, are wary of becoming embroiled in potential controversies.

Conclusion

In exploring the regulation of food and consumption rights we have drawn attention to the parts played by key actors: government, retailers and consumer groups. We have shown how their strategies can be interpreted through two competing notions: an individualised freedom to consume goods and a collective freedom from adverse effects. In practice these perspectives can be found operating alongside one another. Moreover, although these may be competing notions they are not mutually exclusive. Government can have a role in promoting food choices and also protecting the consumer.

Over time, as the nature of food supplies and products shift, so the focus of public sector regulation moves, with a relatively greater emphasis on safety and quality issues and less on security of supply. As a result of the approach to regulation of the Conservative governments of the 1980s and 1990s the public sector retains a role as guarantor of basic food standards. At the same time the Conservative governments devolved new rights for the private sector to utilise in the form of freedoms to consume. Essentially these rights have devolved to the retailers and take the form of assessments of food quality. This in turn means that retailers must be able to exercise considerable influence over those that supply them. The ability of the major retailers privately to regulate their supply chains and thus guarantee food standards has been formally recognised with the Food Safety Act 1990. One of the provisions within the Act is that retailers and manufacturers must be able to show that they have exercised due diligence in their activities in case there should be a problem with a product. The Act, though, simply legitimated what had become commonplace and made due diligence a legal defence. As a senior figure at one of the major retailers commented, well before the Act 'we said to people [i.e. suppliers] . . . we expect you to be operating under quality management systems' and by determining quality within the supply chain the major supermarkets seek to gain competitive advantage.

The restructuring of the regulatory framework will have two further important consequences for food choices. First, the much greater diversity of consumption opportunities, certainly compared to the late 1940s and 1950s, allied to changing patterns of regulation, means that notions of quality are increasingly embedded in where consumers purchase products. This in turn depends on the ability of retailers and manufacturers to engage in supply-chain management, which will vary enormously. There is, therefore, the potential for already significant gradations of food quality between different retail outlets to be further accentuated. Second, for the most part individual consumer problems with food safety (e.g. a strand of hair in a loaf of bread) can easily be resolved by retailers and manufacturers and environmental health officers. Much more problematic are crises in food safety which go beyond the individual and expose both the different imperatives of public and private sectors and the difficulties in managing a coherent response. Government now finds it extremely difficult to marshall a collective response. In the late 1980s the then Minister of Agriculture, John McGregor, claimed that MAFF has responsibility for 'keeping the whole food process safe' (*The Times* 13 February 1989). His successor, John Gummer, similarly claimed responsibility for the entire food chain 'from sowing the seed to selling in the shop' (*Guardian* 3 July 1990). The experience of dealing with food crises such as BSE as well as the everyday management of food safety within the corporate retail sector exposes the hollowness of such claims: food regulation is very much a shared experience between public and private sectors. Together they play a central role in constructing a regulatory framework to structure food choices.

CHAPTER 10

Studying food choice in its social and cultural contexts: approaches from a social anthropological perspective

Pat Caplan, Anne Keane, Anna Willetts and Janice Williams

Introduction

This chapter will consider some of the factors which influence food choice in two very diverse settings in Britain. It aims to show that food choice is not simply a matter of individual taste, but rather needs to be seen in a social and cultural context. In the first section, we outline briefly some of the anthropological approaches to food and eating which informed the thinking behind our research before going on to describe the two locations in which it was carried out – a densely-populated south-east London borough, and a small town and its rural hinterland on the west coast of Wales – and the research methods we used. We then consider the extent to which food choice is socially and culturally constructed by examining four variables – gender, age, class and ethnicity – and demonstrate how they influence patterns of eating (see also Keane and Willetts 1993, 1994, 1996; Keane 1997; Willetts and Keane 1995; Williams 1996, 1997).

Food and anthropology

There is a considerable literature on the social anthropology of food (for reviews see Messer 1984; Murcott 1988; Mennell, Murcott and van Otterloo 1992; Caplan 1994, 1996, 1997), showing clearly that cross-culturally, definitions of what is considered to be edible varies enormously. Much of this work is heavily influenced by the structuralist approach of the French anthropologist Claude Lévi-Strauss (1965, 1968, 1992 [1964]), who treated food as analogous to language, and examined the way in which its meanings can be gained from an understanding of symbol and metaphor. Lévi-Strauss maintained that food was 'good to think with' and that deciphering the codes underlying such matters as food enables the anthropologist to reach 'a significant knowledge of the unconscious attitudes of the society or societies under consideration' (1968: 87). This kind of work has produced important insights into the rules underlying everyday life, perhaps most famously in Lévi-Strauss' own work on the raw and the cooked (1965, 1992).

A compatriot of Lévi-Strauss, Roland Barthes, also utilised a linguistic analogy in his attempt to understand food. His basic argument is that where there is meaning, there also must be system. In other words, if we argue that food stands for more than itself and, indeed, serves as a medium of communication, then inevitably it will form patterns or systems. Such patterns may not be obvious to the people eating the food, but they are amenable to analysis by social scientists, in the same way that language can be analysed by linguists.

The British anthropologist Mary Douglas was influenced by both Lévi-Strauss and Barthes, but developed their work in slightly different directions. Douglas has published work on food throughout her career, beginning with an analysis of the Jewish dietary prohibitions laid down in the book of Leviticus (1966) and showing that these were linked with cultural notions of pollution and purity. Later she tackled the topic of British food and the composition of a meal (Douglas 1975, 1984; Douglas and Nicod 1974). In her work, food and eating stand for much more than themselves: they are symbolic of a particular social order.

Such anthropological work, which focuses on food as an aspect of culture, remains important and influential, but it does not tell us everything we might want to know. For example, it does little to explain historical changes in food habits, and also has a tendency to ignore political and economic questions such as who gets what and why. Conversely, while much of the literature on the political economy of food, including that by non-anthropologists, does take an historical approach and reveals differences in entitlement to food, it has little to say about culture and meaning (Walker and Cannon 1984; Cannon 1987; Lobstein 1988).

More recently, some anthropological and sociological work on food has fruitfully combined these various approaches (Goody 1982; Mennell 1985; Mintz 1985), as indeed we have done in our own research. It is thus the argument of this chapter that an understanding of both culture (patterns of meaning) and political economy (the interrelation between economic and political processes), as well as history, is vital if we are to answer the question 'Why do people eat what they do?'

Research locations

The London borough of Lewisham was formed in 1965 from the old metropolitan boroughs of Lewisham and Deptford and covers an area of 13.7 square miles. Its population of just over a quarter of a million (235 700 in the 1991 Census) is ethnically diverse, with the two largest self-defined groups being 'White' (78 per cent) and 'Black Caribbean' (10.1 per cent), and it was on these that the study concentrated. Within Lewisham there are a number of different areas, each with its own character and history, but a broad division between the relatively poor areas in the north and the more affluent areas to the south may be distinguished (Hyde, Balloch and Ainley 1989; Deptford City Challenge 1993, 1994a, 1994b). Research was conducted in both the northern and southern areas of the borough.

Newport provides a striking contrast, being a small seaside town situated in an area of outstanding natural beauty in the Pembrokeshire National Park. Its history spans several millennia and has left monuments dating back to the Stone and Iron Ages. The current population of just over 1000 (1166 in the 1991 Census) quadruples in the main summer tourist season.

Although at first sight the two areas could scarcely be more different, there are factors which they have in common since both have suffered from economic decline. In the last century Newport was much bigger than other west Wales towns which have since outstripped it in size and population and, until the middle of the last century, had its own shipbuilding yards. Today it contains no major employers, apart from a small bus company, and the local economy is heavily dependent on agriculture and tourism, both industries which have suffered a number of vagaries in recent years. Unemployment is high, and the wages in the county are the lowest in Wales, which itself has a much lower average than the rest of Britain. There is a long tradition of outmigration by young people in search of higher education and employment; this is countered to some extent by the immigration of retired incomers, many from England, leading to an usually top-heavy age structure.

Lewisham too flourished during the period when Deptford was a centre of shipbuilding from the sixteenth century on, but has suffered economic decline since the nineteenth century, especially after the closure of the docks in 1869. Today the borough offers relatively few employment opportunities, and many of its residents have to travel outside its boundaries to work. Like Newport, it has a declining population, probably because of outmigration by those of working age, although it has also received many newcomers, especially from such areas as the West Indies, West Africa, Greek and Turkish Cyprus, Vietnam, India and Pakistan. Its age structure is relatively balanced by comparison with that of Newport, for most incomers have been young adults.

Methods used in the research

Since the aim of the studies was to examine food in its social and cultural context, the primary emphasis was on in-depth qualitative data: empirical material gathered through interviews, food diaries and participant observation. Quantitative techniques have also been used through the administration of food-frequency questionnaires. Steps have been taken to place this micro-level data in a wider context, which has meant drawing on existing material on labour markets, access to housing and land, health policies and campaigns, as well as the availability of supermarkets, shops, cafés, restaurants and fast-food outlets in the areas of fieldwork. The work has also been contextualised historically not only through the use of published and archival material for both areas, but also through the collection of oral histories from older interviewees. Below we discuss briefly our research techniques.

In order to elicit people's own views of what they ate and why, the most important technique in both areas was to carry out semi-structured interviews with a wide variety of men and women of varying ages and socioeconomic and ethnic backgrounds who were contacted through social networks of families and friends and through community groups. The interviews covered shopping and expenditure, food preparation and consumption (including the division of labour), hospitality and eating out, dietary changes, views on food manufacturing and processing, and on health and healthy eating, including diet and body image. Background data on participants' household composition, socioeconomic and educational status, age and ethnicity were also sought. The interviews were designed to be flexible and people were given the opportunity to discuss their own concerns. Interviews lasted from 45 minutes to three hours and were audiotape-recorded and transcribed verbatim. Some participants were interviewed more than once and, in several households in each location, more than one member was interviewed. It is from such interviews that the bulk of the data for this chapter is drawn.

Interviews were also carried out with health and food professionals, the former category comprising doctors, practice and community nurses, health visitors, dieticians, health and welfare advisors, and alternative health practitioners, while the latter included food retailers working in supermarkets and shops, and caterers running cafés, restaurants, pubs, hotels and guest-houses. Here the aim was not only to obtain 'expert' views on food and eating, but also to subject such views to a critical analysis similar to that conducted on the interviews with lay people.

To supplement interview data, a selected number of interviewees were asked to record details of their food and drink in a seven-day food diary. The diaries provided valuable information on the contexts of eating and the extent to which consumption varied throughout the weekly cycle. Just over half of the interviewees (53 per cent) returned completed food diaries in Newport and almost one-third (31 per cent) did so in Lewisham.

At the end of the fieldwork period all interviewees in both locations were asked to complete a questionnaire which was divided into five sections: food-frequency, health concerns, time allocation, food budgeting and income and expenditure. In Newport, they were administered both to people who had already been interviewed, and to many other local residents who had not, with the major means of distribution being local voluntary organisations, and the families of children at the local primary school; the response rate was 66 per cent. In Lewisham, the questionnaire was used only with interviewees, just over a half of whom responded. Additional shorter and simpler questionnaires were also filled out by local schoolchildren.

Researchers also engaged in anthropology's most important ethnographic technique of participant observation. They joined or observed a variety of groups which had a focus on food and health. In the case of Lewisham these included dieting organisations, fitness groups, cookery classes and health workshops; researchers also attended meetings of community groups such as pensioners' and women's organisations, advice centres, job clubs and environmental pressure groups. In the case of west Wales, there were also coffee mornings/evenings, festivals and carnivals, agricultural shows, fairs and fêtes, fund-raising events, and local planning meetings.

Each of these different methods provides a slightly different angle of vision on the question of food and eating. For many households, we have a multiplicity of data of various kinds, enabling not only a certain amount of cross-checking, but also in-depth analysis.

What determines food choice?

It is often thought that people are free to choose what they eat out of the enormously wide range available in the contemporary West. This notion of free choice is one which, while having a long history in Western thought, has recently been further encouraged by the adoption of a particular discourse around the market economy. Yet such an individualistic view of why people eat what they do fails to take account of social and cultural constraints on people's eating, which may range from lack of money to buy, time to prepare, or unwilling-ness, perhaps on ethical or religious grounds, to consume certain kinds of foods.

In our work, we made every effort to elicit the reasons people themselves gave for eating or not eating certain foods. However, there are limitations attached to a stance which relies only on people's conscious reasons. It is one of the tasks of social science to reveal patterns and meanings which are often hidden, and to articulate the manner in which they may influence everyday behaviour surrounding food. Thus we follow standard anthropological practice and seek to make manifest some of the implicit and recurring themes and patterns which are beginning to emerge from a preliminary analysis of the data collected.

It is commonly said that 'you are what you eat,' yet one of the premises of this study is that the reverse is also true – you eat what (or who) you are – and that people's food habits are central to their identities. One way of establishing this is through comparison, which has been built into the study from the start, not only in terms of the differences between an inner-city area of London and a semi-rural area of Wales, but also in terms of the differences between people within each area. In this section of the chapter, we demonstrate some of the ways in which what people buy and eat can be correlated with who they are. Using some of the preliminary results from the two projects, we consider in turn four variables: gender, age, class, and ethnicity. The underlying premise is that people are cultural and social beings, and this needs to be explicated in understanding food 'choices'.

Gender

Since much previous food research in Britain and indeed the West generally has concentrated on women (e.g. Murcott 1982, 1983a; Pill 1983; Charles and Kerr 1988; DeVault 1991) we considered it important that this study should include men among the interviewees. It did, however, prove somewhat more difficult to recruit male informants and, in the end, approximately one-third of the interviewees in each area were male (32 per cent in Lewisham and 35 per cent in Newport). Many men tended to consider food a female topic and, particularly if their wives or female partners had been interviewed, thought they would have little to add.

Cross-culturally, there is a large amount of literature on the differential entitlements to food of women and men. Although there are particular cultures, especially in South Asia, in which women's entitlement is notably less than that of men (Harriss 1990; Sen 1990; Papanek 1990; Rizvi 1991), some of the literature on food in the West also suggests that there is a long-standing and widespread expectation that women will not only eat less food than men, but also eat food which is different in certain ways (Delphy 1979; Bourdieu 1984; Charles and Kerr 1988). Our findings were similar in both respects.

While few of our respondents stated that men needed more food than women, it was clear from some of the interviews that there were often contradictory, albeit implicit, assumptions about gender-related appetites and dietary needs. Men who worked 'outside' needed more food than women who remained 'inside', even if the former were doing sedentary work, and the latter heavy housework. Food was often seen as a kind of fuel of which the male body required greater quantities, and which it was women's job to supply.

Women were far more likely than men to monitor their food intake for aesthetic reasons. Most of the women interviewed in Lewisham described themselves as having 'been on a diet' for most of their lives, or else as perpetually 'watching what I eat'. A significant minority of women living there also had personal experience of eating disorders. In Wales, too, women were more likely than men to undertake a weight-loss diet, but here there was much less concern with body image than was the case with London interviewees and, according to local medical practitioners, virtually no incidence of eating disorders.

Our research also confirms gender differences suggested in other literature on the types of food eaten. Several men and women in both areas thought it was important for men to have meat, and women were much more likely than men to be vegetarians (Willetts 1997; Fiddes 1991). On the whole, women ate more salads (although certainly in the Lewisham study, this was related to a concern about body image and weight loss), but men tended to be less keen, as shown in an extract from an interview with a Welsh farming couple:

Q: Is there something that you avoid because of your health?
Husband: Oh yes, lettuce and things like that. They tend to make my stomach bad.
Q. They don't agree with you?
Husband. No, not a lot.
Wife. And I'm cross about that because I love them.
Husband. I'm not keen on them. I haven't ever been very keen on lettuce and I'm not keen on tomatoes either, as far as that goes.

Not only does this extract indicate a difference in food preferences between a husband and wife which are fairly typical of many other interviews, but the implication is also that the husband's food preferences take precedence over those of the wife. Frequently, women reported that they would like to have vegetarian food more often, but that their husbands or partners insisted they must regularly have meat.

The findings from both areas were that in most households with adult couples, it was usually the women who were responsible for planning meals, shopping and cooking. In spite of an oft-professed ideology of sharing whch was more marked in Lewisham than in Wales, it was relatively rare for men in either area to cook on a regular basis. Further, although decisions about shopping and preparation were largely made by women, male preferences as well as those of children were very significant in the purchase and preparation of food. The dominant ideology, then, remained one in which feeding the family was seen as women's work, and even if women themselves objected to the inequality of the domestic division of labour, they felt there was little they could do about it.

Gender cannot, however, be discussed without reference to other factors such as age. Couples under 40 would be much more likely to profess an egalitarian ideology, and in some instances, go part way towards realising this. Older couples frequently noted that 'things are different today', and gave examples of their own sons or grandsons who were able to cook. In the next section, we consider the topic of age in greater detail.

Age

In Lewisham, more than half of the interviewees (60 per cent) were below the age of 40, while in Wales, the figure was much lower, at just over a quarter (26.2 per cent). Conversely, in Wales, the over-fifties comprise more than half of the interviewees (53.8 per cent), but only just under a quarter (23.8 per cent) in Lewisham. In large part, this reflects the top-heavy age structure of Newport already discussed. One of the questions asked during the interviews in both areas was whether there were particular foods which were suitable for old people. Very few, whether old or young, thought that this was the case, although many older interviewees commented that they noticed themselves eating less as they moved into old age. However, it was apparent from interviews and food diaries in both areas that older people tended to eat in a more structured way than younger ones, with set mealtimes, usually eaten at the table, and at least one cooked meal a day; in such households there would be little snacking, although there might be consumption of tea or coffee between meals. Further, it was mainly older interviewees who still cooked a 'Sunday dinner' with roast meat, although a few said they had ceased to do so when the household numbers fell to one or two persons, on the grounds that it was uneconomic. Many younger families, on the other hand, had either abandoned, or else adhered irregularly, to the traditional Sunday dinner, often because of the time needed to prepare it; in a few instances, it was revived once the children were older and could help in its preparation, or because it served as a focus for an otherwise dispersed family.

'Traditional food' was an important category for older people from all ethnic groups. Older interviewees of British, English or Welsh origin in both areas were less likely than younger people to incorporate 'new' items into their diets, such as pasta, rice, curries or Chinese food. Indeed, some expressed strong resistance to such 'foreign' culinary innovations. Similarly, older interviewees from an African-Caribbean background who had been born in the West Indies were likely to continue cooking traditional West Indian food.

There were also age differences in receptivity to convenience foods. In both areas, take away food was seen as unhealthy even by those who consumed it regularly because it was not home-cooked, and older people in particular tended to regard increasing takeaway and convenience food consumption as symbolic of worrying social changes. One 69-year-old Lewisham woman said:

> You see them eating along the road. You see them standing at bus stops, they throw the carton down. With all these McDonald's and Burger King's. Drinking out of these plastic cups standing at the bus stop. It's horrible, but there you are, I'm in a generation where we didn't do that.

Some of these differences between the generations can be perceived as historical changes, but they can also be linked to changes in both the individual life course and the domestic household cycle. The notion of the 'proper meal' remained important for family households, and mothers in particular considered them important for children's health.

Indeed, many interviewees reported only having seriously considered the health implications of their diets when they became parents.

Young people in their teens and early twenties, on the other hand, when away from the parental home, or living on their own, were likely to feed themselves on snacks, convenience foods and takeaways (Chapman and MacClean 1993). Our data suggest this does not mean that they will always do so – rather that they will do so at particular stages of the life cycle. Getting married or moving in with a partner, and particularly acquiring responsibility for the health and welfare of children, often meant a change in dietary habits and the resumption of more structured meals (Murcott 1997).

Furthermore, although young people, especially males, often voiced a rather blasé attitude to the health implications of their diets, men in their forties and fifties tended to display considerably more concern. In Wales, many middle-aged men had received check-ups ('MOTs') as a result of local health campaigns, and some had been advised to change their dietary habits. Such advice was, however, more likely to be followed if the recipient had actually experienced a problem, than simply as a preventive measure.

Age is, then, a significant factor in food choice, but it cannot be viewed as simply one of chronicity; rather, account needs to be taken of stages in the individual life course and the domestic group, as well as of such factors as gender differences, and broader historical trends.

Socioeconomic background

We turn now to the third variable, that of class. In our studies, we wanted to look at the material consequences of income levels, an issue on which there is already a significant literature which demonstrates that low income has highly deleterious effects on the quality of the diet (Graham 1987; Health Education Authority 1989; Lobstein 1991; National Children's Home 1991; Leather 1992; Dobson et al. 1994; Dowler and Rushton 1994; Stitt 1996).

We also wanted to consider to what extent different dietary sub-cultures are associated with particular socioeconomic backgrounds. Work on food in the West by both anthropologists and sociologists has suggested that higher status groups will seek to differentiate them-selves from the lower ones through a variety of means, including diet (Mennell 1985; Bourdieu 1986), while lower-status groups will seek to emulate them (Mintz 1985; Fitchen 1988), thus leading to a continual process of change and innovation. Food consumption is therefore likely to show class-correlated differences which are attributable to both material and cultural factors.

We used two main methods for measuring class. The first considered people's own definitions of their class background: approximately 40 per cent of interviewees in both locations defined themselves as 'working class'. The second used the Office of Population Censuses and

Surveys (OPCS) definitions of class. This system has a number of drawbacks since it is based largely on occupation (OPCS 1991), and there are often considerable discrepancies between people's actual income and their class background as measured, for instance, by their previous occupations, or by their educational levels. It thus gives little notion of the number of people managing their food budgets on relatively low incomes. People who were unemployed, worked part-time, were students, or supported children on a single salary, as well as some of those who had retired, found themselves juggling food purchases with other needs. Food was often considered to be an elastic part of the household budget, as an unemployed Lewisham woman made clear: 'We have to lessen our food so that we can pay the bills to carry on living here. Food, that's the only thing that's expendable.' Shopping on a low income was time-consuming and often meant using a variety of shops. As an 80-year-old woman commented: 'I know where I can get the cheapest food for the cheapest money.' Interview data indicates that economies were made on the quality as well as the quantity of food, including cutting out what were seen as healthier choices. As one woman said:

> If I had more money I think I'd probably buy different things. I think I'd probably eat more heathily if I had more money. Like [now] I buy squash and things for the kids. I wouldn't buy squash, I'd buy fruit juice ... You buy them squash because it goes further and the children like it. But it's got all the Es (additives) and stuff in it; it's not very good.

In Wales, food tended to be more expensive than in Lewisham, especially if purchased locally, while wages and salaries were lower. Most people interviewed used one of the supermarkets in nearby towns for their bulk shopping, but would 'top up' locally. Many felt guilty for not purchasing all their requirements in Newport, recognising that the shops there needed their custom, but argued that they were simply unable to afford to do all their shopping there.

Although some households on low incomes tended to purchase cheap, calorie-dense foods, many others were endlessly inventive in seeking to maintain proper meals and a healthy diet, like a Lewisham community worker who said:

> I've had to do it on benefit money so it can be done. You haven't got much choice, but you can do your mince and do your spag. bol. and make up a load and bung the red beans in it the next day, cook it as chili con carne or freeze it or something.

In both areas, but particularly in Wales, there were significant minorities, usually with a middle-class background and a high level of education, who had chosen to live an 'alternative' lifestyle. Such people, living on very low incomes, were likely to grow at least some of their own food and be willing to spend time preparing relatively inexpensive dishes.

Those, however, who were unwilling to adopt such drastic measures or who did not have other resources such as families nearby, found it much harder to manage. In Newport, a 40-year-old single mother, living largely on benefit, explained how her options were limited:

> I haven't ever been to Tesco in Cardigan yet, because I know that if I went in there I'd see a lot of things that I'd like to have, and I'm not in that situation at present . . . every penny has to be watched very carefully at the moment.

Problems of eating on a low income were compounded by the presence of children; mothers managing on scarce resources were just as much subject as others to the ideal of giving them what they wanted. One Newport woman in this situation said that while she would be quite happy to live on 'greens and brown rice', her children wanted other foods:

> It's what I've got to cook for the kids, and because I'm the only adult here it means I'm doing these chips, something that they really love, or baked potatoes . . . It's more expensive to be more healthy; it's just very difficult catering for their needs and mine together.

To a certain extent, then, socioeconomic status does explain some forms of dietary differences in the sense that people living on low incomes have very restricted choices. In contrast, those with more comfortable incomes could eat out frequently, buy good quality meats and vegetables, and indulge tastes for more specialised or exotic foods. People in households in Lewisham with two full-time wage earners, or members of affluent middle-class households of retired people in Newport, reported that cost was not a determining factor in their food purchases, and that they did not budget carefully for food. Indeed, many of them were unable to say how much they spent on food each week, and those who did provided surprisingly different amounts, ranging between £15 and £50 per person per week.

Income, then, is significant in determining the extent to which people really have any choice in what they can afford to buy and eat, but above a basic minimum, it does not necessarily allow us to predict what proportion of their budgets people will spend on food, or what they will buy and eat. For some middle-class interviewees, eating (and drinking) well, and perhaps entertaining, were a priority, forming part of their leisure activities, such as a retired professional man in Wales who reported spending £1000 a year on good wine. For others, food was of much less interest: they cooked standard fare, were not very keen to innovate, and rarely ate out.

Ethnicity

There is a relatively small literature on the relationship between ethnicity and food choice in Britain, although some work has been carried out in the USA (Sharman *et al.* 1991) and there is some recent work on Britain by Bradby (1997) and James (1997). Ethnicity was one of the issues investigated in detail in both areas of the current research.

As with class, participants were asked to define their own ethnicity. These definitions were wide-ranging but in Lewisham, interviewees could be broadly categorised as either White British (75 per cent) or African-Caribbean/Black British (25 per cent). In west Wales, ethnic affiliation is complex, and language is important, although not entirely determining. A number of people who defined themselves as Welsh did not speak the language, while several incomers whose first language was English had learned it to high levels of fluency, and some had even switched their ethnic identification from English to Welsh. While two-thirds of those interviewed defined themselves as Welsh, only just over half spoke the language fluently and defined themselves as 'Cymry Cymraeg' (Welsh and Welsh-speaking born and bred).

One of the questions asked in the interviews was about culinary traditions, including what people thought was meant by 'British' or 'English' food (Back 1996; James 1997). In Lewisham the older generation saw such food as plain and wholesome, nourishing and healthy, whereas most of those under fifty saw 'British food' as bland, boring and unhealthy, and in defining it, described stereotypical meals, such as 'roast' dinner, 'meat and two veg', suet pudding, or shepherd's pie, which they themselves rarely ate. Many Lewisham interviewees saw such food as a 'dying concept', recognising that their diets reflected many influences, such as a 34 year-old woman who stated: 'I cook things from a variety of origins: spaghetti bolognese, traditional English breakfast, chili con carne, stir-fried vegetables.' In this area, foods of Italian, Chinese and Indian origin were commonplace in the culinary repertoires of younger informants of both ethnic groups; indeed, they were rarely described as 'foreign', but had been assimilated to a new form of creolised cuisine. It was, however, striking that few White interviewees had ever eaten West Indian food, unless they happened to have friends with that background.

Lewisham residents who had been born in the Caribbean and were middle-aged or elderly at the time of fieldwork had tended to retain their culinary traditions, described by one young African-Caribbean woman as follows:

> Green bananas, breadfruit, yam, chocho, cassava, ackee and salt fish, pepperpot soup, calallo, my God, there's so much. Rice and peas definitely every Sunday. There's a pudding my mum makes, sweet potato pudding. That's kind of West Indian cooking. You could go on for ever.

The younger generation of Black Britishers, however, did not eat such food regularly. Some said they found it 'heavy and starchy' because much of it is fried and salted, although it was also argued that the emphasis on fresh and unprocessed food made it healthy. Some younger women avoided West Indian food because of fears of weight gain; others because it was time-consuming to prepare. Many people ate it only at certain times, as a 32-year-old man explained: 'I go to my Mum's at the weekend most of the time . . . Sundays it's usually traditional West Indian food: rice and peas, carrot juice, pineapple juice . . . Those things I usually have weekends but not during the week.'

Many stated that eating West Indian food was an important part of Black identity, as one woman noted: 'I try to keep a lot of my Jamaican in me. I make myself cook a West Indian meal on Sunday because I like to keep in touch or keep a part of my culture.' Some interviewees described how they had rejected such food as children and teenagers, but started eating it again in their twenties. One man aged 24 stated:

That's what I grew up with and that's what makes me feel more comfortable. I mean when I was a kid I didn't used to like it; it's only nowadays that I can really appreciate the food. I would definitely say it's important to me.

In short, then, African-Caribbean interviewees switched their food codes, depending on time, place and company, although most recognised the symbolic importance of West Indian food for their ethnic identity.

If we turn to the Newport area, we find an even more complex relationship between food and ethnicity. We would argue, however, that a distinctively Welsh cuisine may be discerned in two senses: one is in terms of both particular items and patterns of eating by Cymry Cymraeg informants in contrast with other informants. The second is in terms of the recent creation of a tradition of Welsh food which is presented to tourists and visitors in restaurants and in cookery books (Binns, Davies and Parry 1989; G. Davies 1990; Heard, Heard, and Corder 1994 and Freeman 1996). We suggest that here, as elsewhere, the first may be termed food *in* culture, and the second food *as* culture, and now consider each in turn.

There was a discernible pattern of eating among Welsh farming families which had similarities to other British patterns, but also included items which were seen as distinctive and 'Welsh', such as *cawl* (broth containing meat and vegetables), and Welsh cakes cooked on a griddle (*planc*). Older residents cited such foods as part of their childhood (Tibbott 1976), but they were frequently eaten by many people today. There was also a particular pattern of eating on Welsh farms which had important links with, as well as discontinuities from, the recent past. Here, the meal pattern was chiefly constructed around four food events: *brecwast* (breakfast: an important and substantial meal, often cooked), *cinio amser cinio* (literally, dinner at dinner time), *te* (tea), and *swper* (supper). The same would apply to 'typical' Sundays, except that the 'dinner at dinner time' would, certainly in recent years, generally have been a roast and gravy, accompanied perhaps by a few more vegetables than during weekdays, and usually followed by a pudding. Sunday tea was also more elaborate, with a greater variety of items than on a weekday. Although in some households the main meal had moved to the evening, this pattern remained a template for the structure of meals.

The plainness of Welsh farmhouse food was seen by interviewees as desirable, and a number expressed strong resistance to dietary innovations in terms of what were perceived as 'foreign' foods, as is shown in an extract from an interview with two brothers in their sixties who farmed together:

Q. Have you tried curry or Chinese?
First brother: Oh *Duw*, leave the curry out – I always ask – on the television [food programmes] always they show these things – [they get a] saucepan and they turn it and they pour this in and pour that in – and the only question I always ask is 'Has the stomach been made to cope with things like that?'
Second brother: There's so many different things in the dish.
First brother. I always say if I saw something like that and ate that – phone the undertaker afterwards! [Laughter]
Second brother. That's it!
First brother. I don't know what they call all these things – and people eat them then.
Q. Well, people have travelled so much nowadays and tasted so many different things.
Second brother. Youngsters now go around so much.
First brother. I wonder at what children eat these days, you see. I say 'What have you got then?' 'Oh some Pot Noodle or something like that.' I haven't got a clue what that is. What is that then?

Here resistance to innovations in eating was frequently phrased in a specific and highly localised manner. The extent to which certain themes, such as the emphasis on 'plain' as opposed to 'fancy' or 'exotic' foods, recurred in interviews with Welsh farming families is just one of the ways in which the data reveal the imprint of culture.

In the second context, food as culture, we found that the presentation of 'Welsh foods' to tourists affords a public image of a quintessential and idealised regional culture (Williams 1996, 1997). In restaurants, *cawl*, for example, had ceased to be a main course, and had assumed the status of a 'Welsh soup', while certain items, such as cheese, butter, lamb and leek, were extolled because of their 'Welshness'. Similarly, cream teas were advertised as 'Welsh cream teas', and would invariably include such items as *bara brith* (currant bread) and Welsh cakes. Welsh foods are thus in a sense 'invented' for the benefit of tourists (Hobsbawm and Ranger 1983) as part of a process of Western consumerism echoed in other regions and in other countries. But this cuisine is not only presented to tourists: local people Welsh themselves, on public occasions at which food is served, also have recourse to such a notion of Welsh food, even if it is not necessarily what they themselves would eat at home.

Thus in both areas, food choice is not only patterned and mediated by local culture, but is also significant in terms of identity, including ethnic identity, and social relations with others.

Conclusion

In this chapter, we have argued that the concept of 'food choice' is not just about individuals and their preferences. We have sought to demonstrate that food choices have to be seen alongside constraints, and that often both are in fact contingent on who people are. Here we have focused on only four variables: gender, age, class and ethnicity. While ethnic traditions seem to offer positive points of identity, particularly for those who define themselves in opposition to 'Englishness', other factors, particularly socioeconomic and gender identity, are not simply 'chosen' but can, in the current context, restrict choices and possibilities for change.

Furthermore, while each of these factors is significant in itself, none can be discussed in isolation: each articulates with others in a complex way, leading to shifts in behaviour associated with food according to context and over time. People's priorities change throughout their lives as they adapt to changes in circumstances. Thus patterns of food consumption are emblematic of social changes and also contribute to them.

CHAPTER 11

Food choice and diet change within the family setting

Spencer Henson, Susan Gregory, Malcolm Hamilton and Ann Walker

Introduction

The project described in this chapter set out to explore what happens to food choices within the family when one member unilaterally decides to change their diet. If one member of a family decides to become a vegetarian how do others react? If the change in diet requires extra shopping and cooking, who does it? Who in the family takes responsibility for ensuring the person who changes their diet is eating a nutritionally adequate diet? By focusing on the social ramifications of a change in diet, the project addresses the complex role that food plays in the family context, both in terms of responsibility for the practical tasks associated with the acquisition and preparation of food and in terms of the social functions that food performs.

Food choice within the family

Although the notion of 'food choice' is in common usage among those involved in food-related research, it is clear that individual academic disciplines interpret it in quite different ways. As companion chapters in this volume illustrate, for some, 'food choice' is largely a question of *what* foods people select from the range available to them. For others, 'food choice' involves understanding *how* people decide which foods to select, with a view to identifying the factors which influence the choices that are made. The availability of a range of foods between which choices must be made and the ability and freedom, both economically and socially, to make such choices, appear to be taken as given.

    In effect, much of the existing work is based on a model of food choice which fails to recognise that food obviously has to be acquired and prepared prior to consumption, and that the vast majority of foods are eaten at home and/or as part of a family rather than out of the home and/or in isolation. Though this body of work provides some insight into the factors which influence what individuals choose at the actual point of consumption, the approach ignores the social contexts in which foods are selected and the likelihood that the selection is the product of collective family or household decision-making which may involve negotiation or compromise. Indeed, the way in which familial influence on the individual's food choices tends to be regarded as an external 'environmental' factor (Khan 1981) fails to acknowledge the role of the individual within the family and the complex interrelationships between an individual's food choices and those of the rest of the family.

The definition of 'food choice' adopted in the project described here encompasses all activities involved in the acquisition and preparation of food, taking account of three interlinked features:

1 the majority of individuals purchase and use most of their food as part of a household rather than individually
2 in consequence, food selection is liable to derive from a collective household decision on behalf of its members
3 nonetheless, the responsibility for selecting foods for the household is more often than not delegated to one of its members.

Within the context of the family, food-related tasks are typically performed by one member, whom we shall call the 'home manager', on behalf of all the others as part of the domestic division of labour (Charles and Kerr 1988; Morris 1990; DeVault 1991). Most commonly, the home manager is a woman. She is likely to attempt to reconcile such factors as the financial cost of various foods and budgetary constraints, the time taken to procure and prepare different types of food and meals and the nutritional content of food on the one hand with the preferences, likes, dislikes and perceived needs of different family members on the other (DeVault 1991). In this process a home manager is influenced by the expectations that family members have relating to food and meals, the degree to which she herself derives satisfaction from the pleasure she gives to her family and their appreciation of her skills in relation to the provision of meals as well as her own sense of responsibility to her family and her role within it (Murcott 1982, 1983a). This may not simply be a matter of balancing preferences against constraints, but might involve seeking to provide something different or novel. In this way other family members may be introduced to foods which they themselves would never have considered or been able to choose. In turn, family members may, to a varying extent, modify their demands or requests for different food or meals in recognition of the difficulties of the task of providing meals which are economical in terms of time and money as well as appetising.

Taking all this into account illustrates the manner in which food choice cannot be understood in terms of *individual* preferences. Varying patterns of expectations and relationships within the family/household determine the outcomes to the extent that raise the question as to how

far the term 'choice' is entirely appropriate to capture the con₁ᵣ
involved.

Families and households

The terms 'family' and 'household' are so familiar that at first sight it
appears obvious what they mean. It is, however, useful to distinguish
between them for analytic purposes. 'Household' is a matter of shared
residence, 'family' of relationships of actual and putative kinship
(Yanagisako 1979). The study described in this chapter was based on
households the great majority of which, but by no means all, consisted
of nuclear families, i.e. a married couple with or without dependent
children. It is recognised that this household type now represents only a
minority of all households in Britain. Given the need to recruit cases in
which one person's diet changed, household type could not also
feasibly be one of our selection criteria.

Households and families, food and the role of women

Evidence of the centrality of food in family life is directly reflected in a
number of studies (Murcott 1982, 1983a, 1983b; Charles and Kerr 1986a,
1986b, 1988; DeVault 1991) and indirectly in others (Delphy 1979;
Graham 1984; Calnan 1994). For Murcott (1982) and Charles and Kerr
(1988) this is indicated in the importance of the 'proper meal', its
preparation and the character of the group eating it. Such a meal is
cooked, made up of 'meat and two veg', a meal in itself for all the
family. Mennell, Murcott and van Otterloo (1992) point out that eating
at the same table and sharing the same food expresses boundaries
constituting group identity and highlighting 'togetherness'.

From a different perspective, Charles and Kerr (1988) and DeVault
(1991) suggest that food practices reproduce patriarchal families and, as
such, endorse the principles of capitalism. Thus food and the provision
of meals form part of an ideology of caring as an inherently female
characteristic which serves the interests either of men or of the owners
of the means of production. These and other studies (Delphy 1979;
Graham 1984), have shown an unequal distribution of food within the
family which suggests a 'hierarchy' of access to food. Women defer to
men and to some extent to children in respect of access to both type and
quantity of food, a hierarchy reflecting 'traditional' ideas of men's and
women's needs, but also related to poverty. Equally, there has been
some debate over the relationship between responsibility and control
within the family (Murcott 1983a; McIntosh and Zey 1989; Pahl 1990),
which manifests itself most noticeably in the case of food consumption

(Charles and Kerr 1988). As Murcott (1983a) has indicated, women's responsibility for food-related domestic activities may have to be seen as delegated and thus entailing more limited autonomy, rather than automatically being taken as evidence of her control over decision-making (and see Kemmer, Anderson and Marshall, Chapter 12 in this volume).

The identification of women with practical food-related tasks continues, and is reflected in data collected nationally from various surveys (Nicolaas 1995). One of these indicates that while 66 per cent of employed women and 86 per cent of unemployed/inactive women claim to prepare meals for the family every day, the comparable figures for men are 14 per cent and 36 per cent respectively. Another surveyed 2000 respondents, reporting that 80 per cent of women said they cooked all meals, while 20 per cent of men said they did so. Some 16 per cent of men reported that they never cooked at all.

The link between diet and health and the dilemmas women face when attempting to bring them together have been illustrated in a number of studies. In their study of married women with young children in the North of England, Charles and Kerr (1988) found that they juggled their desire to provide their families with a healthy diet with their need to fulfil cultural demands of the family and the region. In doing so, both the form and content of a proper meal were well established as a 'cooked meal of meat and two veg', as well as the nature of the preparation and the consumption; that is, proper meals were cooked by women and consumed by the whole family sitting round the table together. These arrangements established the relationships between family members, and could be seen to reinforce the existence of the traditional, patriarchal family.

These findings endorse the work done by Murcott (1983a) a few years earlier in South Wales, and developed by DeVault (1991) in her study in Chicago. The latter challenged the assumption that women were merely forced into this position through the unequal economic role they tend to hold in society. DeVault sees this role as part of the social construction of society, which requires the active endorsement of gender roles on a day-to-day basis.

Study design and methods

The aim of our study was to examine the effects on the family of a planned change in the diet of one of its members to either (1) a vegetarian diet, (2) a medically-prescribed diet; or (3) a 'slimming' diet. This assumed that, within a family, there would be a range of attitudes towards food choice and preference, while at the same time established attitudes regarding appropriate food for that family. These views, whether individual or group, generate tasks and responsibilities which might have to be negotiated from time to time. The negotiation might not be formally recognised or overt, but nevertheless establish how tasks are allocated and conducted. The context of dietary change, especially where it is on the part of one family member, is likely to be particularly revealing of the sort of processes of negotiation and compromise and of the constraints and flexibilities involved in the role of home manager as they affect the collective process of food choice. It is precisely when established patterns change that the underlying assumptions and expectations, which may receive little conscious reflection simply because they are so established, become clear. A change in diet by one member of the family group might trigger a number of other changes associated with food choice, for example patterns of food purchase and preparation. This study sought to examine the extent and pattern of change in new circumstances, and to identify factors which affected and were affected by this process of change. This included factors directly related to food and diet, such as nutrition and health, as well as shopping and cooking tasks, but also included indirectly related factors, such as role identity and expectations.

The research was designed in three stages using methods that moved progressively from qualitative to quantitative data collection and analysis. Stage one involved a series of ten focus groups with individuals who had experienced a change in diet within their family, either because they had changed diet themselves or because a member of their family had changed diet. Participants for both this and the second stage were recruited through local vegetarian and slimming groups, health food shops and dietitians/general practitioners' surgeries. This approach was used to explore issues associated with diet change as perceived by participants themselves and to ensure that the language and vocabulary employed in later stages of data collection reflected those of the individuals being studied.

Stage two used semi-structured interviews to investigate further the issues raised in the focus groups with 75 families (see Table 11.1 for details) in which one member had changed their diet and could recollect the impact of the change. In each family the 'diet changer', the home manager and, where these were the same person, one other person, were interviewed (Table 11.2). Previous studies of food and eating in the family context have interviewed only one family member and either only female family members (Charles and Kerr 1988) or have interviewed very few men (DeVault 1991) for which they have been criticised (Mennell, Murcott and van Otterloo 1992). In the current study a major objective was to remedy this by interviewing more than one family member including men whether the diet changer or otherwise.

Stage two respondents first completed a questionnaire which collected demographic data and details of the nature and impact of the diet change. Each respondent was then interviewed using a semi-structured schedule. The aim of the interviews was to examine in depth the process of diet change and its implications for the diet changer and other members of the family.

Table 11.1 Families in stage two of the study, by type of diet change

Type of diet change	Number
Weight loss	31
Medical	37
Of which:	
diabetic	10
multiple sclerosis	11
myalgic encephalomyelitis	6
coeliac	3
other food allergies	7
Vegetarian	7
Total	75

The final stage of the study used a self-completion, structured questionnaire requesting details about the impact of the diet change on the individual and their family which were distributed through slimming and vegetarian magazines. The aim was to establish whether the results obtained from the semi-structured interviews with a small number of people who had changed their diet and their families reflected the experiences of a wider sample of individuals. The questionnaire was completed by individuals who had themselves changed their diet within the last five years, either because they had become a vegetarian (n = 190) or because they had followed a weight-reduction diet (n = 873).

The process of diet change

The extent to which a change of diet affected or was absorbed into the family routine reflected an interplay between perceptions of 'gender roles' and the division of food-related tasks, largely based on gender roles but also to some extent on employment status and work patterns. Where there was a clear division of food-related tasks, there was less incentive for other family members, whether the diet changer or not, to take an active part in introducing and maintaining the change in diet.

Table 11.2 Individuals interviewed in stage two of the study

	Male	Female	Total
Home manager and diet changer	7	48	55
Diet changer	13	13	26
Home manager	6	18	24
Another member of family	25	12	37
Total	51	91	142

For example, in one family interviewed in stage two of the project, the home manager was responsible for virtually all food-related tasks and the diet changer was a teenage daughter who had become a vegetarian. When asked about the impact of the diet change on cooking arrangements the home manager commented: 'I have had to make all sorts of changes to what we eat . . . new foods, new ways of cooking.'

Our stage two sample was drawn from a relatively affluent area of south-east England where, given its class structure and mobile population, we might perhaps have expected to find a less 'traditional' division of domestic tasks. Yet, for the most part, the families in our study maintained the pattern of wives/mothers doing all or the bulk of the shopping for food and cooking. There was, however, a degree of departure from this pattern. Some families reported a greater degree of sharing of tasks than others. Stage three data showed a rather higher percentage of families' sharing cooking, 29 per cent in the case of vegetarians and 15 per cent in the case of slimmers. The lower figure for slimmers probably reflects the fact that since most are female and also home managers they are less likely to expect others to assist them in maintaining their dietary regime. A greater proportion of the vegetarians were not home managers and were perhaps prepared to share the cooking rather than impose extra work on the home manager. The qualitative data from the stage two showed that in families where roles were less clear and tasks were shared rather than firmly divided on gender lines, there was more shared decision-making. For example, in one family in which the home manager had changed her diet for medical reasons, her comments indicated that a number of members of the family had contributed to decisions regarding the extra tasks associated with the diet change:[1]

> We made a collective decision that the extra things that had to be done for my diet should be shared out. It hasn't been down to me. Others in the family have helped out, suggesting new foods and ways of cooking.

In many cases the authority of the home manager with respect to food, in the sense of the capacity to suggest and have accepted proposals for altered patterns of consumption, was the basis, regardless of gender, for a willingness to adopt new foods as part of the family diet, rather than being a jointly negotiated revision of understandings about food and diet. For example, in one family in which the home manager was responsible for all food-related tasks, the diet changer, who was the husband and had changed his diet for medical reasons, commented:

> Before I was a really fussy eater but I knew that my diet had to change, the doctor made that quite clear. My wife is the one who does the cooking and she had read up about my condition. I don't like some of the things she puts in front of me but I don't have any choice any more.

The authority of any household member whom the others considered knowledgeable about food and nutrition was often enhanced and permitted that person to introduce new foods or ideas about food into the family routine. In most cases, this individual was the home manager, whether it was that person who was actually changing their diet or not. Dietary change in the family context may thus play a role in altering traditional patterns of role expectations. It was not at all unusual in our stage two sample to find that the female home manager had considerable authority in such matters: an authority which underpinned her role as carer and guardian of the family's nutritional well-being. This role, and the authority underlying it, often seemed to have been strengthened by the occurrence of dietary change. For example, in one family in which the husband had changed diet for medical reasons, the home manager was responsible for all food-related tasks and had spent a considerable amount of time gaining knowledge about her husband's new diet: 'I spent a lot of time reading about his condition so I would know what and what not to cook.' While this sense of authority may be a reflection of the traditional idea of the woman as carer within the home, there was evidence that authority was frequently endowed on the home manager regardless of gender.

The notion of authority, however, did not preclude negotiation within the family over food choices and the division of food-related tasks. Nor was it always the case that diet change enhanced such authority to the extent it overruled the preferences of other household members. The home manager, whether male or female, generally remained concerned about whether food was eaten or wasted or whether members of the family enjoyed their meals. For example, the home manager in one family in which her husband had changed diet for medical reasons commented: 'I have had lots of ideas for healthy meals but I know he wouldn't like them and so haven't tried them yet.'

While support from other members of the family was not always sought or expected by the diet changers, where there was a desire for support, this was generally in the form of practical changes associated with food and eating. Thus in many cases other members of the family were asked, expected or volunteered to fit in with the new diet. This was apparent for all types of diet and for both sexes of diet changer. For example, in one family interviewed in stage two of the study in which a young child suffered severe food allergies and was required to eat a highly restrictive diet, the rest of the family also adopted the diet – remarkable considering that the alternative strategy of cooking separate meals is available and often preferred in some households. In a family consisting of a married couple with three teenage children and one younger child, both husband and children converted to the wife/mother's vegetarian diet to ease her tasks as home manager with respect to shopping and cooking. In another case, a father and two daughters adopted the slimming diet of the wife/mother while in a further instance the part-time employed wife of a full-time employed man on a slimming diet joined him in the diet. Many more examples could be cited but overall 65 per cent of households in stage two of the study reported that other family members also followed the diet.

In the case of situations of dietary change, however, the data from stage two of this study suggest that it may not be unusual for the whole or part of the family or household to follow the diet of the diet changer even when that person was the wife/mother and home manager. This was also true of the stage three data; 44 per cent of vegetarians and 23 per cent of slimmers reported that other members of the family also followed their diet. It is perhaps significant in this respect that the need for emotional support was rarely mentioned explicitly by diet changers in the stage two sample. On the other hand, 30 per cent of the vegetarians and 48 per cent of the slimmers in the stage 3 sample said it would be helpful to have the family's support in maintaining the diet.

Complaints about the demands on the home manager or the family as a whole as a result of the change in diet were rare. In most cases the change in diet did not involve significant increases in the amount of time spent shopping for food or cooking. Only 10 per cent of the vegetarian and 11 per cent of the stage three slimming respondents reported that extra time shopping resulted from the dietary change and only 14 per cent of the vegetarians and 17 per cent of the slimmers reported that cooking took up more time. Even where the changes in food-related tasks consequent on the change in diet were significant, this was rarely regarded as a problem. Most home managers in the stage two sample regarded such tasks as part of the job and incorporated them into their normal workload. The one exception was in cases where the new diet was considered 'strict' in that it afforded little flexibility in terms of foods eaten and cooking methods employed; in almost all such cases the diet was medically prescribed. The absence of any perception of a major problem for the home manager resulting from the change in diet is perhaps consistent with DeVault's (1991) analysis of the place of meal provision and preparation in the caring role of women in the family and its significance for the emotional and affective side of family life.

Understanding and perceptions

An important factor in the way families and home managers react to dietary change on the part of family members might be the degree of 'legitimacy' that the change has in their perception or which can be claimed for it. Although this term itself was rarely used, it is apparent that specific factors or events were used to legitimate the change in diet. In certain cases the 'legitimacy' was automatic in that all members of the family had negotiated and agreed to the change for the same reasons and according to the same rules. For example, in a family in which the diet changer was a diabetic, it was agreed by members of the family that certain foods, sweets for example, which the diet changer could not eat, would be banned from the house to avoid temptation.

A diet recommended by a health professional enjoyed an authority that an individual decision did not have. If this involved a clear medically diagnosed condition, the authority was even greater. For example, in a family in which a member had changed diet for medical reasons, the home manager who was responsible for all food-related tasks commented that: 'We have to take the diet seriously because it was prescribed by the doctor. We try to stick to the diet sheet.'

In contrast, diet changes were more likely to be challenged in some way in cases where one member of the family had made their own personal decision to change. It is significant, however, that most dietary change was regarded by family members in the stage two sample as legitimate whether a medical, vegetarian or slimming diet. Our finding did not bear out those of researchers such as Amato and Partridge (1989) who found a certain degree of conflict and tension, even if in only a small minority of cases, surrounding the adoption of a vegetarian diet by a family member. The small number of vegetarians in our stage two sample, however, may have precluded our uncovering this sort of finding.

Legitimacy also took the form either of the 'test of time' whereby the new diet had to be sustained for sufficiently long to 'prove' the diet changer was serious about the change, or through a 'proof of commitment', for example, by joining a slimming club, particularly if this involved paying a fee. In one family, in which a teenage girl had become a vegetarian, the home manager initially refused to adapt her cooking to accommodate the needs of her daughter. However, after a period of time it was judged that the diet changer had shown that she was serious about the new diet and meals were adapted for her accordingly.

The process of absorbing a new diet into the family's established practice often involved claims of acceptability which played down ideas of oddness or peculiarity that might be associated with it. In many cases such claims were associated with the introduction of under-standings and explanations which implied that little or no real change had been made to the way in which food-related tasks were organised within the family or affirmed a belief that the change was not too far from what the family 'normally' did. For example, in one family in which the home manager had changed her diet for medical reasons, she commented: 'We didn't have to make any big changes. We ate all right before. We still sit down and have a family meal.'

In some cases, the home manager, whether the diet changer or not, played down the effect of the changes on food shopping and on meal preparation by omitting to tell other members of the family or by suggesting such changes were insignificant. Further, in a number of cases the home manager developed 'expertise' in the new diet and, although initially there was significant disruption to established methods of food preparation and eating, over time new ways were found of incorporating the diet into the usual family patterns.

Strictness and flexibility

Adherence to the rules of a diet may be more or less strict depending on the circumstances. In many cases, it was the source of legitimacy, for example a medical practitioner or slimming club, which defined the rules. Further, considerable effort on the part of the diet changer and/or the home manager was frequently required in the initial stages of the diet change to gather information on what these rules were. For example, in one family in which a young child was required to change diet because of a food allergy, the home manager spent a considerable amount of time finding out about the diet: 'I spent a lot of time reading about foods, which foods I could cook for him. We got a diet sheet from the dietitian. We had to know what he could and couldn't eat.'

When individuals first changed their diet, they were often anxious about failing to abide by its rules. At this stage, many diet changers inclined towards great strictness. For example, slimmers often planned each meal with very great care, weighing everything that was eaten. In the case of medically prescribed diets, foods may be banned from the house altogether in a bid to obey the rules of the diet. The diet and its associated rules must, however, operate within the social setting of the family. Consequently, as well as fulfilling the rules associated with the change in diet, the new eating regime must correspond with the social activities of the family whether associated with food or otherwise. Many people, both diet changers as well as other family members, talked about the compromises and trade-offs necessary to incorporate the change in diet into the family's established norms of behaviour, whether related to food or otherwise. This implies that over time, the degree of strictness with which the new dietary regime is followed may decline and more flexible modes of behaviour are established, though a different research design would be needed to be sure. For example, in one family in which one member had changed diet for medical reasons, the home manager observed: 'To begin with we stuck to the diet to the letter. If it wasn't on the sheet we didn't eat it. But it was really difficult and soon you begin to eat the odd naughty thing. Otherwise life wouldn't be worth living, would it?'

Strategies for coping with a change in diet

The households which participated in the first two phases of the study adopted one of two strategies for dealing with the change in diet and incorporating it into the normal family routines. Either different meals were prepared for or by the diet changer or all/most of the rest of the family adopted the different diet. In either case the consequences might or might not lead to an altered pattern of domestic tasks relating to food provision and preparation. The redistribution and sharing of both food and non food-related tasks between different individuals was a strategy commonly adopted by families faced with a change in diet by one member. The families that incorporated task sharing talked about this strategy in very practical terms. In certain cases the allocation of tasks was organised, or at least justified, on the basis of individual preference, or in terms of individual skills, for example in cooking. In one family, for example, the diet changer who had become a vegetarian commented: 'My partner does all the cooking, she is really good at that. Me, I can't cook at all. But I go to the health shop when we need extra things like tofu.'

As indicated above, in the majority of families one person generally the female home manager, took responsibility for all food-related tasks. When other members of the family cooked meals, for example on special occasions, the female home manager generally still did the shopping. Home managers and other members of the family justified this division of tasks in terms of convenience, e.g. because she had more time. The home manager who was responsible for all food-related tasks in one family in which the husband had changed his diet for medical reasons commented: 'It was easier for me to call into the health food shop, it is on my way home from work. John works the other side of the town and it would have been right out of his way.' In other households food-related tasks were shared among members of the family in various patterns: one person did the cooking while another did the shopping, cooking and shopping together, or, in a small number of cases, different family members catering for themselves.

In the majority of cases, the home manager absorbed the impact of the change in diet on food-related tasks, especially when the home manager was also the diet changer. It was, however, rare for the home manager to complain about the impact of the diet change. Rather it tended to be reported as a minor issue creating few problems and was generally not measured in terms of additional time spent shopping or cooking. Home managers who were responsible for shopping for food also justified this arrangement in terms of 'personal responsibility' for the family diet or that their partner/husband was less 'efficient' or 'expert' at food shopping. For example, the home manager in one family in which the husband had changed diet for medical reasons commented: 'He never comes into the kitchen. I couldn't expect him to cook separate meals for himself because he wouldn't know what to do. It wouldn't be fair.'

In certain cases the diet changer did cook for themselves or there was greater sharing of cooking, yet it was not unusual for the home manager to cook separate meals for the diet changer as well as cater for the rest of the family. For example, the home manager in one family who was following a slimming diet commented: 'I tend to cook a separate meal for myself and the rest of the family. I have to be in the kitchen anyway so it's not a problem. I couldn't expect them to go on a diet as well.'

In stage three of the study, respondents were asked to indicate the specific changes to food preparation associated with a change in diet. These included adopting new cooking methods, using new recipes or adapting existing ones, seeking information on the nutritional content

Table 11.3 Changes to food preparation associated with a change in diet

Change	Vegetarian (%)	Slimmers (%)
New cooking methods being used	64.6	70.8
New recipes being used	91.0	72.6
Adapting existing recipes	77.8	65.0
Increased planning for, and discussion about, meals	50.5	51.7
Finding out about nutritional content of food	78.8	67.3

of food and so on (Table 11.3). In most cases it was the home manager, whether the diet changer or not, who took on the responsibility for implementing these changes. When asked about this in stage two of the study, it was not unusual to find the home manager commenting that the family had not noticed many of the changes. This is a finding which again seems to reinforce DeVault's (1991) claims about the depth of the household manager's contribution to family solidarity.

Although the families in the study indicated that additional foods had to be purchased as a result of the change in diet, this rarely resulted in the use of additional shops. In many cases, the supermarket where they already shopped sold all the additional items they required. In others, where shopping did change it was not to go to additional shops so much as switch to different ones. Even in cases where a new medically prescribed diet required buying a wide range of specialist foods only sold in health food shops or chemists, it was generally claimed that purchasing such items fitted into the established shopping routine without great difficulty. For example, the home manager in one family who was following a slimming diet commented: 'I have to go to the health food shop to get some of the foods on my diet but it is on my way and so no hassle.'

Although a number of families in stage two of the study indicated that they had to spend more on food as a result of the change in diet, cost was not considered a major problem. To some extent this may reflect the characteristics of the families which participated in the study, few of whose income might be considered low. However, in many cases the families found it difficult to separate out the cost of the change in diet from other changes which would have happened anyway and which might have influenced the amount spent on food, for example, the increased consumption of convenience foods.

Conclusion

In changing diet our respondents were obviously choosing a new pattern of food consumption. Our focus on dietary change, however, throws a spotlight on the fact that this 'choice' is not that of a single isolated individual but is made in the context of a routinely collective and negotiated process of food choice. Even more importantly, the choice of the family member who is changing their diet affects the food-consumption patterns of others in the family and, in large part, determines their food 'choices' as well. Ensuring that the new dietary requirements are met and maintained limits the extent to which home managers are able to choose the pattern of food consumption.

The authority of home managers in these respects, however, is always and to varying degrees tempered by the highly consensual nature of family life. It is also affected by the propensity of home managers to take into account the preferences of other family members, and to please them by providing meals they enjoy, thus interpreting their role as one of forging family solidarity via the collective activity of eating. In this sense the 'choices' of other family members are crucial in determining the overall pattern of food consumption. These choices differ between family members, with some prevailing more than others but all prevailing at least some of the time.

The process of collective determination of food consumption patterns, then, is a complex and negotiated one which balances authority against affection, responsibility against the desire to please, varying patterns of preference, mutual concern for one another's welfare, likes and dislikes, work load and pattern, convenience and cost in terms of time as well as money. It is striking that our study families seemed to adapt quite well to one of their member's change in diet and that there is little evidence that the effect is experienced or perceived as entailing any great difficulties. Perhaps this testifies to the fact that family relationships are sufficiently flexible to allow mutual adjustments that accommodate different and new preferences, demands and expectations. It also underscores our contention that food choice has to be understood in collective not solely individual terms.

Note

1 While we might perhaps expect this sort of support in the case of a medical condition suffered by a member of the household it was not confined to such instances. In any case, the literature on compliance with medically prescribed diets shows that it is not high, even in the case of life-threatening conditions, and that one of the primary reasons for non-compliance is lack of support in the family context (see for example Crumb-Johnson *et al.* 1993).

CHAPTER 12

The 'Marriage Menu': life, food and diet in transition

Debbie Kemmer, Annie S. Anderson and W. David Marshall

Introduction

Three complementary approaches, from sociology, nutrition and marketing, were brought together in our study of the 'Marriage Menu'. This research project aimed to examine the nature and process of changes in food choice and eating habits during early marriage, a crucial period in the life course. The thinking behind our aims reflects the call for alterations in the nation's diet that is part of current public health policy (Department of Health 1992). We reasoned that if dietary change is, in some fashion, to be engineered, then understanding how changes occur naturally may reveal the influences at work. Making these influences apparent might then allow planned interventions to take account of what happens *in any case* and thus improve the likelihood of success. Our study focused on marriage as one situation where it was reasonable to expect that dietary change would indeed be occurring naturally. It was also one in which those involved were highly likely to be more than usually conscious of diet, food planning and preparation and, as likely, to be readily able to report and comment on the way any changes came about. Periods of transition can highlight elements of daily life which otherwise often go unnoticed or unquestioned. Choice, according to the *Oxford English Dictionary* (5th edition), is 'the act or power of choosing; preference; variety to choose from, thing chosen'. We acknowledge that choice is not entirely 'free' but constrained by what food is made available via the food system (i.e. production, manufacturing, retailing and distribution). Our interest is in the act of choosing, the power to choose, the ability to choose and the extent to which food choice is negotiated in the transition or 'honeymoon' period. In other words we were looking not only at what was chosen, but why it was chosen and what it told us about how the couple went about it. Food choice, in this project, extended beyond any one instance to a consideration of preceding experiences (including individual preferences, shopping patterns and access to food outlets) and past experiences and expectations.

The investigation focused on marriage/cohabitation (to make it less cumbersome, hereafter we use 'marriage' and its variants as a shorthand that covers both). It sought to examine whether and how food choice changed when shifting from membership of one type of household (an individual living alone, as part of a nuclear family, or with flatmates or friends) to another (as a newly wed couple) and to determine any constraining or liberating effects on food selection. A range of factors, including decisions about the selection of brands or the effect of health and nutrition on choice, was considered, together with the manner in which these were learned, transmitted, shared or negotiated. Throughout, we were aware of the need to consider food choices at various stages from purchase through preparation, cooking and consumption (Marshall 1995).

In our project the collaboration between sociology, marketing and nutrition brought a number of different interpretations to the study of food choice, just some of which are included in this paper. Along with recognising some of our own disciplinary limitations, we achieved a fuller awareness of disciplinary similarities and differences. The sociological perspective on food choice in courtship and early marriage was concerned with the identification and understanding of those social and cultural factors which, first of all, place some of the foods that are generally available within the ambit of the individuals under study, and, second, inform selection from within that smaller range (Mennell 1985; Mennell, Murcott and van Otterloo 1992). It meant asking how couples negotiated and constructed their food selection shortly before and after marriage, and how they perceived, experienced and influenced the processes and outcomes involved.

The marketing perspective provided an insight into food choice at the level of purchasing by examining the reaction to the 'marketing mix', to product, price, promotion and place of distribution and how these might affect what food is bought. This perspective led us to ask whether, why and how shopping patterns change as a consequence of marriage or cohabitation. The nutritional perspective benefited from examining the health beliefs and concerns of couples, and how these might inform food choice, but its main contribution was in assessing and evaluating the food consumption actually reported and the effect of any changes on nutrient intake.

This chapter is written largely from the sociological perspective. We therefore consider the social forces, institutions, organisational features, social routines and social conventions shaping individual food choice, with which sociology is concerned. We discuss food choice in the transition from single to married status, reviewing relevant literature and drawing on some of the findings from our 'Marriage Menu' research project. (For a fuller account of the project and its findings see Kemmer, Anderson and Marshall forthcoming.)

The project: methods and study group

The 'Marriage Menu' research project asked the following questions. What are the shopping, food preparation, eating and dietary habits of single men and women who plan to marry in the near future and what changes occur during the first three months of marriage? What are the influences and processes that lead to changes in food purchase, preparation and consumption during the first three months of marriage? As far as is known, only one similar study, carried out in metropolitan Sydney, is available (Craig and Truswell 1988). However, it benefited from neither a sociological nor a marketing perspective. Our study was, then, inevitably exploratory, seeking to formulate, as well as answer, questions, for which a small-scale, qualitative approach is appropriate.

An intensive recruitment campaign across Scotland's central belt invited individuals who were living apart and planned to move in together to join the study. Twenty-two couples living in and around the cities of Edinburgh and Glasgow volunteered to take part in interviews and dietary assessments three months before and three months after marriage. Their ages ranged from 19 to 33. Notwithstanding a middle-class bias, there was a wide range in terms of occupational status and income. They also varied in the type of household before marriage, including the parental home, shared flats, living alone and halls of residence.

The partners were interviewed separately both before and after marriage, using three main data-collection techniques. One was a semi-structured interview which allowed them to discuss in some depth, both their experiences of shopping, food preparation, etc., and what it all meant in the context of marriage. This method, which leans towards the ethnographic, ensured that the researchers were able to cover a number of important topics with each person, thus providing for comparison between them, at the same time as allowing each informant plenty of leeway to introduce and develop topics that concerned them. The approach (Davies 1990) permits the examination of attitudes, values and feelings as well as reports of actual behaviour.

The second technique was a short questionnaire on purchasing habits relating to specific, core food items rather than general concepts of food and meals. And the third was a seven-day weighed dietary survey in which informants weighed, described and recorded all items of food and drink consumed over a seven-day period (including one Saturday and one Sunday). Information was also sought on where, when and with whom food was consumed. A brief cross-check questionnaire on a few very specific aspects of food selection (for example, type of milk used) and alcohol intake was also presented. Body weight and height were measured after each diary to enable us to assess some of the physical changes which may have occurred over the six-month period. We encountered a major, and unanticipated difficulty, in that a number of couples' lives were changing in other ways in addition to their impending marriage. For example, 17 out of the 44 individuals in the study experienced changes in their employment situation (affecting 15 couples), a factor which is believed to play a part in food choice.

Early marriage/cohabitation: a period of transition

Marriage has been described as a 'decisive phase of socialisation that can be compared with phases of childhood and adolescence' (Berger and Kellner 1974: 122). This process of socialisation, whereby two individuals negotiate (verbally and non-verbally) new sets of norms and values, can be seen in action over matters such as which foods are bought, how they are prepared and served and who is responsible for their preparation.

Marriage continues to be a central institution in Britain, serving key functions in the lives of most people. According to the General Household Survey, in 1993 only 28 per cent of women in the United Kingdom age 18 to 49 had never been married and 22 per cent of the single women in this age-group were cohabiting (OPCS 1995). Clearly the vast majority of individuals marry/cohabit at some time in their lives. Marital status is related to mortality and morbidity, especially for men, and although the extent and nature of this effect is not yet fully understood or agreed on, eating habits may play a significant part (Trovato and Lauris 1989; Wyke and Ford 1992).

Late-twentieth-century families operate as, among other things, units of consumption (Delphy 1979; Jordanova 1981) so sharing food and eating together remains one of the central themes of living in partnership. This focus on food is illustrated by the tendency of wedding presents to focus on kitchen and dining equipment: scrutiny of *Bliss, the Magazine for Scottish Brides* in 1994 and 1995, showed that approximately 75 per cent of gifts in the wedding-present lists were for the preparation and serving of food and drink. Entertaining is often expected of newly weds and food (and drink) is used in celebration of shared experiences such as moving in to the first home and the wedding itself (Charsley 1991, 1992). The married couple has particular significance in terms of dietary attitudes and patterns; they have been strongly influenced by the previous generation and by their own, and they lay down the foundations of the diet of the next generation (Gillespie and Achterberg 1989). Marriage encourages (at least notionally) a commonality of attitudes, values and behaviour between husband and wife (Berger and Kellner 1974; Morgan 1991), and conjugal eating habits can illustrate ways in which these are reached and maintained. They also demonstrate elements of conflict within the marital relationship (Ellis 1983). Even where couples have similar backgrounds and experiences, their food selection, meal patterns and dietary intake may be radically changed after marriage or cohabitation.

Food-related activities can be used to describe ways in which the domestic and the more public worlds of the individuals in a marriage meet and negotiate. Food, from its selection and purchase, through its preparation to its consumption, occupies a place on the boundary between the public and the private (Murcott 1983a). This symbolic importance of food is also recognised by Davidoff (1976), who provides a useful summary of some of the symbolic functions of food and eating: 'who partakes of the meal, when and where, helps to create the boundaries of the household, of friendship patterns, of kinship gradations . . . These eating patterns vary between and help to define the boundaries of classes, ethnic, religious, age and sexual groups.'

Socioeconomic and cultural influences are major factors in food choice, meal and other food-consumption patterns of individuals at the time of marriage. While shopping habits, food preparation, cooking and eating are all likely to be affected by new relationships, they might continue to be influenced by contact with parents and parents-in-law. 'Traditions' held by individual families can have strong effects on individuals after they leave their family of origin and set up another household – some habits are fondly retained, others may be abruptly rejected as a symbolic act of independence. Similarly, childhood habits and experiences can have positive and negative effects. Moreover, the degree to which traditional tastes and habits are adhered to will depend on how adventurous the individual feels (or is able to be) in their new life. Henson *et al.* (1995) have suggested that among the personal factors affecting dietary changes are the attitudes towards food and diet of the primary meal preparer and their attitudes towards change generally. Some intergenerational changes in eating habits are likely to result from the greater range of foods to which the younger generation have access, rather than a deliberate rejection of old habits. In a rare study of perceptions of the value of food to health between generations, a greater diversity of food items was mentioned by the younger generation, reflecting the greater variety of foods which make up their meals (Blaxter and Paterson 1983).

The transition from single status to marriage usually involves moving from the parental home, shared peer accommodation or single accommodation to a new setting of two individuals with responsibility for shopping and cooking. Although there have been several studies describing 'pathways' into marriage and experience of early married life (Leonard 1980; Mansfield and Collard 1988; Clark 1991; Irwin 1996), the influences on food choice and eating habits of cohabiting or married couples have received little attention. Yet sociological studies of food and diet have pointed to the importance of marital relationships in meal patterns and food choice; for example, Murcott (1982) showed the symbolic importance of the content and structure of the 'cooked dinner' in the domestic lives of couples in south Wales. Pill and Parry (1989) point to the importance of men's food preference in family meals, arguing that while women make day-to-day decisions about food purchase these are influenced by trying to please others (and see also Murcott 1983a). Charles and Kerr (1988) reported that of 73 per cent of the women they interviewed in the north of England take male preferences into account when planning meals.

Marriage/cohabitation and food-related activities

Setting up home together is self-evidently likely to affect timetables for work, leisure and household tasks. Further, the amount of time available for food preparation may well have a significant effect on what is served. More time (unless it is associated with unemployment and reduced income) may result in more elaborate meals and more experimentation. Food choices are affected not only by the amount of time available for food preparation and eating but also by *when* this time is available. The extent to which a couples' timetables are synchronised is also liable to affect how often they eat together or separately.

Most of the 'Marriage Menu' couples described breakfast as a light, quick meal which, when eaten at home, was not necessarily eaten with their partner. Lunch was rarely shared and rarely affected by marriage. The evening meal, however, was usually shared and couples would strive to coordinate their activities in order to eat together in the evening. They emphasised its importance as time together, in a relaxed atmosphere, enjoying the same food. A quick snack was generally regarded as inappropriate. The evening meal was usually one which required a degree of care and attention, a number of ingredients and time in preparation and consumption to a degree that was often absent from meals taken alone both before and after marriage. It was often described as a 'proper meal' and, although its structure and content was much more varied and less rigidly defined than those described by Murcott's (1982) and Charles and Kerr's (1988) respondents, there was a clear understanding of the meaning of the 'proper meal' and how it could be distinguished from a snack or light meal (Marshall 1988, 1993). We might expect this variation not only as a result of the increased familiarity with more varied and non-British cuisines but also as related to different stages in the life course. The shift to virtually daily consumption of a 'proper meal' in the evening affected the women more than the men, since the women had been more likely to eat snacks rather than a meal when alone and were also more likely than the men to prepare such a meal for them both.

Turning our attention from the structure and meaning of meals to food selection we begin at the level of purchase. A number of marketing studies have investigated marital roles in the shopping decision process (Davis and Rigaux 1974) but few have focused on family food shopping *per se* (Polegato and Zaichkowsky 1994). While wives remain responsible for the majority of food-shopping tasks there is some evidence of sharing as men appear more willing to take on food shopping (Maret and Finlay 1984; Blaylock and Smallwood 1987). The idea of sharing food shopping seems to be relatively new, and is in line with recent US studies of 'baby boom' couples showing that some of the more 'traditional' patterns of wives doing the household shopping may be breaking down (Lavin 1993). Recent research suggests a high degree of similarity between husbands and wives in their approach to time and task management, store loyalty and in-store shopping (Polegato and Zaichkowsky 1994). One suggestion for this is that wives might teach or guide their partners' shopping behaviour (Blaylock and Smallwood 1987; Charles and Kerr 1988). What is absent from these studies is any investigation of the changes which occur in the transition from single to married status.

While income level is obviously a major factor in food choice, it is the way income is managed and distributed which strongly influences the foodstuffs on which it is spent. This is complex. Concluding her analysis of the different financial arrangements within families, associated with couples'· different levels and sources of income and varying normative expectations about the allocation of expenditure, Pahl (1983) argues that responsibility for spending on specific items of household expenditure does not necessarily correspond to the freedom to spend according to one's own interests and desires. The real power is assumed at the level of 'orchestration'. This is the level at which decisions are made about the allocation of household income for 'house purchase', 'holidays' and 'housekeeping'. Power is then delegated to the level of 'implementation', i.e. the actual purchases. As a result,

> (T)he way in which orchestration power is exercised can leave the spouse with implementation power in the position of being forced to sacrifice her own interests in favour of other more powerful members of the household. (Pahl 1983: 254)

Charles and Kerr (1986b) show that the preferences of men are most favoured where women are given housekeeping money but men retain money for personal expenditure. In her later work on the spending and control of money within marriage Pahl shows that in the case of 74 per cent of her sample of 102 couples, the wife was responsible for spending on food, and that this proportion was even higher than for spending on clothes for the children (Pahl 1990: 126).

All of the 'Marriage Menu' couples were dual-income couples and all operated some version of what Pahl (1983) would describe as 'shared management system' of organising household finances. 'Orchestration power' was therefore not gender-specific. Main shopping trips were generally planned and carried out as activities in which both partners took part. *Ad hoc* shopping patterns or more regular, but unplanned, shopping trips as singles (Marshall, Kemmer and Anderson 1996) shifted to regular trips to the supermarket as a couple, whatever the frequency. The women were, though, more likely than men to take responsibility for the shopping in that they tended to take the lead in the main shopping trip and were more likely to undertake local, 'top-up' shopping and smaller trips to the supermarket. The joint trip was often discussed as a novelty and an enjoyable, shared experience. But some suggested this might be short-lived.

Gender-role influences on diet in marriage

Data from studies on the division of labour between couples with children show that the responsibility for food preparation lies mainly with the woman (Mennel, Murcott and van Otterloo 1992) and three studies which focus on food and food preparation within the family examine the meaning and effect of women's role as food preparer (Charles and Kerr 1988; Murcott 1982, 1983b). One explanation for women's greater involvement in food preparation is their greater likelihood of being at home because of other domestic commitments (Calnan and Cant 1990). However, McRae's (1987) study of cross-class families shows that women are almost always responsible for food, even when they work longer hours away from home than their husbands. Similarly, a study of childless newly weds showed that women took on the responsibility for cooking, and were expected to do so by their husbands (Mansfield and Collard 1988). Although it seems that there was no prima facie reason to differentiate between the value of husbands' and wives' employment, most of these newly weds intended to have children soon after marriage which, along with their parents' example, meant that the women's employment was seen as temporary (Mansfield and Collard 1988). The assumption that cooking is women's responsibility has recently been challenged by evidence from the north-east of England reporting that in 59 per cent of dual-career households men and women shared the cooking (Gregson and Lowe 1993). Clearly, as Ray Pahl (1984) has demonstrated, life-course stage is a significant factor in the domestic division of labour. Since those studies which focus on food are mainly based on economically dependent women at the child-bearing or child-rearing stage, our study usefully provides data on the division of food-related tasks at a stage before this.

Out of the 22 couples, 13 of the women were largely (or wholly) responsible for preparing the evening meal, two of the men could be thus described and in seven cases the task was shared, either by taking it in turns or some other form of equitable allocation. However, it is clear that the relationship between food preparation and power over the choice of food is not straightforward. McKie, Wood and Gregory (1993) suggest that, where involvement of men in food-related tasks is great, so is his level of control. Calnan and Cant (1990) also noted that where the husband was involved (common among the middle classes) he had more say in food issues, whereas where the husband was passive, the wife had more autonomy. However, Murcott (1982, 1983a) and Charles and Kerr (1988) have shown that this seeming autonomy can obscure wives' deference to their husbands' food preferences, which can constitute a weakening of wives' power in favour of husbands' power over the choice of what is eaten.

The 'Marriage Menu' couples who shared the task of food preparation usually discussed what they would eat and arrived at roughly joint decisions. Where the women were wholly or largely responsible for food preparation they showed less deference to their partners' preferences than the women in Murcott's or Charles and Kerr's studies. While his preferences might be taken into account, the woman would tend to encourage her partner to eat what she liked, would ensure that she enjoyed what she prepared and would avoid preparing food which he liked but she did not. This represents a subtle difference from the findings of the previous two studies discussed. This might be accounted for by the different stages in the life course of the couples in these studies (women in Murcott's and in Charles and Kerr's studies were, or were about to be, mothers of young children), by the related economic arrangements of the household in terms of income and expenditure and/or by ideological shifts which have occurred in the 15 or so years between these earlier studies and the 'Marriage Menu' (Collins 1985).

Diet and health considerations

A number of studies have reported on the apparent health of married adults (especially men) compared to single, divorced or separated individuals (Gove *et al.* 1983; Trovato and Lauris 1989). These differences may well be associated with differences in diet and eating habits. However, in the west of Scotland Twenty-07 study, Anderson and Hunt (1992) reported that only 40 per cent of the study's married adults consumed a diet conforming to the advice of local health-education campaigns compared to 51 per cent of adults who had never been married. Current nutritional recommendations promote the consumption of a diet high in fibre-rich carbohydrate and low in fats to prevent the development of coronary heart disease, cancer, diabetes and other diet-related chronic diseases (World Health Organisation 1990; Department of Health 1992). Putting these recommendations into practice means that the quantities of food people eat needs to change, implying in turn, as the Scottish Diet Report notes, changes in meal structures, snack and meal composition (Scottish Office 1994).

Health concerns are most likely to affect food choices among those who have actually experienced health problems: for example, individuals who have experienced a myocardial infarction are known to adhere to dietary regimes to avoid further health problems (Fehily *et al.* 1989). Those marrying for the first time tend to be of an age when they are unlikely to have suffered heart disease themselves, for example, though they might be influenced by the experiences of older family members. They might also have been affected by recent campaigns which aim to promote healthy eating. We might expect a more nutritious diet among those who take an interest in food and health, than among others who are less aware, but this also depends on the accuracy of their information.

A central issue in food choice in marriage is the extent to which, where there is one, the 'healthier eater' influences the diet of their spouse. Recent research suggests that women tend to be more concerned to ensure a healthy diet for themselves (and their partners) than are their partners, and that male partners may block attempts by their wives to achieve a healthier diet (Worsley 1988; Calnan and Cant 1990). Worsley's Australian research showed that, although the men tended to adopt the women's patterns of consumption at first, later in the marriage men and women move towards patterns established by their men when they were single.

The 'Marriage Menu' couples generally thought that, as a result of eating more regularly and having a more 'balanced' diet, their eating habits had improved since they began to live together. However, the men were far more apt to claim that their diets had improved than the women (who had been quite satisfied with the healthiness of their diets when they were single), citing an increase in vegetable consumption as a signal improvement. This finding was supported by the nutrient intake data which showed small (but significant) increases in the intake of vitamin C and iron in men. The reasons for this lie in a number of related influences on the men's eating habits in early marriage: that the event itself (eating together) deserved a 'proper meal', that women were more likely to prepare the evening meal, and that women were more likely to include fresh vegetables in the evening meal, encouraging men to do the same when they prepared it.

Summary and conclusion

The fundamental concerns of the research were to examine and measure the changes in food consumption which occur when couples marry in order to further our understanding of how such changes are negotiated and experienced, and to document their effect on eating habits, diet and nutrient intake. It was found that food and eating were indeed important in the lives of courting and newly married couples, many of whom were surprised at how much time, energy, thought (and money) they devoted to food after setting up home together. A number were also surprised to discover that food selection and consumption, and food-related activities, often had emotional implications for the relationship with their partner.

Some dietary changes accompanied the transition from single to married for all the men and women in the study. These changes were many and varied but were concentrated in meals and on food and drink consumed in the evenings. Other 'food events' such as weekday breakfast and lunch were rarely affected while weekend eating demonstrated a continuation of the patterns which were established during courtship, when many couples frequently spent weekends together. After marriage, shopping and the consumption of evening meals were planned, whereas many while still single had shopped, cooked and eaten in a more *ad hoc* manner. This change occurred in response to a desire to carry out these activities as a couple which necessitated some organisation to take account of the work and leisure timetables of both partners.

The main change observed in the food shopping over the transitional period was the extent to which the relatively unplanned shopping trip of the unmarried appears to have been replaced by a more regular pattern. What is less certain, at this stage in the analysis, is the extent of partners' influence and whether or how it is manifest in the choice of brand, in food expenditure or in concerns about health. Couples were much more likely to shop together for food on a regular basis, but despite the increased participation of men, women were more likely to carry the bulk of responsibility for food shopping. However, the fact that men are beginning to accompany their partners may offer some new opportunities for retailers to appeal to the male shopper both at the store level and prior to the shopping trip. The extent to which this will continue to feature for the study couples beyond the 'honeymoon' period is unknown; evidence from other studies would suggest it may not.

There was a strong emphasis on the appropriateness of eating a 'proper meal' together in the evenings as often as possible. This change affected more women than men, since the women had been more likely to forego a meal in the evening when single. The 'proper meals' described by informants varied in terms of content and structure, but were nevertheless highly significant in the couples' daily lives. Not only was this a shared event in that partners sat down to eat together, but the importance of sharing of food – eating the same foods at the same time – was implicit in their discussions about evening meals. The attempt to discover mutual preferences was therefore an important process, one which began during courtship.

More than half of the couples claimed they conformed to a division of domestic labour whereby the woman was mainly responsible for food preparation. In two cases the men were reported to take responsibility for food-related tasks and the remaining seven to share them. Decisions about the menu were largely made by the food preparer (although taking account of partner's preferences) who frequently took advantage of this position to ensure that their preferences prevailed.

Overall, then, the women were more likely to influence the food choices of the men than vice versa, although this was not exclusively the case. Women were also more likely to register concern about the link between food and health and indeed most of the men (and some of the women) said that their diets and eating habits had improved since they married. This supports the suggestion that early marriage might be an appropriate stage at which to target healthy eating campaigns, when changes are expected and are therefore more readily accepted than at other times, when they are more likely to be felt to be an imposition (Worsley 1988; McKie, Wood and Gregory 1993).

The effects of the presence and of the preferences of a spouse (or partner) are clearly major factors in food choice. At this very early stage in the development of a living-together relationship these factors are brought sharply into focus. Previously held values and behaviours are examined in the context of this relationship and new circumstances, while appropriate values and behaviours are negotiated and gradually established. Throughout this process, food purchase, preparation and consumption are high on the couple's agenda.

The transition from single to married status involves both a new situation and a new set of relationships which have a bearing on food choice. We have presented just a few of our findings showing that getting married is associated with a notable change in eating patterns and an improvement in diet. If these are confirmed in future studies, then it may be effective to target the early period of marriage as part of a 'healthy eating' campaign for both men and women. As we have indicated, a wide range of interrelated elements is involved in food choice at this stage in the life course. We have attempted to identify some of these elements but find that they can be difficult to disentangle from each other and from other factors unrelated to marriage. So the 'Marriage Menu' has been a useful exercise in the social science of food choice in highlighting the complexity of factors which can be significant in food choice at a given stage in the life course. This suggests a note of caution for any enthusiast striving for clarity via simplicity in food-choice research. Food choice is complex, not simple, and any clarity achieved by dint of failing to address this complexity is naïve and of little theoretical or heuristic benefit.

CHAPTER 13

Ethnographies of eating in an urban primary school

Robert G. Burgess and Marlene Morrison

DON'T LET THEM CHEW FAT, ROBIN SQUIRES TELLS SCHOOL
MEALS CHIEFS
Schools can promote healthy balanced choices not only by providing
healthy options for school meals but also through the curriculum and
a whole school approach to healthy education and healthy living.
                    (DfE News Circular 271/94, 3 November 1994)

Introduction

Food, food use and eating have become the focus of growing national
and international interest. Our study aims to advance understandings
about the complex issues that underlie food choices as they are
understood and mediated through the practice of schooling (Burgess
and Morrison 1995) and to develop a distinctive ethnographic approach
to studies of food and eating that draws on expertise more usually
applied to other areas of sociological enquiry. It is at the meeting-point
of sociological and educational interests in food choice that our project
is framed. Issues associated with food choice are central to our research interests in the processes of teaching and learning about food
and eating.

Alongside increased nutritional and social concerns about the quality
of British school children's diets there has developed a commensurate
belief in the ability of education to affect changes in both attitudes
and behaviour towards more 'healthy' eating linked to individuals'
lifestyles. Such a belief, it has been argued, has often been both ill-
founded (Rodmell and Watts 1986) and ill-formulated (Coombes
1989). To date, links between the concept of food choice and the role
of schooling have been heavily reliant on a political ideology of
individualism to underpin strategies that encourage 'individual res-

ponsibility, awareness and informed decision-making' (NCC 1990a: 7). 'Self-empowerment' is the mechanism advocated for enabling pupils to make 'healthy' food choices. The relative absence of perspectives that place individuals within the political, social and economic systems of which they are part could be seen as a form of ideological control over education in which teaching and learning about the individualisation of food choice is given not only as an accurate account of the *status quo* but also a desirable goal for which to aim. Yet what we eat, when we eat and with whom are questions of social and sociological significance where differential access to food choice is linked to relations of power and control, and to notions of inclusion and exclusion. This masking of the structural foundations underpinning inequalities in food choice has, to date, been partially sidestepped within a developing genre of health education that aims to have a 'healthy' influence on young people's choices while they are at school. Results from Scottish research (Young 1994) indicate that while such approaches can and do have a positive effect on school-based eating, they do not as yet appear to alter overall food choices and consumption beyond school. Other commentators have pointed to the negative implications of 'educational' advice that is unaffordable by socioeconomically disadvantaged groups, and its implications for the reinforcement of social exclusion and the denigration of self-esteem (Leather 1994).

Food and eating are interlinked yet distinct features of daily educational experience. Prior to this project, however, sociologists of education had seldom focused on the social and educational contexts in which children and young people learned about food as classroom activity and/or as routinised activity in schools. Indeed, at the start of the project, attention had only recently been drawn to patterns of teaching and learning about food in institutional settings including schools (Purvis 1985; Attar 1990; Young 1994). Food and eating have a special significance both in terms of collective eating rituals and as the focus, context and content of the curriculum. Here, the notion of choice, linked to processes of teaching and learning about food suggests certain courses of action rather than others have multiple investigative implications. Among these are the various interpretations of food as 'official' and 'unoffical' knowledge, and as eating practice.

The methodological contribution

Central to the research task was the importance of making connections not only with the biographies of teachers and learners but also the organisational contexts in which teaching and learning about food and eating took place. The intention was to focus on the visible and invisible influences on teaching and learning within and beyond schools, and to consider how far pupils (and teachers) were passive recipients of such influences. Linked to recent education and health priorities, attention was also focused on schools as micro-political arenas in which wider influences on food choice were reassessed and adjustments made to practice.

A key aspect of the research was the use of a sociological perspective to examine the interrelations between a range of understandings about food-focused education, which included various interpretations of food choice explored through interviews, observations and diary use with teachers, pupils, dinner ladies and parents. The fieldwork for the project was carried out by Morrison who used a combination of ethnographic approaches in order to generate data; an approach which follows procedures that have been discussed by Burgess (1984) and Hammersley and Atkinson (1983). Ethnographic explorations of food use involve 'trading off' depth for breadth and the project illustrates the value of detailed description and explanation in making clear the complex influences on food choice. In recognising that classical views of external validity are of little assistance to ethnographers interested in enhancing opportunities for their work to speak beyond the school situations where investigations took place, we share Ward Schofield's (1993) view of the need to develop a conception of generalisablity that is useful and appropriate for qualitative work (cf. Burgess *et al.* 1994). Accordingly, our study was based on four multisite case studies. Here, detailed attention to what Guba and Lincoln (1982) describe as the 'fittingness' of the case studies was accompanied by a concern to investigate heterogeneous rather than homogeneous sites. The robustness of an approach which allowed for variations along the dimensions of interest identified was balanced by the need for the fieldworker to immerse herself in the micro-systems of the schools, in itself a hallmark of the qualitative approach to sociological research.

In this chapter we focus on an urban primary school and different forms of eating, while 'making strange' some of the familiar practices of daily eating. The range of topics that could be explored in this setting were well summarised by a school lunchtime superintendent when she stated:

I like to see the children eat their dinners. I like to see them behave, and when the infants first come into the reception, I mean, we have to show them how to use knives and forks, and I like to see them appreciate their dinner, you know, when they really get tucked into it and eat up, and I think that's the joy to me to see them really enjoy their meal, and what I don't like is their bad behaviour at dinner times. We have had two boys this week. They tipped a jug full of water over a table up the far end and just walked away. Left it and went and sat at another table and I just got them, made them clean it up. Took them to the teacher and said what a mess they had made. So the next day I stayed behind with them and they wiped all the tables and swept the dining-room. That actually gave me pleasure because I thought well, at least they have done something for the mess that they've made. I mean, they wouldn't do it at home so I don't see why they should do it in the dining-room at school. I like to think that they would treat the school dining-room like they do at home.

This snatch of conversation demonstrates how eating at school is seen as a social event, how age and gender are involved, illustrated by the discussion of the way children in reception classes are inducted into patterns of eating in the school, and how attempts are made to control and develop social behaviour within this setting. To this can be added other topics for investigation: for example, the way in which control is exercised in the dining-hall; the pattern of formal and informal experiences associated with eating within school; the social divisions associated with eating and the way in which food and eating become part of the annual cycle of work within the institution. It is in these respects that our chapter focuses on different ways in which eating and food use were observed in an urban primary school.

The school setting

Within the school setting, adults and children experience food and eating in a variety of formal and informal ways. Indeed, food use can be explored in relation to the formal curriculum and also in relation to the day-to-day activities of the institution. It was our intention to focus on the experiences of food use and eating by examining them in the context of our first primary school case study: a coeducational urban primary school.

Brook Street Primary School was located in a former boys' secondary school. It consisted of a series of multistoried buildings in which the classrooms were located. The school was surrounded by terraced housing, corner shops, council flats and various factories. The catchment area was, according to the headteacher, more than 50 per cent Asian, and in recent years he considered that 'problem' families had been decanted from other parts of the city to the area surrounding Brook Street School. Indeed, the head argued that among his pupils' parents were those with drink, drugs, social and economic problems; as a result many established Asian families had moved out of the area. Those who remained were not considered to be in an economic position to move. In turn, the head maintained that some 'White families' had moved in from other parts of the country with higher unemployment and in turn brought a series of social problems with which members of the school had to deal. Several of the school's sub-sites were selected to examine food use: first, formal and informal food use; second, the use of breaks and lunch hours; third, the school dining-hall; and fourth, festivals and food use as classroom topics.

The food curriculum – teachers' views

Our evidence suggests that adults and children learn most about food through daily experience, and much of what is learned is cultural and practical. Part of children's experience is mediated through schooling. For educators, the link between teaching and learning in classrooms is critical. Our interest in food extended beyond the classroom, curriculum and pedagogy as we focused on its formal and informal aspects. The juxtaposition of the formal and informal, and its intended and unintended dimensions emerged as a critical theme at Brook Street.

Recent legislation and subsequent analyses (Weston, Barrett and Jamieson 1992; Morrison 1996a) provided frameworks for reviewing the formal curriculum for food. From this perspective the National Curriculum could be seen as 'a set of Chinese boxes' (Weston, Barrett and Jamieson 1992: 13) in which a curriculum to include food might be diffused or concentrated within core and foundation subjects, and as 'extra' activities. This located food and nutrition within a science core, and food, as resource or industry, among foundation subjects that included technology, geography and history. Early guidelines (NCC 1990a) promoted cross-curricular themes, dimensions and skills as critical bonding to fuse the National Curriculum into a 'whole'. Health education (NCC 1990b) is, for example, one of those themes, and has a prominent food and nutrition component. The extent to which such coherence or bonding was possible during a quick-fire succession of curriculum demands has been challenged (Weston, Barrett and Jamieson 1992; Stitt 1995; Morrison 1996a). Others have warned against assumptions about common responses among and within schools (Ball, Bowe and Gold 1992), seeing practice as 'mutations' (following Corwin 1983) which include gaps between intentions and outcomes in a range of classrooms in the same school.

At Brook Street, as elsewhere, the formal curriculum was circumscribed by National Curriculum documents. This had several major implications. A curriculum for food was viewed increasingly by teachers as theoretical (rather than practical), subject-focused and fragmented. Curriculum links were mainly with science, but also history and geography. Discussing what 'you can actually cover in the time', deputy head Mike Newley considered that:

> It's a question of whether we look at the curriculum as an academic curriculum or do we look at it as learning experience . . . it's much more going back to basics and though I appreciate that food is very important I wonder if that side of education will become more firm when they've finished school. I'm not saying it's desirable . . . We're going to be faced with let's say slightly more abstract scientific treatment of food . . . rather than the social aspects.

Where references to food were not explicit they tended to be ignored, as indicated during an interview with reception teacher Sylvia Kern who was asked whether food and nutrition was included in the curriculum. She replied:

> No, it didn't cross my mind to do it and it isn't part of, you know, we work very closely with the National Curriculum now, so it isn't sort of major in that until later on. I think it figures more when the children get older.

Within these curriculum boundaries, food-related classroom activities also depended on the specific inclinations and expertise of individual teachers. Not surprisingly, this led to diversity, but beyond the classroom, experiences were more uniform. In three-year 5/6 groups, food topics linked to healthy body/science themes tended to be the province of one teacher; in three-year 3/4 groups, one teacher linked food to art; and a religious education coordinator offered 'hands-on' food activities mainly to infants as an introduction to different religious events and customs. Resources, for example for cooking, were also unequally distributed and used. A small transportable cooker available for infants and an older model for juniors were apparently neglected even before the recent theft of the school's microwave oven.

Fragmentation of interest was accompanied by an ambivalence among teachers about whether or not food education should be the responsibility of teachers or parents; what constituted healthy eating and its promotion; and a reluctance by several staff to 'get involved' in 'sensitive' issues of culturally diverse eating patterns and contrasting levels of parental income. This was partially reinforced by a lack of knowledge about non-Western diets, and a view that time spent on food-related education was more affordable or appropriate in all-White, middle-class schools. While Sylvia Kern pondered whether 'it's [educating children about food use] not up to teachers, we ought to be looking towards parental responsibility', comments by another member of the teaching staff were also instructive:

> What I can do in this school is totally different to what I've been able to do in other schools and unfortunately you have to ride your horse according to your course. I mean there's a richness in terms of cultural diversity here but unfortunately the bottom line in this world today, if our children can't read and write they're not much good to themselves, their families, or society . . . at the moment we are struggling between a curriculum designed for basically middle-class, let's say White middle-class, and we're trying to apply it to children it isn't really suitable for.

This teacher considered his views corresponded with 'commonsense' parental expectations of a 'basics' approach to primary education. Subsequent parental interviews tended to favour the inclusion of food-focused education in the curriculum but there were exceptions:

> I don't think they should learn about it [food]. I don't think there's

much to learn unless you are going into cooking. It's like explaining to somebody 'oh, you know it's a bar of chocolate', I don't think they want to know how it's made.

If concentration on the 'basics' was prioritised over an emphasis on cross-curricula diversity, insufficient knowledge was, on occasion, the reason given for neglecting food. As the Deputy Head commented:

I do not know enough about what foods they [Asian children] would eat at home and I find it very difficult for them to tell me what it is . . . I get the impression that they have a sort of Eastern–Western diet and generally they pick up the worst from both diets.

Negative perceptions about urban living and the effects of low income on wider experiences were also considered responsible for the educational gaps between children's knowledge and understanding. One class teacher said:

I think there's a large number of children in this school, quite a high chronological age, who will not be able to tell you where milk comes from and yet that will have been dealt with in farming . . . So there's a difference between teaching and learning . . . I know that when we made a visit to a farm . . . last year it was the first time that some of these children had actually been out of [the city].

None of these remarks detracts from the efforts of individual teachers. Year 1/2 teacher Mary Holt, for example, made connections between early science activities and children's experiences of food outside school by using a variety of foods, Western and non-Western, to engage children in stepped learning activities. Here, a 'hands-on' approach to food explored early conceptual themes like touch and taste, growth and development, each linked to the encouragement of linguistic skills in a class where, according to the class teacher, an estimated quarter of parents experienced some difficulties with the English language.

At Brook Street, there was no written school policy on food and eating, although there were mixed views among staff and parents as to whether this was desirable. In addition to the absence of a written policy, there were interesting contrasts in practice at the classroom/school interface. Snacking was widespread before school, during breaks, and after school. In some classrooms, snacking was part of some children's 'social' activity in contact time and not in others; certain foods were restricted by some teachers but not by others. A tuck shop served the year 5/6 groups; in selected classes tuck was sold, and among younger children there was a 50p weekly charge for squash and biscuits. In assembly, more widespread concern about litter disposal than healthy eating was noted, although the school had held 'healthy eating' weeks or 'happy heart' days, usually at the instigation of individual teachers. Previous attempts to introduce 'healthy' food, according to the head, had floundered when sales dropped, and children brought food from outside. Tuck-shop funds were important in providing supplementary financial support for outings and substitute breakfasts for some children. Meanwhile, an unintended consequence of the widespread availability of food in classrooms was its potential to encourage furtive eating, noted regularly in a year 1/2 class.

Since the industrial action of the mid-1980s and subsequent legislation, lunchtime activity had been excluded from 'official' interpretations of educational experience by teachers at Brook Street. This was reinforced by the physical separation of the dining-hall from the main school buildings and a disinclination by teaching staff to eat there. While recognising the nutritional benefits of the school lunch, staff were unanimous in viewing lunchtimes as negative experiences for children that were felt to contribute to an escalation of discipline problems and lack of concentration in the afternoon. Some of that concern is captured in the following comments from Sylvia Kern: 'Lunch has caused a lot of misery . . . dreadful, dreadful'. Referring specifically to the needs of young children, she felt that school dinners did not:

> look like what they've had at home. The chairs and tables are too big. The knives and forks are too big. The children can't reach . . . I think the ideal would be to have them sitting down at tables with an adult or older children at each table . . . I don't feel it's pleasant there at all. I feel like it's get in, eat your lunch, and get out as quickly as possible.

A management viewpoint was summed up by the Deputy Head:

> It's [lunchtime arrangements] largely an inconvenience in a large school . . . it's a drain on resources, it is much better without lunchtime . . . Children do not come in after lunchtime particularly prepared to start the afternoon well and that may be our fault as a school . . . that lunchtimes now seem to be almost getting in the way. At the moment we've got the worst of all worlds, we've got an *ad hoc* system where many dinner ladies are very good, but basically they're not trained.

In such ways, food, eating and educational experience were interwoven at Brook Street. In the myriad of understandings and experiences, observation and interviews indicated connection and disconnection in the formal and informal processes of teaching and learning about food and eating.

Food, fasting and festivals

As already noted, food and eating was part of the curriculum provided under the heading of health education (NCC 1990b). This includes the ways in which schools can utilise the topic of food and eating in order

216

to generate a sympathetic understanding of different cultures and races (DES 1977: 41) and a 'view' that Britain is both multiracial and culturally diverse (DES 1981: 6). Indeed, many schools within multiethnic areas of Britain have engaged in food-related events that make links between cultural and religious festivals, and as such these links have been used to develop collaboration between schools and their communities. Such approaches have their critics (Troyna 1983; Troyna and Williams 1986; Troyna 1989). Indeed, Troyna has remarked:

> Multiculturalists have tended to concentrate on the expressive and historical features said to represent particular cultural groups . . . this has often resulted in . . . what I have termed the three s's approach: saris, samosas and steel bands. (Troyna 1989: 161)

In particular, he challenged the notion that multicultural approaches can be used in favour of an antiracist education whereby teaching and learning about food and nutrition would need to be incorporated into, and integrated with, the formal and informal aspects of the curriculum. It is to some of these issues that we now turn in the context of Brook Street School.

Discussions of food and food use can be incorporated into the curriculum throughout the school year. Indeed, in Brook Street this was well illustrated by the Deputy Head who commented:

> There are times in the year, and obviously the major time in this school would be around the Ramadan period, when many of our children seem to be suffering because they are fasting and we see in many ways, for example, children go swimming find it very difficult, perhaps don't go swimming, can't take part in physical exercise, very tired, although all our children always seem to be very tired – they go to bed too late and perhaps their food quality is not particularly good, watch too much television. Particularly this period of Ramadan in the spring, and I mean I can think of a case this present spring where one girl had been fasting, got up in the middle of the night, had eaten a lot of fruit which is the normal custom, and then promptly proceeded to bring it up all over the stairway coming up into school.

In this example, the school curriculum was influenced by the annual religious cycle (cf. Burgess 1983) but in this instance food use was associated with it.

While this teacher focused on one particular festival, others were able to provide illustrations of the way in which food, festivals and schooling became linked together. As one teacher explained:

> It depends on what you are talking about at the time. If you
> are talking about festivals, then the children remember what they eat.
> They remember the sticky stuff, they remember food things and they
> remember savoury and the fried stuff because that is special and is

made on certain occasions. Like at Christmas you'd have mince pies and Christmas cake, but you wouldn't normally have it, although some children may not eat it at home, but they remember that. It is like children, they remember food things and sticky things from Diwali, but like a Samosa it might be too hot for them, they might not eat them, but they remember that as part of their celebration. But when we do a topic on food, we think about healthy eating, what foods are good for you, what foods are bad, that's a topic. We have done that and we have talked about food that is good for you that you must eat plenty of, food that is bad for you, and then you have gone into why they are bad for you and too much sugar will harm your teeth, and if you eat too many sweet things you put on weight and how you eat healthily and do exercise.

Here, food, food use, festivals and the formal curriculum were brought together as the teacher explained how they were incorporated into discussions during lessons. However, discussions about food did not only coincide with festivals, but also with the lifecycle, as this teacher continued:

Sweetness is because it's a richness, because it is any sort of occasion in India. If it is a happy occasion, you have sweets, the sugary stuff you will have because it is something that is nice, something that you celebrate, whereas if it is a sad occasion you don't have them, like at a funeral you wouldn't see them. Sweets are given out on the dates of birth and they are given out as presents, and if there are weddings sweets are given out . . . they are given out to people after the wedding as presents and it is a significance of happiness, whereas if it is a funeral you wouldn't see them you would have a savoury, but you wouldn't see any sweets unless there is someone who is very old, then you'd well, well he had a long life, so you can celebrate that he had a long happy life, and so you can celebrate that, but otherwise you couldn't celebrate so you wouldn't see any sweets. You would have very, very simple food, not very expensive food at all. You would have very simple food and you wouldn't have variety either. You would have a Dahl and maybe some veg, they wouldn't see any need for anything, and at the house where somebody had died they wouldn't even cook until they have had the funeral, and then after the funeral the ceremony after 16 days after the funeral they have the temple ceremony. They wouldn't cook meat until after that ceremony is over, they wouldn't have any richness of food, say meat or anything. That is associated with weddings or births, they wouldn't have anything like that until that time is over and they can start. They will go through that time if anybody does come in mourning. They will have simple foods as well. A lot of the time they don't cook at home either, other people cook and bring it to you. You don't cook at home because it is sad. If you cook for yourself then you know how you would like something, so you are not sort of eating for tasting it, you are eating because you need to eat, because you are sad you shouldn't be eating because you enjoy eating.

Links between way of life and food use were re-emphasised. Other teachers also drew our attention to the way food is used when celebrating festivals associated with the lifecycle. For example, one teacher talked about how food was used primarily as a social rather than an educational activity in relation to parties, when children brought cakes or sandwiches or biscuits and drinks into school. In turn, this same teacher indicated how parties and birthdays were also linked with regulatory concerns about food use. She used these situations to control children's informal food use in the classroom setting, as she remarked:

We do limit children bringing sweets to school to birthdays only. They are allowed to bring sweets to share with their friends on their birthdays. They are not allowed to bring sweets at any other time, so I mean that does interfere in that way because we are making a statement then by saying 'Don't bring sweets except for birthdays'. Sweets are not something that you encourage children to have every day, but I know that when I go out and stand out there are a lot of mums from here, as the first thing they do is hand over a packet of sweets.

Here we see the way in which birthdays were celebrations that were linked with particular foods, and in turn with foods that would not normally be approved by the teacher. However, birthdays also had gender-specific meanings within particular communities that Brook Street School served. One teacher described the way in which a parent had used a boy's birthday to celebrate and drew a distinction between boys and girls. He remarked:

Some parents have on occasions brought in food for the staff to share. The last time I can remember was a fairly well-to-do family, and to their way of thinking they were fortunate that now at last they had a boy in the family after so many girls, and when he was five the food that they brought in for the boy, although we joined in with them and they thought there was a strong feeling from the staff who didn't say so, it was very unfortunate for the girls who had gone before in the same family that they weren't treated in the same way. The food that was brought in, it was amazing. I think the family had a restaurant somewhere, but they supplied so much food the staff couldn't eat it all and they were quite prepared for us to take it away home at the end if we wanted to, but that was because the boy was five, and obviously it was more important than any of the girls. That sort of thing has gone on in schools, probably still will do occasionally in the future.

Food was used to separate different social occasions, and to celebrate particular events and particular circumstances. Food could also be used in a divisive way to create social distinctions in terms of marking out particular cultural attributes.

Food and social divisions

During the early part of the fieldwork in Brook Street School, a number of different events in the school dining-hall was observed. An early fieldnote describes the event:

> Queuing into the dining-hall. This can't be pleasant in the cold or rain. Children take plastic trays with a place for different items. One child offers me a knife and fork. The menu includes carrots, mash, fried chips, baked potatoes, cheese and onion pasty, beans, salad, cooked meat in a roll. Pudding – scone with jam, cream yoghurt and fruit. As on previous days, chips are popular and scones. A girl joins me with three kinds of potato chips, mash, jacket potatoes plus beans. The notion of a balanced diet goes awry when children select what they will eat across the menu range. Packed lunches vary in quantity and quality, but quantity is the most obvious dimension along with crisps in just about every box. Some children keep their lunch box lids firmly closed and are secretive about revealing the contents. I observed a child I had seen last week with bread and margarine sandwiches and a dry biscuit. This week she is minus the biscuit and once again only water to wash it down. The contradictions are extreme. Opposite her a boy with a plate full of pasty, beans, chips, milk drinks and jam scones is reeling off the list of games he professes to possess for his Nintendo. Discussion centres on ghosts, aliens and Sonic the Hedgehog. My friend with the margarine sandwiches looks on. Talking to me slows down their pace of eating as the children ask me about my family. They are urged to eat up by the patrolling dinner lady.

This extract from fieldnotes (see also Morrison 1996b) highlights several themes: first, children who have school meals as opposed to those who bring packed lunches; second, the divisions between those who have a range of food and those who do not; third, the control exercised by dinner ladies who worked in the dining-hall. Some of these themes were subsequently followed up during the fieldwork. Indeed, it was found that children in reception classes were encouraged to bring 10p per day for a sugar-free orange drink and biscuits. Not all children, though, were in a position to participate in such a scheme. Indeed, so much so that the educational assistants who worked alongside teachers were dividing biscuits in order to give those who had not brought money for food, some biscuits or parts of biscuits to eat.

In following up the observations in the dining-hall, it was found that the kind of food the children ate was used as a means of organising both seating and the flow of children through the dining-hall, thus acting as a mechanism for social division. For example, children were told when they could go to lunch, as one teacher was reported as saying:

> If you eat meat go to the toilet and wash your hands and then line up.
> If you don't eat meat go to the toilet, wash your hands and line up.

The same procedure was extended to those children who brought packed lunches to school, and in turn those who were going home for dinner. Children were thus identified in the classroom according to what they ate and the ways the classroom was organised in preparation for lunch according to what children were eating. This was repeated in the dining-hall:

> Reception children were lined up into those who eat meat and those who do not. They take their trays. When they get to the hatch their meat/non-meat preferences are rechecked. Packed lunches sit separately. The emphasis is on eating everything up and speedily to await the entrance of the older children. (Morrison: fieldnotes)

In this particular setting, distinctions were sharply drawn between what the children ate. In turn, the kind of food that children ate was used to reinforce social organisation and also social divisions within the school. Older boys were separated from girls, sometimes of their own volition and sometimes because they had misbehaved in the dinner queue or at the dinner table. They had to sit at one end of the dining-hall under the watchful eye of a dinner lady. 'Packed lunches' were kept separately from others, and in turn the importance of control was emphasised. On one particular occasion, a boy was observed trying to avoid eating part of his lunch:

> All the food around me is being eaten except for the fish on Jason's plate. 'It's horrible,' he whispers to me. He puts his hand up. Dinner lady approaches. He asks if he can leave the fish. Permission is refused – 'You shouldn't take it if you don't want to eat it.' Jason looks increasingly fretful. He cuts the fish. Ignoring me he throws the fish, tiny pieces at a time, on the floor. Just when he thinks success is his, a dinner lady comes alongside and steps on a piece of fish. He has to pick every piece up, put it in the bin and remain behind. The canteen gets noisier as the older children begin to queue. (Morrison: fieldnote)

Here, several elements come together: first, the extent to which children had choice over the food they ate; second, the notion of eating up; third, the element of control that dinner ladies exercised over children's eating habits; fourth, subversion and the way in which it was dealt with. In these respects what happens in the school dining-hall at lunchtime is not only a social event, but an occasion when a wide range

221

of social behaviour is played out in terms of school organisation, school ritual, social division and social control. In this sense, food use and eating involves much contradiction and conflict in the school system.

Food as a medium of control

Evidence from the case-study schools indicates that the significance of food appears in different forms according to the type of institution. What they have in common is the propensity for food whether available or scarce, uniform or varied, used as punishment or reward, to become part of a struggle for control. For example in Brook Street School, previous references to snacking have already suggested that, apart from its timing, adults allowed children considerable discretion. While one teacher used sweets as a reward for good behaviour, another used them as learning tools. In such cases teachers were given substantial (if partial) control over food choices and uses.

Nowhere was the issue of control more visible than in relation to lunchtime arrangements (Morrison 1996b). At Brook Street 230 children out of 326 on roll stayed for lunch. Of these, 58 brought packed lunches and the remainder ate meals provided by the city's School Meals Service. Seventy three per cent of children received free school meals. Adults, that is dinner ladies, supervised by a lunchtime superintendent, were in charge. Ultimate responsibility lay with the head, to whom the most serious misbehaviour was reported. In the most severe incidents, suspension was the punishment. Children were not allowed to save spaces for friends. The superintendent would also oversee the quantity and quality of packed lunches. Where either or both were thought to be lacking, the head was informed. While this did not happen often, it resulted in an interview with parents, occasionally combined with home visits for other purposes, and liaison with health or social services.

The non-involvement of teaching staff reinforced the segregation of lunchtime as 'non-educational' activity. Lunchtimes were staggered, allowing the youngest children to enter the dining-hall before the majority. The sociability of eating resembled a conveyor-belt system, with queuing, eating at speed, a minimum of talking, and emphasis on 'through-put', its salient features. While most dinner ladies ate at the same tables as children, stewardship was exercised with minimal discourse and included patrolling to maintain order. 'Eating up' was of paramount importance. Queuing served as a control as well as a labelling function, and daily lists of children in receipt of free school meals reinforced a perceived need among adults to encourage children to 'eat up'.

The process of individualised eating in an institutionalised setting had specific features at Brook Street. Because dinner ladies viewed eating and conversation as incompatible, the latter was discouraged, and persistent offenders were isolated at separate smaller tables, as is illustrated in the following:

> Observe Natalie isolated in the corner of the canteen. As usual slowly rolling her sandwiches around the mouth and playing with a beaker of water. I ask one of the dinner ladies about Natalie. She has been ushered into the area in advance of her class because she is such a slow eater. (Morrison: fieldnote)

'Deviant' children were those who resisted rules about queuing, eating up, talking or fighting. Control was maintained, with differing degrees of success, by dinner ladies who befriended, joked, cajoled, ordered, shouted, and in one case, ranted at children. An extreme case is recorded:

> The dining room is noisy. Screaming Mrs B [a dinner lady] adds to the noise level. She doesn't differentiate her screaming for different levels of reprimand. Consequently, at times her screaming is ignored by the children ... I find it more and more difficult to ignore her. (Morrison: fieldnotes)

On difficult days, the superintendent used her whistle. Children could be isolated from each other – but for very different reasons: because they were rowdy, or quiet, or slow eaters. Among the latter were several young children who seemed quite happy with these more confined arrangements. The rationale for keeping control was dominated by practical and institutional concerns to feed large numbers in a relatively short time span. Dinner ladies also invoked other kinds of rationale. These included the view that children who had 'free school meals' should 'eat up' not only because it was 'their only meal' but also because 'other people's taxes' paid for them. Those whose parents paid were also chivvied to 'eat up' to fulfil parental expectations and in the belief that to waste food and money was wrong.

The practice of isolating slow eaters had implications for children which sometimes extended beyond the meal. On one day, Thomas from the reception class was observed as follows:

> Thomas eats all his meals (eventually) ... but breaks the cardinal rules – he eats slowly and wants to talk. Sit next to Thomas. Reprimanded four times for talking ... Reception children told to sit outside on the grass once they have finished. I ask Mrs C [the dining-hall superintendent] why. Slow eaters, humid weather, high noise levels in the hall. So young children wait outside for others to finish. This doesn't work for Thomas because as older children enter he's still there and Mrs C's getting exasperated. He finally leaves the dining hall at 1 pm (plate still not empty). I shadow him across the playground. Thomas has a problem since detention in the dining-hall has meant that friendship and play groups have already been established and he finds it difficult to break in ... finally he finds two

> boys who are playing hide and seek – he joins them before the bell.
> (Morrison: fieldnotes)

Children tried to resist control, the older pupils with more success. Among the latter, attempts to keep 'packed lunches' separate from 'school dinners', for example, had been resisted, and segregation abandoned. They did talk, sometimes very noisily; some water play was also seen to take place in the dining-hall toilet area. Because of its potential to disrupt and cause damage, fighting and horse-play was most strongly combatted by the dinner ladies, and persistent offenders were sent to the head's office.

Control extended to what was eaten at a school meal. The School Meals Service made central decisions about the choice of menu which included attention given to cultural food preferences. In the dining-hall, such decisions were reinforced *and* thwarted by counter staff and dinner ladies, and by the children. Membership of the 'meat' and 'no meat' queue was rigidly enforced. Omnivores had to state a preference and remain consistent. Blanket 'no meat' assumptions about mainly Asian diets could pose problems for children, as the following field note indicates:

> Ravi (year 2) joins me at the table. Tells me dinner ladies are – points a finger to the head and twists finger. I look quizzical enough for him to continue 'They keep telling me I'm "no meat" but I do eat meat'. Anyway, today he has secured some chicken pie. Do you eat meat at home? I ask. We establish that meat at home comes from a special shop.

This conversation highlighted another issue; some 'no meat' children said that food at school – for example, curries or samosas – tasted 'different' from home-cooked food. This tended to restrict choice even further, usually to cheese, beans and chips.

Adults and children also thwarted central attempts to control the nutritional balance of meals. The overriding adult view was that eating something was preferable to not eating at all, and so children's food trays might contain a combination of supplementary dishes rather than any 'main' dish on the menu. This could mean an abundance of chips on nearly every plate, and in regular instances combinations of boiled, mashed and chipped potatoes. Being labelled 'meat' could also restrict choice. In theory, children could choose a vegetarian dish. In practice, adults controlled choice by discouraging specific categories if it was felt that the vegetarian allocation might be used up.

Lunchtimes also included supervised play. How this was interpreted by dinner ladies varied and was interwoven with issues of training, low pay and relatively low status. Several dinner ladies organised games with the older children, but the most usual practice was to walk round the playground, sometimes hand-in-hand with children, and deal with them one by one. The lunchtime superintendent commented that on rainy days, children:

go inside. Usually the teacher's got a box with spare paper in and crayons and they get that box out and then the children draw, make aeroplanes, and all sorts . . . They used to go in the hall but we just don't have that now so children go into the classroom. Some of the teachers don't take them in at all unless it's really bad weather because they can't stand them inside because there's control and control isn't really there . . . without saying too much about the dinner ladies, there's some got more control than others and one that hasn't keeps them outside as much as she can . . . some of them have got 30 odd children which is quite a lot to look after on your own.

Through an exploration of lunchtimes it was possible to learn about control strategies and resistance among children and adults in school. At Brook Street a conveyor-belt system was reflected in patterns of adult and child behaviour. This showed degrees of opposition to, and some accommodation with, the more widely recognised familial model of meals as social events.

Contradictions

An introduction to various aspects of food and eating at Brook Street School has indicated diversity, contradiction and ambiguities in understandings about and experiences of food choice and eating. These may be mirrored in the wider adult population, where questions about whether food knowledge is acquired primarily through information received, or is heavily influenced by income, culture and food availability, are critical to other research investigations in 'The Nation's Diet' Programme (see especially Caplan *et al.* Chapter 10; Warde and Martens Chapter 8; Williams *et al.* Chapter 16, all in this book). Schools are sites where the various preferences, interests and options available to adults and children (however limited) intersect. At Brook Street we have illustrated that adult interests in school were not always complementary, and might include the 'invisible' influence of adults who, beyond the school gates, provide evidence, in terms of snacks, pocket money and lunch, of practical and cultural control over food choice and consumption.

Among teachers, formal and informal understandings about food, eating and nutrition were fragmented and, in individual cases, peripheral to teachers' professional and pastoral concerns about children's learning. Classroom observation provided some specific examples of innovative and imaginative approaches to food-linked teaching. But in the absence of a whole school policy on food and eating, these were localised. Teachers' strategies were made more complex by disparate understandings and knowledge, and ignorance about Western and non-Western diets. Broaching food issues was seen by several staff as culturally and racially 'sensitive' and therefore best avoided. Understandings were further complicated by recognition of widespread socioeconomic deprivation as a central feature of the school catchment. Among several staff was the view that knowing what was 'good to eat' was an indicator of middle-classness and therefore hardly appropriate to Brook Street, and subject to a degree of controversy and debate, which should not be prioritised as long as other demands, like the National Curriculum, were predominant. In such ways teachers lived with contradiction within and beyond classrooms. Among observed outcomes was formal concentration on diet in science at Key Stage 2 and the acceptance (sometimes reluctantly) of widespread snacking, and of lunchtimes as negative aspects of children's daily school experience.

At lunchtimes, the activities of non-teaching staff responsible for regulating eating experiences were governed by the need to encourage children to 'eat up' at speed, and control the most boisterous aspects of children's behaviour. When school activities like eating replicated activities occurring in the domestic sphere, control was maintained by adults whose status and pay was generally lower than that of other school-based colleagues. Yet, as has been noted, their influence extended not only to the speed and form of consumption but also to what was eaten and its nutritional balance. One result was to transform the meal event into a process more closely resembling a factory than a home setting.

This study also began to explore the extent to which children were not necessarily passive recipients of such influences. Attempts to resist control were recorded, as were strategies to live with contradiction. For example, teacher Annie Drew felt that, in relation to a 'healthy body' project, her children (year 5/6) were not always 'telling the truth' when they completed food diaries. In this case, the children's written expression of their propensity to eat lettuce and fruit, and to drink milk, was contradicted by observations of widespread snacking or lunchtime patterns of consumption. Here, acceptance of contradiction was possible through a separation of 'real' experience from the expectations children had about 'acceptable' school knowledge. In similar ways, a visit and talk from a local dentist did not discourage children from purchasing penny sweets at the start of children's club, using money provided by parents, or deter the club from selling them. (Brook Street School had, according to the Head and confirmed by a health service official, one of the worst dental decay records for young children in the city.) In such ways, contradiction existed among Brook Street pupils in relation to their food choices.

Conclusion

In this chapter we examined a number of different settings within a coeducational multiethnic urban primary school where food use and eating takes place. In particular, we focused on different sub-sites to examine the different themes that occur in relation to food choice. In this sense, the fieldwork experience is being used rather in the way in which Geer (1964) used initial fieldwork to examine a set of themes that were used throughout our study in a number of other school sites where food use and eating were examined using an ethnographic approach.

Overall, the study highlights a range of features that are distinctive in relation to teaching and learning about food and nutrition in school. Among the important elements identified in the data were those which relate to *curriculum issues*, in particular the fragmentation and marginalisation of food-focused education; *whole school approaches* to food and nutrition; recent developments in *institutionalised eating*; and the *social construction of meanings about food and eating* by teachers and learners, adults and children, as they intersect with the policy and practice of schools. The process of disconnecting the nutritional and welfare issues of school eating from its educational significance made the prospect of coherence between the formal and informal curriculum both challenging and contentious. In this sense, food choices were becoming increasingly personal and parental matters, yet subject to discipline, containment and control, as well as financial resourcing, on educational premises. Juxtaposed with the latter was the institutionalisation of eating in Brook Street School as day-long as well as lunchtime activity. Such data challenge the myth of food consumption choices in school as 'free', 'independent' or 'non-political'.

What is distinctive about this study's approach is that it privileges adults' and children's understandings about food and nutrition in school over any assertions about what they *ought* to eat or learn about food. Ethnography produces findings that have major implications for policy and practice in schools. This study demonstrates the ways in which schools are important arenas for addressing understandings and contradictions about food choice and consumption. In educational institutions overtly committed to clarifying a range of positive options for enhancing the well-being of future adult citizens and consumers, much work on food use remains to be done.

CHAPTER 14

Food choice, food scares, and health: the role of the media.

Sally Macintyre, Jacquie Reilly, David Miller and John Eldridge

Introduction

The background to the study reported here was the observation that some concerns about the health-related properties and safety of foods receive widespread publicity in the mass media and appear to influence the public's buying and eating habits. Meanwhile, the health and safety risks of other food products, with perhaps greater consequences for human health in the long run, seem to receive comparatively little coverage and not to influence food buying and eating patterns in so marked a fashion. For instance, Figure 14.1 shows marked peaks in press reporting of salmonella enteritidis and bovine spongiform encephalopathy (BSE) in the UK. In December 1988, the junior health minister, Edwina Currie, said on ITN news that 'most of the egg production of this country, sadly, is now infected with salmonella' (ITN 1700, 3 December 1988). Egg sales fell by up to 50 per cent following this widely reported statement, and were still only around 75 per cent of earlier levels by early 1989 (Mintel 1990; Commons Agriculture Committee 1989). Beef sales fell by 20 per cent between May and August 1990, following massive publicity about the possible risk to human health (Spencer 1990). The risks of salmonella in eggs and chicken had been well known for some time, so why did such extensive media coverage arise at that particular time? And why did this apparently cause a dramatic downturn in the buying and eating of eggs among the general public, when 'health warnings' about the link between eating eggs, cholesterol and coronary heart disease (the dietary hypothesis) did not appear to have had similar effects (Davison 1989)?

Similar questions can be asked about the effect on beef sales of publicity about BSE. Although the consumption of red meat had been gradually declining in the UK, partly in response to health concerns, the decline in the consumption of meat products and saturated fats had not been as fast as health promoters might have wished. Why was publicity about the remote possibility of harm to human health from BSE

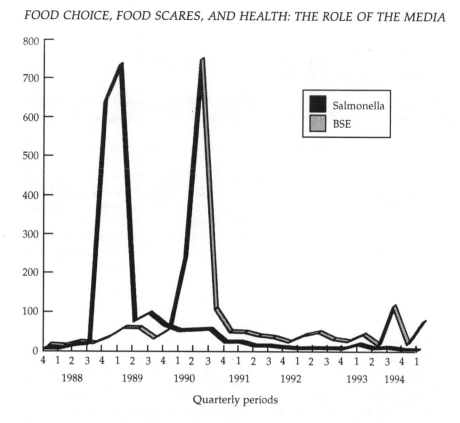

Figure 14.1 British newspaper coverage of BSE and salmonella 1988–94 (number of items per quarter)

apparently so much more effective than health-promotion attempts to reduce fat intake?

The aim of our research was to compare the production, content and public lay understanding of the mass media coverage of 'food scares' (focusing in particular on salmonella, listeria and BSE), with that of coronary heart disease (CHD). An important question for health promotion, and indeed for the food industry, is how the public understand the messages they receive about the healthiness and safety of foods, and whether their understanding of media messages about foodstuffs has any impact on the purchase, preparation and consumption of food.

In this chapter we focus on public understandings of, and reactions to, mass media messages in relationship to food scares and CHD. While there has been some previous work on lay understandings of CHD and dietary risks (Davison, Frankel and Davey-Smith 1989, 1992; Lambert and Rose 1996), there has been surprisingly little on lay understandings of food scares. As Mennell, Murcott and van Otterloo have commented:

Detailed sociological investigation of popular belief systems in the face of the British 'scares' is rare . . . Instead, attention has tended to focus on the role of the media in heightening public anxiety (Mennell, Murcott and van Otterloo 1992: 46)

Neither media coverage of, nor public concern about, public health risks mirrors the incidence of disease or the severity of the health problem. While widely recognised, the reasons for this apparent mismatch remain poorly explained. Some commentators have tended to explain this in terms of inadequacies in human perception (Covello 1983), sometimes allied with 'irresponsible' or 'sensational' reporting by the mass media (Anderson 1986). Previous work in the sociology of the science, the sociology of the media, and the sociology of health and illness suggests, however, that such explanations may oversimplify the complex social processes which combine to produce news media accounts and public perceptions of social problems. The 'deficit' model of public understanding starts from the premises that expert assessments are based on straightfor-wardly objective evidence, and that public responses are based on ignorance (Royal Society of London 1985). This has been shown to be an inaccurate model of both expert assessment and public understanding (Macintyre 1995; Irwin and Wynne 1996; Wynne 1996). Similarly, the idea that the mass media always exaggerate certain dangers has been shown to be inaccurate (indeed the media are often blamed for underestimating specific dangers compared to the assessments of experts) (Kitzinger and Reilly forthcoming). The notions of irresponsible or sensationalist reporting have also been shown to ignore the role of particular news values (types of topics in which journalists and editors believe their viewers or readers are particularly interested) in influencing the media reporting of specific topics (Miller and Reilly 1995). The idea that people do not follow health or safety guidelines in their food purchasing, preparation and eating practices because they are unaware of these guidelines has also been shown to be inaccurate, and incorrectly to assume that health, or official advice on enhancing health, is the prime motivator in people's dietary habits (Davison 1989; Davison, Frankel and Davey Smith 1992).

In this project we wished to test the hypothesis, derived from previous empirical research in the sociology of science, media sociology and medical sociology, that the public's understanding of salmonella, listeria, BSE and CHD is actively constructed in social interactions within specific social contexts. These contexts are both at a macro- (national or international) level (for example, the prevailing system of food production and distribution, the current state of scientific knowledge, the national political scene, the structure and culture of the news and entertainment media, and at a more micro- or local level (for example, workplace settings, friendship groups, families, the newspapers people read and the radio or television programmes they watch).

230

Food (and media) choice

Foods are 'chosen' by individuals, but there is a variety of constraints and influences which requires us to qualify any notion of choice that implies it is 'free'. First, a finite range of products is available in shops and restaurants; we can only buy what is on sale. Many commentators emphasise the very wide range of foods available in contemporary supermarkets (Miller 1995), but there are limitations to this range. If we wish not to consume (both in the sense of purchase and eat) the products of the agrochemical industries or the by-products of the oil industry; or want to avoid sugars, sweeteners or salt in processed foods, then our choices in a typical supermarket are limited. This is not to say that what is supplied in such shops is not responsive to consumer demand; the range available is clearly subject to change in the medium or long term, as illustrated by the rise in the provision of brown and wholemeal bread, 'lite' products etc. (Heasman 1990; Henson 1992; Dawson 1995). However, in the short term there is a finite range of products available; for example, in Britain we cannot buy yoghurt flavoured with savoury vegetables or yoghurt with added fruit but no sugar, and in the USA it is hard to buy full-fat yoghurt. There are also many theoretically edible products which are simply not regarded as being within our culinary repertoire at all (we can buy frogs' legs but not cats' legs) (Mennell, Murcott and van Otterloo 1992; Fiddes 1995).

Second, the 'range' is not equally wide for all consumers. Products are differentially available according to where we live (for example, the Western Isles of Scotland compared with Hampstead, or a peripheral public housing scheme compared with an inner-city area), and according to our sociodemographic characteristics, such as employment, family structure, income, ethnicity, religion, access to transport, physical ability or disability (Leather 1992; Straughan 1992; Sooman, Macintyre and Anderson 1993).

Thus the availability of products is influenced by the supply-side dynamics of the agrochemical or food industries, and food choice exists in the context of the systems of provision of the 'food system' (Fine and Leopold 1993). But there is also a need to examine the role of demand/consumption in influencing what is produced, or in 'addressing what makes products acceptable to consumers' (Fine 1995; Ritson and Hutchins 1995). Our concern in this project was also to consider the reverse: that is, to assess what makes specific types of products unacceptable to consumers in particular historical circumstances.

There is a second way in which we might think of limits imposed by systems of provision: in the provision of information via the mass media or the promotional strategies of the food industry. Both the government and the market can influence not only food provision but also the production of information. Just as the range of food products available is finite and limited, so is the range of information available about the health damaging properties of foods. This is true both of the products of the news and entertainment media, and of the promotional activities of the food production, manufacturing and retailing industries.

First, the production and distribution of information by the news and entertainment industry (including commercial and public service media) tend to follow the logic of the market in the pursuit of mass audiences (Golding and Murdock 1996). In the mainstream media this tends to mean similarity rather than diversity in what is presented to the public: for example news bulletins follow a similar format and often have similar content on different television channels; there are certain times of the day when soaps are shown and other times when foreign movies are shown; it is impossible for us to choose to watch expensive costume drama in the afternoon.

Second, government departments routinely produce large amounts of information which is selectively communicated to the public, and the government has considerable power to police disclosure (Ericson, Baranek and Chan 1989) and thereby set limits to the information available in the news and entertainment media. It has been argued that the ability and willingness of government departments to withhold information from the public compromises the ability of the public to judge the safety or otherwise of foods (Leigh 1980; Cannon 1987).

Third, food industries are continually trying to promote their products and persuade the public to buy them, in a context of secrecy justified by commercial confidentiality (Bolesworth and Waller 1997). It is in the interest of the food industries to emphasise the desirability and health-enhancing properties of their products and to gloss over any less desirable or health-damaging properties. For example, to revert to a previous example, the reduced fat content of yoghurt is emphasised rather than its sugar content. In the absence of any sustained 'balance' to marketing or advertising campaigns (except in the form of health warnings on one or two types of products), the weight of such information is somewhat one-sided and may be a further key factor in limiting and shaping the content of the information available to the public (Gardner and Shepherd, 1989)

Food and media production processes coexist and influence each other. For example, foods are material goods, but they also have symbolic values which are expressed and represented in the media. The supply and price of foods can be affected by the circulation of information, just as the circulation of information (both in terms of advertising and public issues) can be affected by the production and price of foods. Thus we would argue that in practice the interaction between the production of foods and the production of information influences and poses limits on what is thought and what is bought. We further argue that in this context we need to think of 'choice' as a heavily qualified notion, constrained by the limitations of the food, information, production and marketing systems.

Design and methods

The study design involved three components. First, focusing on recent press reporting of salmonella, listeria, BSE and CHD, we interviewed journalists, editors and their news sources (e.g. civil servants, PR professionals, members and staff of pressure groups), and collected primary and secondary documentation such as press releases, official reports, survey and opinion data, and confidential minutes. Second, we analysed mass media output on these four topics, and on food more generally, between 1973 and 1994. Data on the 'food panics' stretched from 1986 to mid-1994, and data on the coverage of food safety compared with CHD between 1973 and 1991. For two separate three-month periods we examined the coverage of diet, lifestyle and health in the English national press, Scottish national press, Network News and Scottish television news and popular magazines. During another period of two months we examined all radio and television coverage (both factual and fictional) of food issues; this ranged from *Farming Today* and *The Food Programme* on BBC Radio Four, to Channel 4's *Food File*, the BBC's *Food and Drink* and the drama *Natural Lies*, to the children's programme *The Attack of the Killer Tomatoes*.

Third, we used focus-group methods to investigate how media messages about food are received, understood and acted on by the public, and what other (non-media) factors influence food choice. We studied 'pre-existing' social groups (people who knew each other through work, friendships or family connections), in order to preserve the elements of the social context within which people actually receive media messages (Eldridge, Kitzinger and Williams 1996). The fact that group members knew each other also permitted useful insights into what people said; for example, as we show later, some people's statements about their own eating habits were contradicted by other people in the group, on the basis of their knowledge of the speaker.

The sampling for the groups was purposive, and was designed to ensure the inclusion of a range of sociodemographic characteristics and of experiences of food or of health, rather than to generate a sample representative of the general population either of the west of Scotland (the area in which the study took place) or of the UK as a whole. When we approached the initial contact we simply said that we wanted to talk to people about food, and did not mention health or food safety. There were 26 focus groups involving 171 individuals, 69 male and 102 female. Table 14.1 lists the groups and the respondents.

Within each session, respondents filled in three questionnaires (one on biographical details and their use of the media; one on food in relation to health, safety and the media; and one on the impact of the group discussion), and participated in a 'News Bulletin Writing Exercise' followed by a period of discussion. The sessions lasted between one and two hours. The discussions were audiotaped and transcribed.

In the 'News Bulletin Writing Exercise' respondents were split

233

Table 14.1 List of focus groups

Groups	Number of participants	Number of females and males	
		F	M
1 Members of a keep-fit class	8	8	0
2 Amateur footballers	7	0	7
3 Members of Glasgow's Healthy Cities Project	8	5	3
4 Mothers attending the same health clinic	6	6	0
5 Work colleagues (shopworkers)	6	5	1
6 Work colleagues (administrators)	6	1	5
7 Neighbours from a lower middle-class area	6	4	2
8 Neighbours from a middle-class area	6	5	1
9 Males 30–40 years old (friends)	6	0	6
10 Females 30–40 years old (friends)	6	6	0
11 Middle-class people over 50 (neighbours)	6	5	1
12 Working-class men over 60 (friends)	7	0	7
13 Restaurant staff (waiting staff and chefs)	9	3	6
14 Professional bakers	6	3	3
15 Friends who are all vegetarian	7	5	2
16 Postgraduate catering students	6	5	1
17 Amateur body-builders	6	0	6
18 Friends who eat regularly at a local community cafe	8	6	2
19 Members of a social club in a working-class housing scheme	7	5	2
20 Health-promotion professionals	6	5	1
21 Addiction counsellors	5	4	1
22 Students, university level	7	4	3
23 Unemployed young people	7	4	3
24 Middle-class young people 18–24 years (friends)	6	4	2
25 Working-class young people 18–25 years (friends)	6	5	1
26 Members of the Chinese community	7	4	3

into two sub-groups, each of which was given an identical set of photographs taken from television news bulletins and asked to construct a television news item about food. The photographs included pictures of government and opposition politicians, government officials, scientists, pressure-group representatives, animals, and different food types, all of which had appeared on TV news footage, and as many as possible of which were potentially relevant to both CHD and food safety (e.g. photographs of eggs, red meat and cheese, and of the current chief medical officer). Of the 52 bulletins written, 11 were based on food-poisoning outbreaks, 16 on food scares in relation to salmonella, listeria and BSE, and 25 were about CHD. Examples of the different types of stories created from using the same photographs are as follows:

BSE Beef in Bargain Basement Britain
Jane Noakes, Environmental Health Officer, today claimed that the government was failing to take seriously the continued dangers of BSE in beef and dairy products to the general public. Despite the initial outcry two years ago and action taken at the time, current lack of media attention has enabled the government to reduce its efforts to counteract the spread of BSE. Thus policy continues despite recent evidence of an increase in BSE cases throughout the UK. This has wider implications for the British population since no British beef is exported to the EC. Currently the EC operates within guidelines restricting the import of British beef, an indication that the EC takes the matter more seriously than the British government. (Group 22)

A report released today states that many young families living below the breadline are unaware of the potential danger they could be causing to their health due to their poor diets. Sir Donald Acheson claims that such families are constantly eating greasy fried foods and are not consuming the vital nutrients essential for a healthy diet. Families which fall into this category include the unemployed, single parent families and those living off state benefits. Robin Cooke MP, opposition spokesman for health, said today that the government was entirely to blame. 'These families do not receive enough money from the government so cannot be expected to maintain a healthy diet. They are being forced to eat cheap, unhealthy foods.' This was opposed by William Waldegrave who claimed that money is not the problem and that healthy foods can be bought on low budgets. He said that these families need better health education which has now been introduced into the school curriculum. (Group 11)

This exercise showed that respondents were familiar with the basic language and structure of news bulletins, and that they had good recall and understanding of a number of specific concerns about food. After each sub-group had read out their news story, the researcher (JR) asked questions about the stories – Why they had been chosen? Did they remember that type of story appearing? What was their reaction to it? – followed by general discussion. The researcher controlled the conversation when it was about to deviate too far from the main point of the discussion (e.g. 'I'm on a diet because we're going on holiday,' 'Oh, where are you going?' 'Well, we've booked up for Spain,' 'Really, I went there last year) and ensured that specific questions about salmonella, listeria, BSE and CHD were covered if they did not emerge naturally. Respondents are identified only in terms of gender and the group of which they were a member.

In this chapter we concentrate on the data collected from these focus groups, although in order to provide a context for public understanding we first briefly describe the mass media coverage.

Mass media coverage of food scares and coronary heart disease

Food scares tended to appear in the news sections in newspapers (both broadsheet and tabloid), and on news programmes on television and radio, whereas CHD was mainly covered in features sections of the same mass media.

We found there to be five 'news values' which seemed to be relevant to the appearance of any mention of links between health and diet in general, or specific foods, in the news sections of newspapers, television and radio. These were 'scientific advances', 'divisions among experts', 'matters of state', 'division in the government', and 'government suppression'. Listeria in soft cheeses rarely seemed to fit any of these criteria of newsworthiness: it was generally agreed by experts, the government and journalists that it could be health-damaging to vulnerable groups such as pregnant women, but was not of major significance beyond that. It was therefore covered mainly in health-advice pages or programmes during the period studied. Salmonella in eggs and BSE seemed to fit all these news values at various times; the former involved the resignation of a government minister, suspicions voiced by some commentators that the true extent of infection among poultry was being suppressed by government, disagreements among experts, and apparent conflicts of interest between the Department of Health, the Ministry of Agriculture, Fisheries and Food, and the egg industry. It is thus not surprising that it received so much prominence as a news story albeit over a relatively brief period. BSE involved all these criteria of newsworthiness to an even greater extent, and for longer, and was frequently reported in the major news sections of national media outlets (main evening BBC and ITV news bulletins, front pages of national newspapers). For example, between 1988 and the end of 1992, BBC Network television news broadcast 128 items on food safety issues, and between 1973 and 1991 food-safety stories made the front page of *The Times* or *Sunday Times* 90 times.

By contrast, stories about dietary risks for CHD appeared only 25 times on BBC Network news, and on only ten occasions on the front pages of *The Times* or *Sunday Times*, during the same period. Fifteen of the BBC news items were straightforward reports of scientific advances. The other occasions on which it appeared in news pages or programmes were characterised by either a 'government suppression' angle (as in allegations in the *Sunday Times* of censorship of the 1983 National Advisory Committee on Nutrition Education (NACNE) report (Cannon 1983; Gillie 1985)) or the 'disagreement among experts' angle, as in the following example:

Newscaster: British scientists are still divided over whether or not eating polyunsaturated fats can help prevent heart disease. Some have put their names to a new national advertising campaign which defends the use of polyunsaturates in margarines and other products.

The campaign comes after a claim from researchers in Cambridge that eating too much of these fats could actually increase the chances of heart disease. (BBC1 2100 21 September 1989)

If the CHD orthodoxy is here defined as suggesting that a high intake of dietary fats, particularly saturated fats, is causally implicated in the genesis of coronary heart disease, then typically assaults on this orthodoxy – as distinct from reporting divisions of scientific opinion, as above – were featured at the margins of broadcasting (for example Channel Four documentaries, opinion programmes), rather than in major news locations such as front page newspapers or television news. Between 1988 and 1991 the only broadcast by BBC television news citing potential disagreement with this orthodoxy was the one described above. Critiques of this orthodoxy were more common in the tabloid press and the more right-wing broadsheets, especially the *Sunday Telegraph* and the *Sunday Times* (the BBC news item quoted above was in part a response to an article in the *Sunday Times* headlined: 'Scientists do an about-turn over polyunsaturates' (*Sunday Times* 3 September 1989)), while being reported but played down by the more liberal broadsheets such as *The Independent, The Times* and the *Guardian*. Tabloid newspapers were much more likely to pick up attacks on the scientific orthodoxy and to feature disagreement among experts, for example: 'Butter can slice heart attack risk' (*Daily Express* 27 February 1991); Butter best for hearts say experts' (*Evening Standard* 28 February 1991); 'Healthy diet is pure tripe' (*Daily Record* 4 March 1991); 'Eat, drink and be merry . . . it could save your life' (*Daily Mirror* 23 December 1991); and 'Fatty food not a killer' (*Daily Express* 23 December 1991).

Thus coverage of the dietary hypothesis for coronary heart disease was comparatively rare in news pages or programmes, and only tended to appear when it was challenged (or when celebrities were reported as having heart disease). It was much more extensively covered in features or lifestyle articles in newspapers, or in non-news programmes on television and radio. Features dealing with healthy eating, diet and lifestyle markedly outnumbered news stories exclusively about CHD; they accounted for up to 87 per cent of press items on CHD in the London tabloids and 60 per cent in Scottish broadsheets. While such widespread availability of information about the causes of CHD and the health implications of diet might influence public belief and dietary behaviour, it does not lead to banner headlines, passionate editorials, ministerial resignations or noticeable changes in government policy in the way that the 1980s–1990s coverage of food scares did.

Public understandings

We identified a number of factors which have a bearing both on the interpretation of media information and on food choice. Here we give some examples of the way in which these shaped judgements on media information and food choice.

The public is not a homogeneous mass, but comprises many different groups and individuals who use different contexts and experiences when making decisions. We found that age, gender, income, personal experience, national identity, and broader aspects of identity (such as desired body image or persona) were associated with respondents' reported eating habits and with what they said about diet and health.

The younger the respondents the less concern they expressed about CHD or long term health maintenance; a majority aged between 16 and 25 agreed with a statement in the questionnaire to the effect that youth made people feel invincible and that lifetime decisions were not important. Younger respondents claimed to reject media-based health education information (which all of them could quote), but reported actively engaging in behaviours (such as sports and weight-reduction diets) encouraged by that information; they were concerned less with the prospect of future CHD and more with current fitness, physical exertion and 'looking good'. As one 18-year-old put it:

> Everything encourages you to try to be your best, to look your best. From adverts on TV to the shops selling clothes . . . the message is clear, if you don't take part you're a loser, if you don't wear these clothes you're not in. I suppose food is part of that. But it certainly isn't the initial thing, I mean I would eat anything but I don't because I want to be a particular type of person . . . what I mean is, there's no point me wearing expensive sports gear if I'm fat. (Male, Group 24)

For both males and females a link was perceived between diet and 'looking good', but there were gender differences in ideas about how to achieve a desirable appearance: the men tended to participate in sporting activities such as playing football while women tended to concentrate on dietary intake.

Most respondents (84 per cent) associated the word 'diet' with weight loss rather than with usual food intake, and all of them associated slimness with health. In the media, too, 'diet' predominantly means dieting, and many of our respondents reproduced information and advice on dieting which they attributed to 'lifestyle' features in the press and magazines. Only a few of the women had not attempted to reduce their weight by dieting. The conflation of weight loss with healthy eating in mass media (and health-education) coverage and among our respondents affects how new information about food is perceived. How this affected eating habits differed. While some reported becoming very disciplined about food intake, consuming (both buying and eating) only very low calorie products, others reported simply altering their normal diet (e.g. eating only once a day, or cutting out meals in favour of snack foods). These changes were reportedly made to lose or maintain weight and to acquire a desirable shape rather than to become healthier or reduce the risks of CHD. There was lot of discussion about the relative advantages of different weight-loss programmes, usually derived from women's magazines and diet books.

Women were more concerned about food safety and hygiene than were men, particularly if they were pregnant or had young children. This was especially true of salmonella and listeria which were remembered as mainly being risky for particularly vulnerable groups such as pregnant women, babies, or the sick and elderly.

Official advice and media information caused a great deal of resentment among respondents on low incomes, who felt that the advice ignored the difficulties of managing on a low budget:

> The leaflets say eat lots of vegetables and fruit and salad. But you know, the price of most fruit and vegetables are sky high and you can't afford them. (Female, Group 3)

> We all know what to do and basically would get on with it. I mean, I'd love to eat good food all the time but I have five mouths to feed on one income and that is not a very easy thing to do. That should be recognised by those who are handing out all this advice. Instead of telling me to buy lots of this and that they should, in reality be taking into consideration different income levels and, well, perhaps offering more realistic ideas about how to feed a family nutritionally. (Female, Group 18)

There was a tendency to see the media (and more specifically, health-education campaigns) as consistently blaming the individual for poor health, while ignoring the importance of material circumstances. Health-education advice was, on the whole, seen as middle class.

Respondents with higher incomes tended not to mention lack of money as an important factor in food choice. Some students from better-off backgrounds were an exception in that they had experienced a sharp change in their material circumstances on starting university. One commented wryly that 'if you go to Safeway you can tell the first years (students) 'cause they are the ones buying chocolate digestives' (male, Group 22). Those only temporarily on low incomes suggested that when their incomes rose again it would not affect the basic components of their diet but only its quality:

> What I aspire to when I actually leave and get a reasonable income is not a radical change in diet but the ability to buy better products. The basis stays the same but you can go and buy expensive little fancy vegetables and decent cuts of meat. (Male, Group 16)

National identity seemed to be important. Advice on food safety and CHD was widely perceived to be English in origin. Edwina Currie (of whom there was a photo in the 'News Bulletin Writing Exercise') was widely remembered for her statement in 1987, when junior health minister, on the unhealthy diets of 'northerners', which respondents interpreted as including Scots. They knew that BSE was less common in Scotland than in England, and some reported having stopped eating English meat or meat products, but continuing to buy Scottish versions because they believed them to be safe. Such views may have been encouraged by the Scottish media. Seventy-nine per cent of our respondents reported buying Scottish newspapers. The Scottish media were clearly differentiated from and preferred to their English counterparts:

> We have our own papers, our own news and other programmes here. I prefer to watch and read these than the British counterparts because we have different politics and politicians up here, different social issues which are reported by Scottish papers and TV. If you want to keep up with what's going on in Scotland you certainly wouldn't get far by watching the *News at Ten* or reading the *Guardian*.' (Male, Group 19)

Many food products in Scotland are advertised as being 'Scottish' (e.g. cheese, water, tea, beef), and respondents claimed that they bought these versions for that reason. Those who originally came from outside the west of Scotland had no such loyalty to local dietary habits, some of which appalled them:

> I thought Scotland was bad, graveyard of Europe and all that, but I think I always assume that these things are slightly exaggerated, especially by the media or people on it – like remember what Edwina Currie said about northerners eating badly, that type of thing. But then I went with my friend into a chip shop here and I couldn't believe it – it was then I thought that what went on here wasn't exaggerated at all. I mean I just stood in stunned amazement as the lady stuck a meat pie in batter and then deep-fried it. God, why don't they just inject the fat straight into the body. My pal swore to me that these things actually tasted very good – yeah right. I just couldn't bring myself to eat stuff like that, it's so totally disgusting. (Male, originally from Newcastle, Group 9)

Our respondents appeared knowledgeable about salmonella, listeria, BSE and CHD. They were sometimes surprised at how much they did know, and at how much of what they knew seemed to have come from the mass media:

> *Respondent:* I don't know that much about salmonella, but I do know that if you boil eggs for seven minutes until they're really hard they should be safe, and you shouldn't ever eat raw or undercooked eggs or use home-made mayonnaise and stuff.
> *JR:* How do you know that?
> *Respondent:* I don't know really, I suppose it just seems like commonsense really. But now that I think about it I must have got it from somewhere because really, when you think about it, we

shouldn't have to cook eggs for ages at all to make them safe, should we? But then I suppose at the time I picked up a lot of things from the magazines that I read and there were a lot of people saying things on TV about how to cook eggs. There was that medical man, what was he called . . .

JR: The chief medical officer?

Respondent: Yeah, that's him, he said it all the time on TV, said how we should be cooking eggs and keeping them and I thought oh well, that's what we have to do to keep on eating eggs, fair enough, that's good advice to follow. Isn't that funny, I just thought I'd always done that naturally. (Female, Group 10)

I suppose you maybe don't think you are watching but the fact that you can regurgitate it means that you have actually taken it in and thought about it, and do alter to some extent. I mean I only eat margarine now, it wouldn't dawn on me to touch butter or full-fat milk. Where did all that come from, how did I know that was the thing to do to cut down the risk of a bad heart? Advertising I suppose and watching programmes and seeing more leaflets about diet. I read a lot of magazines so I suppose they have had an influence as well, particularly when you're contemplating cutting down on food. (Female, Group 1)

One possible hypothesis to explain the apparently different response to media reporting of CHD as compared with the food scares is that the public has been made aware of the risks of salmonella in eggs, BSE in beef, etc. by extensive press coverage, but has not been similarly made aware of dietary risks for CHD. This hypothesis was not supported in our data. We found our respondents to be very familiar with official advice on CHD and able to describe in considerable detail dietary and other guidelines for reducing its risk. However, this knowledge had no consistently direct relation to their likelihood of either believing in or adhering to the guidelines. Information on CHD risk factors was seen as being a constant background feature, and accessible in many different forms; so much so that some argued that its very familiarity meant it could be ignored:

There always seems to be something cropping up especially on Scottish news. You're pretty aware that Glasgow has got a bad health record, but to some extent you are so used to that information coming out that you don't pay much attention. (Male, Group 9)

A frequent comment about official advice on CHD was that 'If you believed everything that you read and everything you heard you wouldn't eat at all.' This attitude attributed to ideas about 'commonsense' in relation to personal eating habits. A crucial issue seemed to be balancing different criteria for selecting food, such as the role of preferences and tradition versus healthiness:

Respondent: At the end of the day you have to make some decision on what to do or not do about bits of new information, and I think that's when you call on other things to help you make up your mind . . . so if they say that you have to stop using lard to cook food, it's better to use vegetable oil or something, then I'd probably do it. I mean it's not a big deal, just means picking up a different item in the shop. But if they say, well, you have to stop eating chips forever or you'll cut ten years off your life, then that would be different.

JR: In what way?

Respondent: Let's start with the fact that I love chips, I can't imagine not ever eating them again, so that's abstinence out. What do I do? Well, I'd say, really I don't eat them that often, so I'm OK. Maybe if I was thinking I'm a bit tired or want to get fit or hear that someone I know has been told to watch out, I'd think maybe I need to cut down on the old favourites.

JR: So you'd stop eating them then?

Respondent: Oh no, I'd just cook them in vegetable oil instead of lard and think, well, that's me done my bit for the cause. You have to understand with things like this you might be prepared to compromise in certain circumstances but giving up altogether is not a realistic option.

JR: Why not?

Respondent: Because it's like I told you, I love chips. (Male, Group 12)

Our respondents demonstrated a general scepticism about official advice and the pronouncements of politicians, scientists, 'experts' and the media:

The reports contradict themselves, don't they? I mean they come out one year and say don't eat this, don't eat that because your cholesterol is too high, you've got to watch cholesterol. Then they come out the next year and say no, no your cholesterol is OK, you don't need to worry about it. (Female, Group 8)

Some combined this scepticism with a desire for balance:

I think you have to take a lot of this stuff with a pinch of salt. One minute one thing is bad for you and the next it's good. You have to make your own mind up and use your own commonsense. Like, for instance, I love butter and I know the experts say I'd be better off eating margarine because it's better for me. Then somebody says something different. And I think, hold on a minute, nobody really knows anything for sure, and really, is it going to kill me. I just don't believe that and probably never will. But even if a scientist came out and said, look, its 100 per cent true that butter will harm you, I'd think, well, I eat other things to balance my diet, I think I'll be alright, and I'd carry on eating butter. (Male, Group 21)

Distrust of experts was most likely when respondents had some

242

countervailing source of information, particularly one that could be regarded as credible because of personal or technical knowledge:

> With the mad cows thing, I just didn't pay any attention to it at all and now I think about it that was definitely because my uncle is a butcher and he said it was a lot of nonsense and that meat was perfectly safe. I assumed he would know if there really was a problem and he wouldn't tell lies . . . so yeah, it was him talking about it, saying it was all rubbish that made me not bother about it at all even though it was all over the TV and papers at the time. (Male, Group 2)

The role of personal experience in mediating the understanding of and responses to media and health-promotion messages seemed crucial. For example, all of the members of one group had stopped eating eggs (and had not returned to them) because a colleague had been seriously ill with food-poisoning from salmonella. The seriousness of the illness (the man in question had been off work for over a month) seemed to have had a major effect, and initial decisions not to eat eggs or dairy products within the workplace had spilled into life outside work. The affected man's colleagues said they were still less likely to buy from fast-food shops, were more conscious of hygiene in particular food outlets (small corner shops, takeaways), were more aware of sell-by dates on fresh food products, and made more efforts to cook foods thoroughly:

> We suddenly realised how easily it could happen, and how dangerous it could be. This was more than feeling a bit queasy after a dodgy takeaway, this was a life-threatening situation and it could have been any one of us. We all became very careful after that, more watchful, you know. (Female, Group 6)

Such incidents seemed to have changed some people's information-seeking, as well as food-purchasing, preparation and eating, behaviour. For example, they described more actively seeking out information than they would otherwise have done, listening to reports or reading stories about food-poisoning with heightened interest, picking up leaflets on food hygiene/cooking practices, and watching cookery programmes on television (particularly those such as *Food File* or *Food and Drink* which went beyond normal cookery formats and offered advice in different areas). Others used personal experience as a reason for not fearing food-poisoning:

> I have never been terribly concerned by safety issues to any great extent. I haven't got the time to be bothered and I haven't had food-poisoning. I mean, I've never gotten poisoned by eating an egg even though they said I would, and I don't think I'll die from eating sausages. I'm not really frightened by that kind of thing. (Female, Group 3)

Many respondents seemed to view food-poisoning as an almost inevitable consequence of eating certain foods, particularly fast or takeaway foods, especially those bought late at night (usually when alcohol was involved). Experiences of being ill on at least one occasion after eating food from mobile vans and the like were commonly described. But instead of blaming the vendor or food-hygiene practices, they tended to blame themselves (and their lack of good judgement because of alcohol) for going there in the first place. None of the incidents of food-poisoning described in this way was particularly serious; all were transient and seemed to be regarded as analogous to hangovers rather than being potentially life-threatening (note that all the fieldwork was conducted well before the 1996/7 E. Coli outbreaks in Scotland).

Many of our respondents believed that the media had their own motives, such as sales or scaremongering, for creating scares. Those working in the catering industries (bakers, catering students, restaurant workers) were highly critical of 'panics' such as those over salmonella, listeria and BSE because they affected their work, and potentially their jobs. Restaurant staff in particular said that they received a large number of queries about the source of their beef, whether their eggs were free range, etc. Eighty-four per cent of our respondents blamed food-poisoning on poor hygiene or inadequate cooking (those working in catering were especially likely to do this); only 10 per cent mentioning food production or distribution. The exceptions were a vegetarian group who discussed food production in detail, and members of a local community-health project who received foodstuffs from European 'food mountains' which they claimed were inedible, particularly meat products. Even when respondents stated that, for example, salmonella was caused by 'feeding dead chickens to live ones' (around 50 per cent), they also said if it were cooked properly and stored at the right temperature chicken would be safe. A new problem was thus understood in relation to already accepted knowledge about food safety and food hygiene.

Our respondents perceived scares as having a clear beginning and end, which meant that eating habits were, in general, only altered for a short space of time. Once the scare was seen to be resolved or disappeared from the news, there was a general return to former eating habits:

> You do think about it for a day or two but go back to normal habits pretty quickly. You assume, I think, that if there's a problem it will be dealt with; if there's a bad product on the shop shelves they'll take it off immediately. (Male, Group 11)

> You do forget, move on. It's like, one day you won't eat eggs because you think, no, I won't take that risk, there must be something in this if everyone is arguing about it. But then slowly you go back to it. Other people are eating these things and they aren't getting sick so you think, well, it must be OK again, these experts are probably arguing

for the sake of it again. We stopped eating eggs just in case after Edwina said they might be dodgey. But then, oh, I don't know, a few weeks later I suppose, there they were, back in my shopping basket. And that's because, well, we like them and I didn't know anyone else who was keeping off them. (Female, Group 21)

Because salmonella stopped being in the news, people thought that the public health problem had been resolved, and went back to eating eggs. BSE similarly stopped being covered so extensively in late 1990 but our respondents were aware that there were remaining doubts about its possible links with human health. Even so, many reported making conscious decisions to take the risk:

> *Respondent:* Some of them on the TV say we're going to get a hideous disease from eating beef and some of them say that's nonsense. So, what do you do? Well, I think they all like to hear their own voices too much and dramatise things and talk about things which they don't really know anything about. So I have to say to myself, do I think eating sausages will kill me, and I don't think they will, so I eat them.
> *JR:* What if you turn out to be wrong?
> *Respondent:* 'Well, *c'est la vie,* I suppose. You have to make decisions based on something you understand at the time, and the experts argue away so much that you say, for God's sake, I've had enough of this. I'm not going to stop eating what I like because somebody says there just might be a chance that it might or might not harm you, it's silly, you'd end up eating nothing at all. (Male, Group 17)

An important aspect of food choice was habit: many respondents described themselves as having lifelong eating patterns which had developed in childhood, and with which they felt comfortable:

> You eat what your mum gives you, you trust your parents and you automatically assume that what they fed you was healthy and good for you. (Female, group 8)

> I can tell you . . . Sunday, as I said, would be like your rolled pork or your beef brisket . . . Monday is mince and potatoes, Tuesday is steak pie and potatoes, Wednesday is a wee treat, you know, it's when my mum goes shopping with her friends in town and she usually just buys something quick. Thursday is like, make up whatever you've got left cause that's pay night and Friday it's shopping and it'll be cold meat and a bag of chips or something like that. Then Saturday you'll get the big fry-up and it's always the same. I know it off by heart and it's still exactly the same. (Female, Group 21)

When they described changing their eating habits, either in order to lose weight or enhance health, most people did not describe radical reworkings to the basic elements of their habitual eating patterns, but, rather, minor or balancing changes:

> It's weird because if I ever go on a diet which is quite rare but if I do go on a diet I never change the kind of food I eat. I'd never start buying fruit and vegetables. I'd just decide how many calories to eat that day like 1000 or whatever and just eat what I like, you know. So, I'd have a fish supper and two creme eggs the whole day rather than having a, like, a big salad. (Female, Group 1)

Some balancing was not always between different foods, but sometimes between food and other important aspects of life. Group 12 consisted of men who had experienced heart disease; all had been in hospital and been given special diet sheets. They reported that their wives enforced these dietary guidelines by removing 'good' or 'tasty' foods from their diets, and that steamed fish and chicken, brown bread, vegetables, raw salads, high-fibre breakfast cereals had replaced 'favourite' or 'traditional' red meat products (sausages, steak mince, burgers), pies, fry-ups, chips and the like. These men unanimously agreed that their wives were 'taking things too far', but that they had to accept these changes because, first, it was the wives who did the cooking and, second, a balancing act was involved. Six out of the seven were smokers and all seven drank alcohol; all had been told to cut out smoking and reduce drinking. They described a process of weighing up which of an 'unhealthy' diet, smoking and alcohol would be easier to give up and it became apparent that they felt that changing dietary habits was the lesser of several evils, and easier to do since it was being taken care of by the wives. None of the men had as yet stopped smoking, and while they reported drinking less alcohol, none had stopped completely. As one put it:

> some habits are harder to break than others. I can't give up everything, it would take all the fun out of life, so I'll eat whatever the missus puts in front of me, as long as I can have a pint. (Male, Group 12)

Another reason given for not adhering to guidelines for healthy eating to avoid CHD was that it was easier not to cook, not to make food 'from scratch', even though convenience foods tended to be high in fat. The reasons for not cooking included work patterns, the demands of family, wanting food instantaneously, and living as a single person:

> the kids torture me to buy basically what they see on the TV, micro-chips, pizza, frozen burgers, because apparently it tastes better than home-made food. (Female, Group 4)

> I would cook for someone else but not just for one person, not when I'm on my own. (Female, Group 1)

> People are too busy these days to be standing cooking all the time. It just takes too long starting from scratch, especially when you've just come in from work and you're tired. (Female, Group 8)

Respondents said that they felt they were being encouraged by advertising to buy convenience foods, and even those who claimed not to use convenience foods said they were sometimes tempted to, especially if they could be seen as being compatible with healthy diet guidelines:

> I wouldn't buy this stuff, but I did stop once when I saw a low fat version of a ready made frozen meal, one of those healthy options things. (Female, Group 14)

Respondents in studies such as this probably misrepresent the content of their diets by over-reporting socially desirable and under-reporting 'unhealthy' foods. The use of pre-existing groups provided several illustrations of this, via 'misrepresentations' being made public by other members of the group. For example, one woman said:

> I eat melon in the morning for breakfast, and something like steamed chicken and vegetables at dinner time. I rarely eat sweet things at all, that box of Maltesers on the table has been there for months. I know all about proper diet from the food and health magazines I get regularly. I follow the advice religiously. (Female, Group 11)

> When she briefly left the room her husband said:
> Listen she's telling the truth about the melon and the chicken and that, and that box of sweets has been there for ages. But what she didn't tell you is that she buys big bags of these Maltesers in the supermarket every week and fills that box up, and never passes it without putting her hand in. She eats them when she's reading these low calorie recipe ideas, for god's sake. (Male, Group 11)

This incident illustrates not only how people may represent their diets in a socially desirable way, but also how accurately their misrepresentations follow current dietary guidelines.

Conclusion

The research reported here confirmed that food choice is constrained by a number of factors, some practical and material (for example, perceived lack of money or time), and some less tangible (for example, the perceived need for balance and for using food to express personal identity). It was clear that our respondents were knowledgeable about the food scares on which we were focusing, and also about dietary risks for CHD; it was also clear that much of their information came from the mass media, in the form of news, features and advertisements (although some initially did not appreciate how much they did know, and how much they obtained from the mass media). The deficit hypothesis (that lack of adherence to healthy dietary guidelines is attributable to lack of information or understanding) was not supported. In this respect our research is consistent with other research on diet and health (Davison 1989; Davison, Frankel and Davey Smith 1992).

It was also clear that our respondents had some tolerance for uncertainty, and appreciated the need to make dietary decisions on the basis of a balance of probabilities rather than on absolute certainties. Indeed, part of their scepticism about the dietary admonitions of experts seemed to stem from the certainty with which certain 'expert' dietary views were expressed, only to be contradicted by other equally certain views at a later date. In this regard they were similar to the people at high risk of heart disease interviewed by Lambert and Rose, who, for example, noted that at one period olive oil was regarded by experts as increasing the risk of heart disease, and at another period as decreasing the risk (Lambert and Rose 1996). They were also similar to the sheep farmers studied by Wynne, who distrusted expert views on contamination in the Lake District by radioactivity from Chernobyl partly because the experts expressed their views so definitely (Wynne 1996).

'Balance' seemed to be an important element of descriptions of food choice in the context of risks to health. Health or safety risks were balanced against other criteria for food choice such as habit ('what I grew up with'), preferences (the desire for chips or creme eggs), practicality (time and money), and identity (as a young person, a man, mother, sportsman, or Scot). In some cases this related to a broader idea of a healthy diet being a balanced diet, or of the importance of dietary moderation, an underlying principle that has also been reported from other studies (Blaxter and Paterson 1983; Homans 1983).

Another key element that emerged strongly from this study was personal experience, whether of working in the catering industry, having heart disease, or knowing someone who had experienced food-poisoning. Even here, however, the influence of personal experience varied according to how it was perceived and integrated into other aspects of people's shared understandings in particular contexts. Knowing someone who had experienced CHD or food-poisoning did not necessarily lead to dietary behaviour change.

The media can make people think about what they eat, and data on sales and the reported consumption of certain food products make it clear that press-reporting of some risks can cause dramatic shifts in buying and eating behaviour. The media can influence what issues people think about in relation to food: that is, they can 'set the agenda' for public discussion. However, the media can also influence both what is thought and what is bought. Our data show that the public can be influenced by media-reporting and by advertising, but that they exercise judgement and discretion in how much they incorporate media messages about health and safety in their diets. Their choices are constrained by personal circumstances (age, gender, income, family structure, etc.), other people (such as wives who cook for their husbands), personal identity, and by the foods and information available, which are limited by the food and information-production systems. As we had hypothesised, our respondents seemed actively to negotiate their understandings of the health and safety of foods, and their diets, in interaction with other people in both a micro context (of their immediate social networks) and a macro context (of the food production and information production systems).

Acknowledgements

We are grateful to Rory Williams for comments on an earlier draft.

The grant-holders were John Eldridge and Sally Macintyre and the researchers were David Miller and Jacquie Reilly.

CHAPTER 15

Food choices for babies

Elizabeth Murphy, Susan Parker and Christine Phipps

Introduction

The working title of our study is 'Food choices made by mothers on behalf of infants and young children'. As such, it reflects the overall objective of the ESRC programme which was to answer the question 'Why do people eat what they do?' The food choices referred to in our title are decisions about what someone else will eat. Ultimately, adults decide whether to offer or withhold food from babies. Babies may contribute to such decisions, but their contributions are largely negative. They may express dissatisfaction, or refuse to eat what is offered, but their awareness of alternatives is constrained by what is made available. Hence, while babies may decide what is eaten, it is adults, usually mothers, who decide what is offered. The focus of this study is, therefore, on the proxy decisions made by mothers about what, when and how their babies are fed.

Decisions about infant-feeding are characteristically self-conscious and overt. Mothers are recurrently faced with decisions, such as whether to breast or formula-feed,[1] whether to feed on demand, when to introduce solid food, what kinds of food, whether to use commercially or home-prepared baby foods and whether to offer the baby sweets or other treats. Such decisions face first-time mothers not just with novelty but with potential difficulties. The baby's birth means that an urgent decision must be made, since the baby's survival requires an immediate action. This initial decision is usually between breast and formula-feeding. The first two years of a baby's life are a period of rapid change and development and mothers are faced with recurrent decisions about infant-feeding. As the baby develops, mothers must re-consider recently made decisions in the light of changing circumstances. Thus, mothers are repeatedly faced with the need to reflect and make decisions.

Such overt, reflective decisions about infant-feeding contrast with many decisions adults make for themselves. The latter are often routine.

Adults may simply buy and eat what they usually buy and eat. Innovation may be the exception rather than the rule. For adults, it may only be when something disturbs their assumptions (such as illness, exposure to a new product, or food scares) that decisions become overt. Thus, adults may be passive rather than active 'choosers'.

This contrast between active and passive decisions about food reflects Mead's argument that, in familiar situations, many of our responses are habitual rather than reflective (Mead 1934). Reflective behaviour is most likely to arise in novel or uncertain situations. Reflective actors consider present behaviour in the light of alternative future scenarios. Infant-feeding decisions are characteristically reflective rather than habitual. They are routinely explicit, overt, conscious and reflective and hence open to study in ways that more habitual decisions are not.

Our study seeks to capitalise on the reflective nature of infant-feeding decisions to increase our understanding of how babies come to eat what, when and how they do. A sample of 36 first-time mothers was followed from late pregnancy until their babies' second birthdays. Since large-scale surveys report that infant-feeding practices vary with both occupational class and age of mother (White, Freeth and O'Brien 1992), quota-sampling was used to achieve heterogeneity in respect of these two variables. Twelve mothers were recruited from occupational classes one and two, 12 from occupational class three, and 12 from occupational classes four and five, using the Registrar General's classification of the women's most recent occupation. Half of the women in each occupational class grouping were below the mean age, at birth of first baby, for that grouping, and half were above. Using 1991 Census data, and information from the Family Health Services Authority, we identified a sample of ten general medical practices, within a ten-mile radius of Nottingham, with contrasting occupational class profiles. Women from the birth registers of the practices were invited to participate and recruitment continued until each sample cell was filled.

Six depth interviews were carried out with each mother, one before the baby's birth, and the remaining five at intervals up to the baby's second birthday. Interviews with 33 women were audio-tape recorded and transcribed. At their request, interviews with the remaining three women were not taped but notes were taken and fully written up immediately after the interviews.

Choice in infant-feeding

Carrying out this research has led us to question the appropriateness of treating women's feeding practices as choices. Our unease with the concept of choice relates both to the concerns and orientations of our discipline (sociology) and to our analysis of women's own accounts of their feeding experiences. Throughout the chapter, we discuss the concept of choice in relation to both our disciplinary assumptions and to our data.

Three elements of the dictionary definitions of 'choice', are particularly relevant here. These are:

1 choice as 'deciding between possibilities'
2 choice as the 'act of choosing'
3 choice as 'the power, right, faculty of choosing'.

In the context of our study, only the first is straightforward. The mothers in our study did make decisions about what to offer their babies. Both initially and recurrently, mothers, indeed, decided between possibilities. In terms of this rather weak definition, mothers do make food choices. However, the second and third definitions raise significant problems in relation to both our data and our sociological perspective. In this chapter, we discuss, in some detail, difficulties raised by the second definition, before suggesting, in conclusion, some of the ways in which the third definition may be equally complex.

Choice as the act of choosing

The second definition of choice ('the act of choosing'), risks obscuring the dynamic, processual nature of mothers' decision-making about infant-feeding. Our concern, in this study, has been with the process by which decisions about infant-feeding are made, rather than with the act of choice. This reflects Schutz's distinction between 'act' and 'action':

> The term 'action' shall designate human conduct as an ongoing process which is devised by the actor in advance, that is which is based on a pre-conceived project. The term 'act' shall designate the outcome of this ongoing process, that is the accomplished action. Action may thus be covert – for example the attempt to solve a scientific problem mentally – or overt, gearing into the outer world. (Schutz 1973: 67)

For Schutz, choosing involved not only an outcome (the act of choice) but the process or action which leads up to this act. Such action incorporates both external behaviour and mental processes (covert action).

In studying decisions about infant-feeding, our focus has been on mothers' processual choosing (action), rather than on their choices (acts). We are engaged in that style of sociology which is less concerned to enumerate feeding acts (for example, what percentage of women breastfeed) than with studying the mechanisms by which women arrive at such acts (Mennell, Murcott and van Otterloo 1992). Feeding 'acts' are already well documented in infant-feeding surveys (e.g. White, Freeth and O'Brien 1992). The design of this study differs in so far as it also allows us to study the process by which women arrived at such acts.

It was our orientation towards choice as processual 'action' rather than as static 'act', itself derived from our sociological perspective, which dictated the longitudinal design of this study. Repeated interviews with a small number of women allowed us to study the processes by which particular feeding decisions were made over time. For example, in the antenatal interviews, we investigated women's preferences for breast- or formula-feeding, before they could translate such preferences into acts. Thus, we were able to study their 'projecting' (Schutz 1973) or 'deliberating' (Dewey cited in Schutz 1973), before the associated act was possible. Dewey defined deliberation as 'a dramatic rehearsal in imagination of various competing possible lines of action . . . to see what the resultant action would be like if it were entered upon' (Schutz 1973: 68).

Eliciting women's preferences, before they were in a position to act allowed us to examine the decisions which women anticipated making, 'all things being equal', and to identify the factors they presented as relevant. In later interviews, we compared projected acts and actual acts, and examined the factors invoked as relevant by women when accounting for departures from their original intentions. Other feeding practices including, for example, the timing of the introduction of solid food, the use of commercially prepared foods and the division of labour in infant-feeding were investigated in the same way.

The discrepancy between projected feeding acts and those which actually happened was substantial. Schutz (1973: 69) argued that both the action and the act of choice are based on the individual's 'knowledge at hand', at a given time, and differences between actual and projected acts reflect shifts in such knowledge. He specified two elements of such 'knowledge at hand', in relation to which we present our data in this section. The first is our knowledge of 'previously performed acts which are typically similar' to the projected act. The second is our knowledge of 'typically relevant features of the situation in which the projected action will occur'. For Schutz, the 'intrinsic uncertainty of all forms of projecting' lay in changes in individuals' 'knowledge at hand' as they moved through deliberation to act. We have investigated the shifts in mothers' 'knowledge at hand' which mediated between projected decisions and eventual acts. In this section, we illustrate such shifts in 'knowledge at hand' in relation to just one decision confronting mothers; that of whether to breast- or formula-feed their babies.

Antenatally, a substantial majority (29 out of 36 women) intended to breast-feed, and six intended to formula-feed. The remaining woman intended to combine breast- and formula-feeding. However, two months after the births, less than half of all mothers' feeding practices were consistent with these antenatal 'projections' (15 out of 36). The difference between the antenatal 'projections' and what actually took place was entirely accounted for by women who had intended to breastfeed (or, in the one case, to combine breast- and formula-feeding) but who had stopped breast-feeding earlier than intended (21 out of 30). Thus, while all six women intending to formula-feed their babies had done so, only nine of those who had planned to breastfeed had continued to feed their babies in line with these antenatal 'projections'. This shift, among those who intended to breastfeed, between the acts projected antenatally and those which happened in the event is consistent with infant-feeding survey findings (White, Freeth and O'Brien 1992). We discuss this discrepancy between 'projections' and 'acts' (or 'choosing' and 'choice') in terms of the shifts in the women's 'knowledge at hand' between the first and second interviews.

Antenatally, these first-time mothers engaged in something akin to Dewey's 'dramatic rehearsal in imagination of various competing possible lines of action'. They drew on the 'knowledge at hand', which was available to them before their babies' births. At the second interview, when the babies were eight weeks old, the 'knowledge at hand' used to explain feeding practices was systematically different from that found antenatally. We present these differences in women's 'knowledge at hand' in terms of Schutz's two categories of 'previously performed acts which are typically similar to the projected act' and 'typically relevant features of the situation'.

Typically similar acts

Schutz argued that, in projecting, we anticipate the future by placing ourselves in our 'phantasy' at a time when the projected action will have been accomplished (Schutz 1973: 69). One of the resources available
for doing so is knowledge of previously performed acts which are considered similar, though not necessarily identical, to the projected act:

> It is not necessary that the 'same' projected action in its individual uniqueness, with its unique ends and unique means has to be pre-experienced, and therefore, known. If this were the case, nothing novel could ever be projected. But it is implied in the notion of such a project that the projected action, its end and its means, remain compatible and consistent with these typical elements of the situation which, according to our experience at hand at the time of projecting, have warranted so far the practicability, if not the success, of *typically* similar actions in the past. (Schutz 1973: 73, emphasis in the original)

One problem confronting the mothers antenatally was, in fact, the lack of 'typically similar acts' to draw on in deciding whether to breast- or formula-feed. As first-time mothers, they had no experience of acts which were directly comparable to breast-feeding and this inexperience was reflected in the tentativeness with which many expressed their intention to breastfeed. In the absence of direct personal experience, they emphasised their inability to predict how feeding would 'work out', whether they would be able to 'do it' and whether it would be 'the sort of thing for me'. A number presented their intention to breastfeed as a provisional decision which might need to be overturned in the light of more reliable knowledge. One woman said, 'I think you've got to keep an open mind on these things because you can't predict these things.' Their sheer inability to guess what it would be like to breastfeed their babies was perhaps best summed up by one woman who said, 'I can't imagine the feeling of it.'

Women who were contemplating breast-feeding were troubled by the lack of such typically similar acts'. None who intended to formula-feed expressed similar uncertainty. Rather, they presented formula-feeding as straightforward and unproblematic. They took it for granted that they would be able to formula-feed their babies successfully and that their babies would be both willing and able to cooperate. This may reflect the availability of acts which are 'typically similar' to the preparation and delivery of formula-feeds. Formula-feeding involves following a series of instructions and is not dissimilar to other familiar culinary procedures such as preparing instant soup or custard. There are fewer everyday activities which can be treated as 'typically similar' to the processes involved in the production and delivery of breast milk.

In the absence of direct personal experience of infant-feeding, the women drew on two alternative sources of potentially 'similar acts'. First, they considered the feeding experiences of others. For a few women, all of whom intended to breastfeed, observing others' experiences increased uncertainty. One woman contrasted one friend who breastfed successfully with another who developed mastitis and stopped breast-feeding. Another contrasted one friend who 'got on really well' with another whose baby breastfed continuously and who felt 'tired, depressed and sore'. For these women, such conflicting observations raised further uncertainties about whose experiences could be treated as 'typically similar' for the purposes of their decision-making.

Other women appeared more confident about the implications of the experience of friends and family for their own 'projecting'. A number, including both intending breast-feeders and intending formula-feeders, drew on the positive experiences of others. Although the logic employed by both breast- and formula-feeders was identical, the terms in which they described other women's experiences are significantly different. Intending breast-feeders used the experiences of others as evidence that breast-feeding was possible. One woman said, 'I shall go for breast-feeding. My sister tells me there's no reason why I shouldn't be able to do it.' The emphasis is on demonstrating that breast-feeding is feasible. By contrast, intending formula-feeders, emphasised favourable outcomes for formula-fed babies. For example, one woman reported that all her friends had formula-fed their children and commented 'They're all perfectly healthy'. In both cases, the women are using others' experiences to defend their decision against potential challenges. Intending breast-feeders are addressing the idea that breast-feeding is difficult and potentially impossible to achieve. Intending formula-feeders displayed no doubts about the feasibility of their plans, but addressed themselves to the potential criticism that formula-feeding implied compromising their baby's future health. Thus, both groups of women used the 'typically similar' experiences of others as a resource in defending themselves against the charges to which their intentions were potentially vulnerable.

Others' 'typically similar' acts were also drawn on more negatively by those intending to breast- and formula-feed. Both groups described the negative impact of breast-feeding on the mother's lifestyle, in terms of social isolation, frequent feeding and the dependency of the baby. For example, one intending formula-feeder described a relative's experience, 'I have seen how my auntie's stuck . . . she's got to limit herself to how long she can be away . . . I'm still young and I'll want to be going out a lot.' Others were similarly concerned but intended to breast-feed, albeit differently from their friends and relatives. They would not allow breast-feeding to 'dominate' their lives, or to be a 'total imposition' in the way that they had observed among others. Although they intended to follow friends and family in breast-feeding their babies, these women were pointing to the ways in which they would nevertheless ensure that their own practices differed from the potentially 'typically similar' but disvalued practices of others.

The second source of 'typically similar acts', drawn on by women in deliberating about infant-feeding, was their own experience of situations which were potentially similar to infant-feeding and therefore potentially relevant. For example, one woman described her sense that her body had been taken over during pregnancy: 'I've found that with being pregnant . . . one of the main things that I've resented was the fact that . . . it's not my body any more. It's the bloody baby's body.' She saw her experience of pregnancy as indicating how she might experience breast-feeding. The women also drew on generalised descriptions of the 'kind of person' they thought themselves to be to predict how they would respond to the novel experience of infant-feeding. For example, another woman, in describing her reluctance to formula-feed, explained, 'I'm not very good at fussy things.'

Thus, in the absence of direct personal experience which could have been treated as 'typically similar', the women we interviewed made use of two resources which were available to them – their own experiences in related areas and the feeding experiences of friends and family – in considering whether to breast- or formula-feed their babies. However, while such experiences were identified as potentially 'typically similar', they were not treated as entirely satisfactory, particularly by those hoping to breastfeed. A number of those intending to breastfeed made comments such as, 'I don't think you can really say until you've started to do it and see how you get on.' Their unborn babies were seen as playing a critical role in facilitating or obstructing their plans. Such doubts were entirely absent from the talk of those who intended to formula-feed, who voiced no doubts about their babies' cooperation.

At the second interviews, the mothers reflected on the decisions they had made during the first eight weeks of their babies' lives and the resources which they had drawn on in arriving at such decisions. Each woman now had direct experience of feeding her own baby, by whichever method, and the focus had shifted to what was typical for her particular baby. Her 'knowledge at hand' now incorporated her experiences of her own baby's previous responses and her assessment of what was feasible was grounded in these experiences. Feeding decisions could be contextualised in individual babies' typical feeding behaviours. The 'typically similar acts' which now informed women's feeding decisions were those which were typical for their baby.

The 21 mothers who stopped breast-feeding earlier than originally intended described how this decision related to what they had come to understand as typical for their particular baby. Their babies' typical responses to breast-feeding were interpreted as making it impossible for them to continue. These babies 'cried incessantly', were 'never satisfied', did not 'know how to suckle', were 'stressed' by breast-feeding, 'lost weight' or did not 'gain it quickly enough'. These mothers did not reject breast-feeding *per se*. Rather, they identified features of their own baby's response to breast-feeding which suggested it was inappropriate for this particular baby. They acknowledged that other babies responded differently but these babies were no longer considered sufficiently similar for such comparisons to be helpful. Where other women's experiences were cited, it was now either as a contrast to their own experience or as a demonstration that their experience was not unique. In the latter case, other women who had experienced problems with breast-feeding were presented in support of their decision to change to formula-feeding.

This focus on the baby's individuality had implications for the way mothers evaluated advice from health professionals. Some professionals were criticised for trying to impose generalised 'rules' about feeding, ignoring the individuality of particular babies. These rules were drawn from theoretical knowledge of 'typical' babies, rather than from understanding what was true for this particular baby. The resultant scepticism about professional advice is illustrated in the following comment: 'They think, you know, that all babies are the same and they all grow at the same rate. But it don't work, especially with Mary.' The mothers had come to privilege their knowledge of their baby, drawn from daily interactions with that particular infant. The mother's expertise lay in first-hand experience. As one woman said, 'Obviously you know your own baby.' In Schutz's terms, the women's 'knowledge at hand' had shifted as they moved from 'deliberation to act' and the experiences deemed potentially 'typically similar' antenatally, were found to be largely dissimilar in the event.

Typically relevant features

The second element of 'knowledge at hand', identified by Schutz, is our knowledge of typically relevant features of the situation in which the projected action will occur' (Schutz 1973: 69). Just as there was a shift between the antenatal and postnatal interviews, in the acts considered 'typically similar', there was a parallel shift in the features of the situation which the women deemed to be 'typically relevant' to feeding their babies.

At the antenatal interviews, two kinds of features were treated as relevant to the decision to breast- or formula-feed. The first related to the baby's welfare and the second to the impact of feeding on the mother. Both breast- and formula-feeders related their decision to the baby's welfare and, in particular, the baby's long-term health. Those who intended to breastfeed stressed factors such as the transfer of antibodies and the development of the baby's immune system. Breast-feeding was described as 'better' and 'more healthy for the baby' and the phrase 'breast is best' was often used (the title of Stanway and Stanway's (1978) popular book on the subject). Those intending to formula-feed also cited health and nutrition as relevant factors. Some (and, indeed, some who intended to breastfeed) expressed concern that they might not produce 'good' milk, because of dietary deficiencies or conflicting demands on their energy.

The second kind of features which the women treated as relevant concerned the impact of different feeding methods on the mother. The impact of breast-feeding was seen as largely negative, even among women intending to breastfeed. Concern was expressed about breast-feeding limiting the mother's autonomy, about 'over-dependent' breast-fed babies and that breast-feeding might mean that women, rather than their partners, bore the brunt of baby care. There was anxiety that if breast-feeding led to women taking prime responsibility for caring for the baby in the early months, this might lead to longer-term patterns of child care which were inimical to the ideal of 'shared parenting' to which a number of the women aspired. There was considerable unease about breast-feeding babies in front of others, whether inside the home, in front of family and friends, or outside the home, in public places. While some intending breast-feeders identified some positive aspects of breast-feeding, including the convenience and cheapness of breast milk which was 'on tap', compared to the complications of preparing bottles, and the tendency of nursing mothers to regain their figures more quickly after the birth, the impact of breast-feeding on the mother was generally seen as restrictive and negative. In contrast, formula-feeding was seen as bringing flexibility, freedom and, particularly among those intending to formula-feed, relief from an embarrassing and even distasteful responsibility.

Thus, in Schutz's terms, both those intending to breastfeed and those intending to formula-feed, treated two kinds of factors as 'typically relevant' to their decision about infant-feeding. These were baby-related features, on the one hand, and mother-related features on the other. Those intending to formula-feed presented the decision as straightforward. The interests of mother and baby coincided. Formula feeding protected babies against the risk of 'poor' milk, while freeing mothers from the constraints of breast-feeding. Formula-feeding was in the best interests of both the mother and the baby. By contrast, for intending breast-feeders the situation was more complicated. The positive benefits of breast-feeding for the baby's long-term health were in potential conflict with the mother's own autonomy and quality of life. Antenatally, the decision to breastfeed, albeit tentative in some cases, can be seen as a decision to prioritise one set of 'typically relevant features' (the baby's well-being) over another (that of the mother).

In discussing changes in the features which the mothers deemed 'typically relevant', between the first and second interviews, we concentrate on the women who had intended to breastfeed at the antenatal interview. There was no evidence of a shift in either the 'knowledge at hand' or in the practice of those who had intended to formula-feed. By contrast, by the second interview, some features which those originally intending to breastfeed had deemed 'typically relevant', in the first interview, had changed. There was continuity in so far as the women still discussed two categories of features: baby-related features and mother-related features. However, within each category, the particular issues treated as relevant had changed markedly, as had the relationship between mother- and baby-related features.

In the case of baby-related features, the long-term health benefits of breast-feeding were now marginalised. This is not to suggest that the women no longer believed that breast-feeding conferred such benefits on their babies. Rather, in the light of experience, many of the women now believed that the pursuit of such long-term goals was incompatible with, and had to be subordinated to, other, more immediate concerns. A number, who had stopped breast-feeding their babies, expressed their regret or guilt. For example, one said:

> I really wanted to try hard at breast-feeding . . . because I knew that it was the best thing for her . . . I'm quite upset now that I can't do it any longer, but I think it's better for her to be on the bottle if she's gonna grow better and be happier.

All those who had stopped breast-feeding cited their inability to satisfy their baby's hunger. Contrary to their earlier belief that breast-feeding would be 'best', their babies appeared unsettled and hungry or had not gained weight in line with their own expectations or those of health professionals. The following description, from a woman who introduced formula milk two weeks after her baby's birth, illustrates how the features of the situation which she prioritised had changed over time:

> I just wanted him to be satisfied, not crying all the time . . . I had to stop. I had terrible cracked nipples and then I had mastitis. So I persevered through all of that, but he was just too hungry all the time . . . and he lost weight as well. Well, he obviously lost weight but he didn't regain his birth weight . . . I really did want to breastfeed . . . I just wanted to. I just didn't have enough milk to fill him. He was just too hungry.

This woman, who was a nurse, had stressed the long-term health benefits of breast-feeding at the antenatal interview and, as she describes, had continued to breastfeed in the face of considerable personal discomfort. However, faced with her baby's distress and the objective evidence of weight loss, she had changed to formula milk. For her, as for others who turned to formula, making sure that her baby did not 'starve' had replaced longer-term health concerns as the priority. In both cases, the baby's interests were the central concern.

This shift in the 'typically relevant features' element of 'knowledge at hand' between the two interviews extended to the small group who continued to breastfeed. These women also treated their ability to satisfy their babies' hunger as of central relevance to their continued commitment to breast-feeding. In contrast to those who had stopped breast-feeding, however, they pointed to evidence that their babies were indeed satisfied and that their growth and development was not being compromised. The following statement is typical of the women in this group: 'I mean it's very straightforward and, you know, she seems quite happy and she's obviously growing.' These women described breast-feeding as 'straightforward' and 'fine' and their babies as 'good' and 'content'.

We have suggested that, for both those women who continued to breastfeed, and for those who did not, satisfying their babies' current needs had assumed greater relevance than promoting the babies' long-term health. It seems, from the evidence presented so far, that women who continued to breastfeed were able to reconcile these two relevances. They saw satisfying their babies' short-term needs as compatible with promoting their long-term health through breast-feeding. For the women who had given up breast-feeding earlier than intended, these two factors appeared to be irreconcilable. For them, breast-feeding appeared incompatible with satisfying their babies' hunger and they prioritised the latter.

There was, however, one woman who did not seem to fit this pattern. At the antenatal interview, she had declared her intention to breastfeed and, at the second interview was continuing to do so. However, unlike the other breast-feeding mothers, she seemed less than convinced that breast-feeding was meeting her baby's needs. She described the early difficulties she had experienced in feeding her baby. In hospital, the baby appeared uninterested in feeding and, later on, her milk supply did not seem to satisfy him, 'With him being a big baby, there was nothing there.' At the eight-week interview, her concerns were unresolved: 'Then the colic started and I associated that with the feeding, thinking, "Well, perhaps I'm not doing it right, you know. Why is he getting so upset in between feeds?" . . . I got to the stage of thinking he might be allergic to my milk.' Nevertheless, unlike the other mothers who were concerned about whether their babies' needs were being met, she was continuing to breast-feed, eight weeks after her baby's birth. However, when we returned to interview this woman two months later, it became clear that, within days of the previous interview, she had introduced formula-feeding. For her, as for the other mothers, once she came to interpret the baby's behaviour as indicating that he was hungry and that she was unable to satisfy this hunger, the baby's short-term needs became more relevant to her decisions about feeding than concerns about his long-term health. In effect, at the time of the second interview, this woman had been involved in the same attempt to reconcile two conflicting relevances as was described by the other women. Like them, she had ultimately felt unable to do so and, in the end, the long-term benefits of breast-feeding had been eclipsed by the shorter-term concern that her baby should be 'satisfied'.

We identified two kinds of 'typically relevant features' of infant-feeding which were discussed in the antenatal interviews. We have shown how the first of these, features which relate to the baby, underwent a shift between the first and second interviews. Turning to the second kind, features related to the impact of feeding on the mother herself, there is both continuity and discontinuity between the features which were treated as 'typically relevant' in the two interviews. On the one hand, at the second interview, mothers continued to discuss their concerns about the impact of breast-feeding on personal autonomy and social isolation. On the other, in the light of their experience, they now gave more attention to the practical and emotional problems they associated with breast-feeding. These included physical discomfort arising from the birth itself, the seemingly constant and unpredictable demands of the babies, difficulties in persuading the babies to feed, painful breasts, negative reactions of partners and other family members and anxiety about whether the babies were being adequately fed. For most of the women, it was the combination of a number of these problems which had proved particularly difficult. The description which one woman gave of her breast-feeding experience illustrates the point:

> You don't know what you're doing . . . she was so hungry. She was waking up every two hours for a feed . . . I was absolutely shattered . . . I wasn't planning for it to hurt so much . . . I found it really difficult to feed. It was hurting all the time . . . I was so sore and it hurt all the time and I was sort of in tears because I couldn't feed her . . . She was waking up every couple of hours, every hour sometimes and she woke up at three o'clock in the night and I was still feeding her at six and she was still screaming because she obviously wasn't getting it . . . My nipples were so sore that she just got blood all in her mouth because they were bleeding . . . It never stopped hurting . . . I'd had stitches and you're really uncomfortable anyway.

The somewhat abstract concerns about autonomy and freedom which were discussed in the first interview were translated into rather more concrete experiences of pain, discomfort, sleep loss and exhaustion in the second.

In both the antenatal and postnatal interviews, the women treated both baby-related and mother-related features of infant-feeding as 'typically relevant' to their decision about whether to initiate and then sustain breast-feeding. In the first interview, women who intended to breastfeed saw a conflict between the interests of the mother and those of the baby, and prioritised the latter. In the second interviews, it was not only the features which were deemed to be relevant which had changed, as discussed above, but also the relationship between mother- and baby-related features. The women were less likely to see the needs of the mother and the baby as being in competition. As one woman put it, 'If it's good for the mother, it's good for the baby.' This applied to both the mothers who had given up breast-feeding and to those who continued to breastfeed. While those continuing to breastfeed acknowledged some inconvenience and temporary loss of autonomy, they saw breast-feeding as bringing pleasure and satisfaction to both mother and baby. Doing what they considered to be in the baby's best interests coincided with meeting their own needs. Similarly, the women who had changed to formula-feeding presented this as a solution to both parties' needs. A number described the ways in which the incessant demands and sleep deprivation, which they had experienced while breast-feeding, compromised the care which they could give to their baby. Introducing formula was a solution not only to the babies' problems but also to their own. Both groups of mothers had arrived at a solution which, while it was not always their preferred option, or the one which they would have taken 'all things being equal', was presented as being in the best interests of both parties. It was no longer a question of setting the baby's interests against those of the mother, as it had been in the first interview.

We have taken issue with the second definition (choice as an act) since it fails to do justice to the dynamic and processual nature of women's decisions about how to feed their babies. We have made use of Schutz's concept of 'knowledge at hand' to show how the constituent elements of such knowledge ('typically similar acts' and 'typically relevant features') change as women move from deliberating about infant-feeding, before they are in a position to act, to acting on the basis of their deliberations, and subsequently reflecting on their acts.

Choice as the power, right or faculty of choosing

The third definition raises further doubts about whether 'choice' is an appropriate concept for this study of infant-feeding practices. Most initiatives designed to 'improve' infant-feeding appear to be premised on the assumption, implicit in this definition of choice, that women have the power to implement their own preferences about how their babies will be fed. Conceptualising women's feeding practices as individual choices in this way emphasises mothers' responsibility for the outcome of such practices. If women know what is 'best' for their babies and yet feed them differently, they are assumed to be 'choosing' to put their babies' interests second. We are arguing that it is misleading to treat women's feeding practices as the simple expression of individualistic preferences. Rather, such practices reflect the material and sociocultural contexts in which their decisions are made. The risk of defining such decisions as choices is that we camouflage the constraints under which women deliberate and act. Such constraints form part of the 'scheme of reference' within which women come to feed their babies in particular ways (Schutz 1970: 72).

Most obviously, perhaps, women's 'choices' about how to feed their babies are subject to material constraints. For example, one woman described how, having bought one packet of baby food at the beginning of the week, she had to eke it out until her next benefit payment was due. Another, who did not have access to a kitchen, could not prepare fresh foods for her baby. However, the impact of economic factors on infant-feeding was more often indirect. Of the 36 women in the study, 23 had returned to work before their babies' second birthdays and a number saw this as a financial necessity which overrode personal preferences. Returning to work meant losing some power to 'choose' how their babies were fed. In particular, where mothers depended on others to care for their babies, their power to choose what their babies ate was dependent on the carer's cooperation. This was a particular problem where family or friends cared for the baby. As such arrangements depended on good will, it was difficult for women to insist on their baby being fed in the way they chose. Where women purchased child care, they felt in a stronger position to insist. One woman explained, 'When I go back to work I'm hoping my baby's going to a childminder . . . I can dictate and say, "I want them to have this. I want them to have that. Could you do this?" Whereas I feel if it was a relative, or particularly my Mum, you're not in the same position.'

Such material constraints are not the only way in which women's power to choose is limited. Feeding decisions are made in particular sociocultural contexts which incorporate belief systems transmitted by parents, teachers and other members of the community (Berger and Luckmann 1966). These belief systems constrain behaviour 'by means of commonsense notions of what is "natural" as well as through moral precepts of what is good, right and appropriate' (Evetts 1966: 9). Such shared beliefs include not only abstract ideas but also 'trustworthy recipes for interpreting the social world and for handling things and men in order to obtain the best results in every situation' (Schutz 1970: 81). Such beliefs constrain people's power to make individualistic choices at two levels. First, culture is internalised by individuals and literally limits what actions are thinkable. Individuals conform to cultural norms not because they are forced to, but because it does not occur to them to think otherwise – they take them for granted. Such taken-for-granted assumptions have a high degree of moral force. It may simply not occur to those who hold them that it is possible to act differently. The power of such constraints lies in their very invisibility. They predefine our experience. Second, even where individuals challenge such predefinitions and redefine experience, they may be dissuaded from acting on such redefinitions by negative reactions which they anticipate from others. Such reactions include potential disapproval, loss of prestige, ridicule or even contempt (Berger 1963).

This interaction between internalised constraints and the anticipated negative reactions of others is illustrated by the reluctance which women in our study expressed about breast-feeding their babies in front of others. The consensus was that breast-feeding in public was 'not an accepted thing'. While a few women were determined to ignore the reactions of others, most identified some people with whom, or places in which, they would feel unable to breastfeed. For some, this reluctance reflected their own sense that feeding in front of others was inappropriate or embarrassing. They described it as 'flashing your flesh' or 'flicking it out' or 'baring all'. This half-joking use of crude expressions, with ambiguous overtones of sexuality, can be seen as reflecting the unease which was generated as the women contemplated transgressing an internalised cultural norm. However, even where the women themselves felt comfortable about breast-feeding in front of others, most felt constrained by anticipated negative reactions from others. One said that other people, 'still tend to think, "Oh God, look at that woman". You know they sort of find it a bit obscene.' Another resented such reactions and yet felt that she would be constrained by them. She said, 'I feel quite angry actually . . . what is so sinful about feeding your baby? I mean you're actually sustaining it . . . I think it's a very weird society we're in.' However, when she was asked if this meant she would feed her baby in public, she replied, 'No, I don't think I would. I think that's what makes me annoyed.' Thus identifying certain cultural norms as inappropriate did not necessarily free women from their constraining power.

The complex interplay of material and cultural factors in limiting women's power to make individualistic choices about how their babies will be fed is illustrated by the distribution of formula-feeding by material position. In our sample, as in the large scale studies (e.g. White, Freeth and O'Brien 1992), it was the women on the lowest incomes who were most likely to formula-feed their babies. Given the cost of bottles, sterilising equipment and formula-feed, this appears odd. At first sight, we might expect those who have least money to spare to choose breast-feeding. It is only when we recognise the constraining power of both internalised cultural assumptions, about what is proper and decent, and the anticipated reactions of others, if we contravene such assumptions, that these women's decision to formula-feed their babies becomes understandable.

Conceptualising women's feeding practices as reflecting the exercise of women's 'power, right or faculty to choose' how their babies will be fed ignores the multiple ways in which their freedom to choose is constrained. This is not to argue for social determinism. Within the constraints, women do have some scope for manoeuvre. Cultural contexts are not straitjackets. As Schutz (1970: 84) has argued, individuals 'stand at the intersection of several social circles'. Each social circle may have belief systems which differ in subtle or substantial ways. Such inconsistencies can offer individuals space to exercise choice. On the one hand, where, as with friendship groups, membership is voluntary, individuals may choose to associate themselves with groups whose belief system they find most congenial. For example, some of the women in our study who had stopped breast-feeding described how they actively avoided contact with those who might disapprove. On the other hand, where, as with most families, membership is given rather than chosen, individuals may exercise choice about the way in which they rank the 'private order of relevances in which each of [their] memberships in various groups has its rank' (Schutz 1970: 85), privileging the belief system of one of the group over that of another. Similarly, material constraints are rarely absolute. It is usually possible to imagine ways of sidestepping such constraints, although the cost of doing so may be significant. For example, the women who returned to work after their babies' birth were not literally compelled to do so. For many of them, however, not returning to work would involve undesirable consequences, including loss of the family home, lowered living standards and an inability to provide adequately for the baby. Thus, implementing one choice would entail abandoning another. Power to exercise choice is also unevenly distributed. For example, women with high incomes or extensive social support networks, may experience greater freedom to pursue their preferences, and to reconcile competing preferences, than lone mothers with low incomes or little support.

Conclusion

In this chapter, we explored some of the problems with attempting to conceptualise women's feeding practices as choices. We suggested that while women clearly do decide between possibilities when it comes to feeding their babies, conceptualising such decisions as choices runs the dual risks of distracting attention from the processual nature of such decisions and the way in which they are made and remade over time, reflecting the inevitable shifts in women's 'knowledge at hand', and of ascribing to women a power to implement individualistic preferences which takes no account of the material and cultural contexts within which they act.

Acknowledgements

We are grateful to the women and health professionals who took part in this study and to Alan Aldridge, Robert Dingwall, Julia Evetts and Anne Murcott for comments on earlier drafts of this chapter.

Note

1   We have elected to refer to commercial milk feeds as 'formula-feeds' rather than using the more common British term 'bottle feeding'. This is to emphasise the content rather than the method of delivery of feeds. Some study women who breastfed their babies also gave expressed breast milk by bottle. We rejected the term 'artificial feeding' because of its potentially pejorative connotations.

CHAPTER 16

Food choice and culture in a cosmopolitan city: South Asians, Italians and other Glaswegians

Rory Williams, Helen Bush, Mike Lean,
Annie S. Anderson and Hannah Bradby

Introduction: food choice, culture and cuisine

The first question faced by a sociologist or social anthropologist about food choice is whether, and where, it is a choice at all. Fischler (1988) has made much of the existential dilemma created by man's omnivorous capacity, which imposes the necessity of choice. But this is a dilemma from which we may be delivered by culture. By storing up hunting, gathering, agricultural or trading knowledge, by organising production, by elaborating the meaning attached to meals, and by making available a stock of recipes for converting the raw into the cooked, while avoiding the further hazard of consuming the rotten (Lévi-Strauss 1965), culture creates the basis of a cuisine (Goody 1982).

The question of food choice thus becomes a question about the ways in which cultures and cuisines, and the economic systems to which they are related, either create or limit choice. Our 'Nation's Diet' project on 'Dietary change among South Asians and Italians in Glasgow' compares data relevant to this point from two minorities and the general Glasgow population. The marked cultural variation in food choice brought about by migration to cosmopolitan centres of affluence is an underdeveloped but potentially vast topic, and the data available are scarce and uneven (Mennell, Murcott and van Otterloo 1992: ch. 10), though the topic is important to health and health services as well as to the food industry. This chapter seeks to open up the topic, while containing it within manageable dimensions in two ways. First, we use as our main illustrations the situation of the two minorities we studied, both originating in peasant-based economies, but one deriving from the post-colonial Indian sub-continent, and the other from western Europe. This comparison can help to illumine issues that are common to widely differing ethnic minorities. Second, given the patchiness of the evidence, the chapter starts from the relatively extensive world data on body size and shape, which as the product of eating and exercise patterns presents the tangible outcome of many important patterns of

267

food choice. This tactic also has the advantage of linking the sociology of food with an outcome of considerable interest to health (*Journal of the Royal College of Physicians of London* 1983), although we only consider those implications incidentally in this chapter.

The first way in which cultures and cuisines affect choice is through the systems of food production which they employ. Today one of the biggest differences is between those which use peasant methods of production, from which migrants often come, and those characterised by large-scale commercial agriculture, and by capitalist methods of distributing and merchandising food, to which migrants have often gone. Peasant production is adapted to local conditions, and the cuisine is usually formed by a substantial staple (typically high in carbohydrate and limited in other nutrients), a vegetable accompaniment including legumes (beans, lentils, peas) which complete the balance of dietary protein, and a relish of some kind, which may include meat or fish, normally occasional or in small quantities if present at all, and/or a spicy, herbal or other flavoured sauce (Mintz 1992). The major challenge which some form of capitalist economic system presents to such a cuisine is a great increase in the supply of foods with high fat and sugar content, often derived by extractive processes and with long shelf life. One sign of this is a corresponding increase in the percentage of nutrient intake in the popular diet derived from fat. Whether this opportunity for a higher proportion of fat in the diet is taken by incoming migrant groups, and why it is taken by some groups and not by others, is a first important question about food choice that was of interest in our project.

Today few systems of food supply rely solely on peasant production; however, there are many areas where peasants are still the main suppliers, and thus the main influence on the cuisine. Such areas can be identified by their high proportion of smallholding farmers, and by the substantial additional population of tradesmen and small businessmen who are engaged in providing services and retail outlets to these farmers in local market towns. An area in which these two groups form the majority of the population may be described as a peasant-based economy, certainly as a peasant-based food economy. These areas still sustain peasant cuisines which migrants carry with them as their starting point.

Next, once migrants have arrived in a Western city, the economic system of the majority culture also creates or limits food choice through the range of occupations and incomes obtainable – often those at the bottom end of the market. Indeed, in so far as there are social classes which inherit and pass on different occupational chances, there may turn out to be lifelong limits on the diet that unlucky migrants and their children can choose. Responses to these limits may be critical. A classic response of the poor, much discussed by nineteenth-century econ- omists, is to raise the proportion of their income devoted to food, and especially to those foods perceived as necessities. But that means that less must be spent on something else, and the trade-offs between food and other heads of consumption in the family budget must therefore form an important topic. Alternatively, an opposite strategy is to cut down on food in favour of other heads of expenditure, or for particular members of the family to cut down on food.

However, the choice available in a cuisine also depends on the values of the group that shares food. For Max Weber, one of the three founders of the discipline of sociology, sharing food is, together with alliance by marriage, the chief marker of the division of society into communal groups of similar status or ethnic identity (Weber 1948). The meaning of food is thus a topic which is typically very close to the sacred symbols of a community. Just as a meal is the focal sacred action in Christianity, so it is also in Sikhism; and feasts mark the most solemn moments of the calendar not only in these religions but also in Judaism, Islam, Hinduism and many other cases. The meal defines both the group who share and those who do not, and divides the latter into those who are owed a duty of hospitality (Pitt-Rivers 1977), and (only too often) those others who are categorically outside the community (Douglas 1966).

Ethnic divisions are usually in a state of varying tension with the division of society into classes based on the means of production (Hechter 1978). But to the extent that ethnic divisions come to coincide with class divisions, creating a marked ethnic division of labour, as has occurred for example with Black Americans, the strength of collective ethnic identity and its corresponding expression in diet is likely to be reinforced; and the food choices of the excluded minority on low incomes are also especially likely to be limited.

Finally, within the food-sharing group, there is also often a division of labour by gender, typically setting up an exchange relationship, involving food, within marriage or some equivalent of marriage. In sharply segregated forms of this relationship, such as have been documented both in the peasant societies from which many migrants come and in conservative groups in the West, it has typically been the women who preserve and pass on the knowledge of preparing and cooking food, and who make the meal in accordance with the preferences of others, as their primary gift in exchange for the gift of the raw materials deemed to be provided by the men (Murcott 1983a). But this is only one of many possible forms of gender division of labour (Goody 1982), and there are many variants, not least those which have resulted from feminist experiments in the West in the last few decades. Naturally all these arrangements are charged with the emotive symbolism of relations between the sexes.

This brings our introduction back to the point from which we set out: the meaning of food choice within sociology and social anthropology, especially in the context of migration to a cosmopolitan Western city. Perhaps the key issue is that some cultures tend to prescribe food choice, and some to leave choice as open as possible. The latter option – maximum choice – is at least theoretically propounded in many capitalist economies. The former option – a fixed choice, usually invested with collective meanings – is often assumed in peasant societies, and by regional, ethnic or religious communities with strong collective bonds and identities within capitalist economies. Weber described patterns of action determined along these strong collective lines as traditional (Weber 1947: ch. 1.2). Clearly these patterns of action cannot be described as choices in the sense usually assumed under capitalism. Nor is choice in this sense a very appropriate term for the food prescribed by the symbolism of the gender division of labour – for the most part, it seems to fall under what Weber called emotional patterns of action. Rather, the capitalist form of food choice assumes what Weber called rational modes of action, in the limited sense that an apparently rational calculus is undertaken of the pleasures and costs of alternative means of feeding, and of the opportunity costs they imply for other ends, such as the chance to go out to work. In matters of food, this individual calculus is often ethnically, not to say ethnocentrically, specific to Western cultures, if indeed it applies even there.

Otherwise we are forced to consider something more akin to cultural rather than individual food choices. Culture need no longer be seen as something external, rigid and unchanging, passively received by a population of cultural 'dopes' (Ahmad 1996). Instead, a fluid notion of culture is re-emerging, as something in constant movement, collectively negotiated, reinterpreted and reachieved, from stocks of knowledge held broadly in common, through mutual sanctions of approval and criticism (Kelleher 1996). Many situations also now show an interesting mixture of individual and cultural choices, as members of minorities with an attachment to their own natal group, but with a repertoire extended by multicultural contacts, seek to negotiate practices which can both fulfil their individual strategies for living and at the same time receive the sanction of their culture. In this sense, they are engaging in 'cultural strategies' (Bradby 1996).

In what follows, then, we focus primarily on varieties of food choice in the cultural situation of ethnic minorities in the affluent West. This involves considering how different kinds of food choice are influenced by:

1 world patterns of food production
2 social class and occupation
2 ethnic divisions and sense of identity
4 religious ideas and the gender division of labour.

These issues are considered in relation both to the literature and to our own study in 'The Nation's Diet' programme.

The study on dietary change among South Asians and Italians in Glasgow

We compared women with descent from the Indian subcontinent (South Asians), those with descent from Italy, and the general population. The dietary patterns of these groups, the way they used up their food energy in work and exercise, and their resulting body size and shape, were of particular interest because these things are relevant to health, and to heart disease in particular. South Asians in Britain have high levels of coronary heart disease and Italians low, compared with the general population.

Women were studied because they are more involved in food preparation, and at the same time share most of the relevant ethnic differences in diet, exercise and body fat with men. The sample of 259 women was formed in five subgroups:

1 63 South Asians born abroad
2 56 South Asians born in Britain
3 39 Italians born abroad
4 51 Italians born in Britain
5 50 general population.controls

These sub-groups were sampled randomly by maiden name and country of birth from birth registrations in West of Scotland Health Boards, with small supplements by snowballing to complete numbers in the Italian subgroups. Ages were restricted to the range 20 to 42. Data were provided by a structured sociological interview lasting two to two-and-a-half hours, with pretranslated schedules as needed, physical measures of height, weight, waist, hip and triceps skinfold thickness, and a seven-day weighed diary of food intake.

In what follows, we consider the literature on the themes already set out in the introduction to this chapter, present some of our main findings under each theme, and comment on directions for the future.

The influence of food supply on diet and body image

Where food is relatively scarce, fatness is often considered a desirable attribute and an appropriate consideration in food choice, especially among women, on whom our study was focused. It is primarily in the industrialised societies that fatness is disparaged as obesity, though even for Western women thinness as the ideal is a twentieth-century notion. In societies where a woman can only attain status through motherhood, female obesity can symbolise fertility and nurturing, since adequate fat deposits are required for successful reproduction (Brown and Konner 1987). Female plumpness can also act as a symbol of male economic status, demonstrating a husband's ability to provide 'wealth and survival where food is scarce' (Fallon 1990: 84). Similarly some peasant societies equate fatness with health. For example, the Punjabi greeting 'You look fresh and fat today' (Nasser 1988: 574; Fallon 1990: 95) illustrates the positive value that has been ascribed to surplus body fat in some South Asian cultures, while in Greece plumpness has been indicative of well-being and good fortune (Hirschon 1989)

As far as Europe is concerned, Trowell (1975) has argued that obesity was not widespread before the eighteenth century. The food shortages or irregular food supplies experienced in the Middle Ages by the mass of Western Europe's population (Mennell, Murcott and van Otterloo 1992) would have precluded obesity. Even so, though it could seldom have been achieved, surplus body fat was evidently valued since the ideal female shape was full-bodied:

> Between 1400 and 1700, the maternal role was idealized, and fat was considered both fashionable and erotic. Womanhood was equated with motherhood . . . Beauty images portrayed matronly plumpness, full nurturant breasts, and the earthy, fruitful look of a Botticelli nymph. (Freedman 1986)

There is an obvious parallel with the symbolism of female obesity in peasant societies: it demonstrated economic and reproductive security.

By the Restoration it was less easy for the élite to be differentiated by the volume of food they ate (Mennell, Murcott and van Otterloo 1992). The food supply was improving in the next levels of social ranking, so that 'social distinction came to be expressed more through the quality and refinement of cooking than through sheer quantitative stuffing'. Self-control had become important in courtly society, and thereafter in the professions and bourgeoisie who depended on it. As the means to achieve surplus body fat became available to lower-ranking groups, so those of high rank began to distinguish themselves from the rest of society by symbolising self-control in slimness.

Thus by the nineteenth century, obesity was a matter of concern for the upper classes, although advice on how to gain weight continued to be directed through the press to the lower middle classes (Mennell 1985). Similarly, in the United States some women were still anxious about being too thin (Fallon 1990). After the First World War, however, when the means to achieve surplus body fat had become available to the majority of people in the industrialised societies, a boyish figure became *de rigueur* so that there was a virtual absence of female secondary sexual characteristics. Thereafter perceptions of the ideal female body shape fluctuated between varying slim shapes, perhaps the most extreme period being the 1960s and 1970s when Twiggy (the fashion model Lesley Hornby), weighing approximately six-and-a-half stone, was the model for many women. At a time of worldwide concern with overpopulation:

> Slimness became a sign of emancipation, a symbol of nonreproductive sexuality and independence. The accent shifted to looking like a play-girl rather than an earth mother. (Freedman 1986)

It is arguably as a result of these changes in body image that the body size associated with wealth has contrasted markedly in peasant economies and industrial societies. Numerous studies have shown that in industrialised countries, women of wealth and high social standing are likely to be thin. Poorer children are thinner than the better-off before puberty but by mid-adolescence, poorer females become fatter and more affluent females become thinner (Garn and Clark 1976). The relationship between socioeconomic status and obesity is inconsistent for Western men. By contrast, high socioeconomic status is associated with obesity for adults and children in non-industrialised societies, and although there are some methodological limitations, the finding is consistent across several continents (Sobal and Stunkard 1989).

The Glasgow study

As we expected, migrant South Asians and Italians in our study came from peasant-based economies as these are defined in our introduction: they were born predominantly in farming villages or agricultural market towns within one or two specific regions: the Italians in hill country, in the area of Frosinone to the east of the Roman Campagna or the area of Barga in Tuscany, the South Asians in the East (Indian) and the West (Pakistani) Punjab, mostly the latter. Similarly our evidence of property ownership identifies the bulk of both migrant groups as originating either in peasant families working their own land, or in small business families owning their own premises.

The food supply of these regions is not scarce in peasant terms, but it is restricted compared with what is available in capitalist urban centres; and the diet is of the low fat/high carbohydrate type outlined in our introduction. Although contemporary Mediterranean diets are no longer as close to the 'reference' Mediterranean diet of the 1950s and 1960s as they are supposed to be, Portugal remains closest, as indexed by a mean intake of 33 per cent of total energy from fat, followed by Italy at 36 per cent (Fidanza 1990). Percentages of fat in Indian diets are much lower still (Achaya 1987).

Among the migrants to Glasgow in our own project, only migrant Italians, with a mean of 36 per cent of energy from fat, had the same percentage as in their country of origin (Anderson et al. 1995). Migrant South Asians were already taking in a much higher percentage of energy from fat (42 per cent) than is typical of the rural diet in North India, and a significantly higher percentage than migrant Italians, and similarly had higher total energy intakes. Since they also reported low levels of exercise, their waist and waist/hip measures were correspondingly large. This raises in a pointed form the question of our introduction: why one group from a peasant-based economy should have increased their fat intake (and incidentally become subject to high levels of heart disease), while the other continued to restrict it (and remained with low levels of heart disease).

As this section implies, we found that one way in which the two groups differed was in their attitudes to large body size, though this did not come about quite in the way that the literature on these topics would lead us to expect. Migrants in either cultural group identified slim figures as symbolic of social success both in the occupational

273

and the marital sphere. In this respect, any previous experience of a restricted food supply had evidently had little weight. However beliefs about what is healthy, especially what is healthy for the purposes of reproduction, proved slower to change. Many Punjabi migrants continued to regard plump figures as indicative of eating good and healthy food and being likely to have healthy children; the great majority of Italian migrants, on the other hand, regarded slim figures as indicative of these things (Bush *et al*. forthcoming).

Even if slimness as a sign of occupational and marital success is generally accepted among British minorities, therefore, it looks very much as if slimness as a health choice may still be closely related to previous experience of a secure food supply. Among Italian migrants there was no sign that grandmothers had been thin, but among South Asians there was some indication that this had been so. It is plausible that the memory of food scarcity is relatively distant in the highly developed European food market, even in regions which have residual peasantries. Moreover, in the data of 'The Nation's Diet' study, Italian migrants were financially better-off even than the general population, and South Asians were not, while in earlier data South Asians emerged as considerably worse off (Williams, Bhopal and Hunt 1994).

Health beliefs and preferences concerning body size, and their background in experiences of economic insecurity, will therefore be a topic of considerable interest for the future. Our study has made a case for suspecting that these patterns of thought and experience correspond to major differences in heart disease.

Influence of social class and occupation on food choice

In the relationship between social class and obesity in the West, Sobal and Stunkard (1989) see dieting and dietary restraint as probably the most important mediating variable. Women of low social class may not have the money and sense of control needed to use the more expensive foods seen as necessary for dieting, or to join weight-control programmes; they may also be less educated, and so have less knowledge of nutrition and dieting, and be less committed to the view that slimness is desirable. In addition, though, financial insecurity may act to restrict leisure time, recreational exercise and awareness of the benefits of exercise.

Psychosocial stress may also be a factor in body shape associated with socioeconomic position, possibly operating through dietary behaviour at least in part. Fat laid down in the abdominal area – known as 'central' fat – has been found to be associated with low socioeconomic status in Hispanic minorities (Georges, Mueller and Wear 1991). In Swedish women, a higher waist/hip ratio has been found in association with disturbed sleep, tranquilliser and anti-depressant drug use, and with psychosomatic and psychiatric illness, and stress-induced increases in the levels of adrenal corticosteroids and catecholamines may interact to promote the laying-down of abdominal fat (Bjorntorp 1987). These processes could occur in those experiencing feelings of hopelessness and lack of control in 'the poorest sectors of minority and immigrant populations experiencing difficult economic circumstances, cultural change, and discrimination' (Georges, Mueller and Wear 1991).

There are alternative possibilities. Sobal and Stunkard cite studies which show the prevalence of obesity to be significantly lower among women who have been upwardly mobile (Goldblatt, Moore and Stunkard 1965; Braddon *et al.* 1986). Rimm and Rimm (1974) also found that women with the lowest levels of education who married highly educated men were less obese than similar women who married men with low levels of education. Again, family transmission of wealth may coincide with genetic predisposition to slimness, and may in this way contribute to the relationship between social class and obesity (Stunkard 1988; Stunkard *et al.* 1990).

Nevertheless there are grounds for suspecting that in the West a low social class position reduces the chances of controlling obesity and central fat; and determinants of low social class position among minorities are to be found not least in the occupational structure. In Britain, for example, in many cases, migrant workers found jobs in declining industries such as textiles and metal manufacture which were able to stay in production through the payment of low wages. At a time of full employment these jobs were unwanted by the indigenous population (Miles 1982). Service industries such as hospitals and public transport also offered work which by reason of low pay and unsocial hours was unwanted (Maan 1992).

As a result of this history, previous studies of the labour market position of ethnic minorities have shown them to occupy lower level and more poorly paid posts than White workers. The Labour Force Survey (LFS) (Jones 1993) does not describe the present economic circumstances of Italian migrants and their descendants but it does describe those of South Asians. The 1988–1990 Labour Force Survey reveals a complicated pattern of male employment in that some minority groups, African Asians and Indians, for example, now have similar or better job levels than White male employees, while other groups such as Pakistanis and Bangladeshis (who also came later) are likely to occupy considerably lower positions in semi-skilled or unskilled jobs.

Unemployment patterns mirror this picture. Comparison of the 1982 (Brown 1984) and 1988–1990 (Jones 1993) Labour Force Surveys shows that, generally speaking, the gap between unemployment rates of ethnic minorities and Whites has closed, but that the degree of improvement is not shared equally by all ethnic groups. The 1988–1990 LFS shows African Asian (8 per cent), Indian (11 per cent) and White (8 per cent) males to have very similar rates, but Pakistanis (22 per cent) and Bangladeshis (25 per cent) continue to experience relatively high rates of unemployment, as do Pakistani women (25 per cent) compared to Indian (12 per cent), African Asian (10 per cent) and White (7 per cent) women.

However the insecure position we have documented for many Black and minority ethnic groups in the British labour market also elicits strategies for earning a living outside the labour market, which may affect food choice in other ways. Self-employment can be a strategy for survival when waged employment in the formal sector is not available (Morokvasic 1993). With the decline in full employment nationally and difficulties in obtaining better jobs because of racism, self-employment becomes what has been described as 'a strategy to avoid competition with whites in a restricted labour market' (Jones 1993: 153; cf. Miles 1982). It is intriguing to find that Italians in Britain once faced a similar situation:

> Owing to hostility and solidarity from the local trades unions and craft societies, the Italians were only tolerated if they offered something distinctive and non-competitive. Even in the labouring sector, only asphalting, a particularly dirty and arduous job, was open to Italians, since opposition to migrant labour was strong and, in any case, the Irish had a monopoly on most areas of heavy, unskilled work (Colpi 1991: 58)

The Italians found a niche catering to the public, initially through selling chestnuts and ice-cream on the streets and later through the establishment of cafés.

Self-employment may have different sorts of consequences from those of low social class, in terms of long hours worked and related patterns of food consumption. A possible consequence of this pattern of male work is a segregated domestic division of labour which leaves women responsible for the care of the family, housework and food preparation. The Scottish Office Survey (Smith 1991) confirms the comparatively high number (66 per cent) of Pakistani women, and to a lesser extent Indian women (50 per cent), who reported that they were looking after the home and family, compared with White women (26 per cent). This may mean that more time is spent by women on preparing food.

The Glasgow study

We have already noted that in earlier Glasgow data South Asians were relatively poor (though this was not unequivocally so in 'The Nation's Diet' data). There are historical indications that this may also have been the pattern in the early days of the Italian migration. However, our study found that Italian migrants are no longer poor, and it may be that they benefit from the social position now achieved by the generations born in Britain.

Is the tendency of Glasgow South Asian migrant women to bigger waist and waist/hip measures, to a higher energy intake and low levels of exercise, related to their considerably lower income compared with

Italians? This is possible, but in our 'Nation's Diet' study the equally low income of British-born South Asians and general population women is not attended by similar effects. We also need to allow for the concurrent effect in the migrant generation of the different South Asian and Italian attitudes to body size, described in the last section, and for the differing views of exercise, described in the next section. Our analysis of this complex issue is not yet complete. It is, however, already clear that responses to relative poverty in terms of food choice are not simple. For example, migrant South Asians spend a high proportion of their relatively low income on food. Although Italians in Britain have a much higher income, migrants from both South Asian and Italian backgrounds engage in hospitality much more frequently than general population women, and the meals they make are more elaborate (Bush et al. 1996). In these respects their practice corresponds less with income differences and more with the central symbolic im-portance of food in the peasant-based economies from which they come.

This takes us to the other questions of this section: are the meals made by South Asians and Italians more elaborate generally, not only when giving hospitality but also on everyday occasions – and is this connected with a greater household commitment among the women? If so, is this a consequence of long hours of self-employed work among the men? Our pilot study of the dietary habits of migrant South Asian (chiefly Sikh) women in Glasgow already showed the continued importance of home-prepared, traditional food, particularly for the evening meal, in marked contrast to the practices of general population women who seldom prepare a main meal solely from fresh ingredients (Anderson and Lean 1995). Such a meal would consist typically of chappatti and at least one curry dish, and although food preparation might be undertaken by more than one female household member, the nature and quantity of the food would require a considerable input of time and effort, particularly in an extended family. This is borne out by the main study in our 'Nation's Diet' project, which showed that the time spent preparing and cooking food, although it was similar in all ethnic groups at the weekend, was more extensive among South Asians during the week (Bush et al. 1995). This is not to say that convenience foods such as fish fingers, pizza and super-noodles are not common in the middle of the day (Anderson and Lean 1995). But this itself may reflect the care of children and a high domestic work load, especially since domestic appliances to alleviate the work load may not be a common feature of many poorer South Asian households (Brah 1993).

Results from our study show that the extra time taken by South Asian women in cooking is part of a broader commitment to the household. A much smaller proportion go out to work. Where differences exist between women of South Asian background in responsibility for household tasks, they are likely to place more tasks on the woman, for example washing dishes. An interesting exception, though, is that shopping is one task which husbands of migrant South Asian women will commonly undertake, and it is notable that this task belongs to the public, not the private, sphere (Williams et al. 1996).

Whether this relatively segregated division of labour among South Asians is affected by self-employment is a complex issue. Self-employment on its own is not the catalyst, since Italians are equally likely to be self-employed. But Italians are also better-off, which might make it easier to get help in the house; and it may be that self-employment at low levels of income, as among British South Asians, is particularly constraining. Obviously, though, analysis of this topic has also to take into account religious conceptions of the male and female role, and we deal with this in the last section of this chapter.

Influence of ethnic divisions on food choice

Ignorance, discrimination and hostility from the ethnic majority often shape the experience of ethnic minorities, with potential knock-on effects on their dietary patterns. Data on these ethnic divisions are particularly poor. British data are limited by a general tendency in the literature to assume that ethnic minorities are not White. This tendency is a recent phenomenon. Some of the oldest data in the British Census are country-of-birth tables, in which minorities like the Italians and South Asians figure equally. However, the more recent Census and other official formulations of ethnicity single out those from 'new' commonwealth countries. This is indicative of a process of racialisation, similar to that long established in the American Census, but more associated with the concept of 'race relations' (Miles 1982: 168–9). Like Irish and Jewish migrants, Italians have not been the subject of 'race relations' terminology, despite discrimination.

Although Italians are not immune from racism, in the absence of specific data the present racialised context suggests that South Asians must suffer more, and Pakistanis and their British-born families seem to be particularly subject to racial discrimination and harassment, to which they have responded by increasing their self-reliance and autonomy (Werbner 1990). While members of the Indian Workers Association have been encouraged by their leaders to participate in some British institutions, Pakistani organisations have highlighted 'nationalistic, religious and cultural aspects and so had a somewhat negative effect on the degree of participation in indigenous institutions' (Anwar 1979: 182). Thus discrimination may lead to a re-emphasis of South Asian, particularly Muslim, cultural and religious traits.

Within this context of action and reaction, any ignorance, discrimination or hostility from the ethnic majority may have an impact on dietary balance and the effects of food choice in various ways. First, there is the fact that the ethnic majority's culture has a dominant influence on the food supply, both in the shops and in institutional menus (Bush and Williams forthcoming). The assumptions unconsciously built in to the food supply are illustrated by the difficulties experienced by Muslims in decoding information about additives to determine whether food is *halal* or not (Bradby 1996). Second, there is the fact that the majority culture dominates the food information which is made available by health professionals, and the assumptions built in to this apparently scientific process are illustrated by the incapacity of many health professionals to give appropriate advice to minorities on food (Bush and Williams forthcoming). Factors such as these tend to keep minority diets compartmentalised; then if in addition ethnic divisions do lead to a re-emphasis on cultural and religious traits, the collective symbolic values attached to food may be reinforced at the expense of individual preferences.

Again, changes in exercise levels may have drastic effects on body shape if there is no corresponding change in diet, and in this respect choices about food and exercise are two halves of a conceptual whole. Several studies like ours have shown that British South Asians take low levels of physical exercise and there may be two possibly interdependent explanations for this: discrimination on the part of the majority culture, or different priorities among South Asians.

Discrimination may influence every aspect of the lives of ethnic minorities. At one level, for example, it may lead to the attitudes and unofficial policies Anwar (1979) describes, which discourage minorities from using social facilities. At a more extreme level, discrimination may be manifested in verbal and physical abuse, resulting in:

> an individual or family living in fear, subject to humiliation, stress and physical danger . . . What was a home becomes a prison . . . options are reduced as lives are reorganised to minimise the number of dangerous journeys. (Home Affairs Committee Report 1986, cited in Clark, Peach and Vertovec 1990).

When an individual is denied even the simple exercise of walking outdoors, travelling to sports facilities may be unthinkable.

At the same time, there is little tradition of Muslim or other South Asian women participating in leisure activities outside the home, other than visiting family (Jeffery 1976), and external hostility would tend to re-establish this pattern in Britain. Given the arduous nature of the work of rural South Asian women (Jeffery *et al.* 1989) there would be neither the need nor the time for recreational exercise. This would apply equally to women in the villages of southern Italy, for whom leisure exercise is not an accepted notion (Colpi 1991), and indeed to much of the indigenous British working class. Even when the idea of leisure exercise takes root, special arrangements for women may be necessary for reasons of modesty. If, however, the exercise formerly taken in agricultural or other work is not replaced by leisure exercise, either dietary intake has to change quite drastically, or body shape changes drastically instead.

These are all ways in which ethnic divisions in urban centres may affect food choice in ethnic minorities. However, the direction of influence in an ethnically complex society is not all one way. Members of the majority culture also begin to perceive options for their way of living which are created by the cultures of the minorities, and food is one of the areas where minority influence is first felt, as the frequency of restaurant work in minority occupations testifies.

The Glasgow study

In our Glasgow study, the collective symbolic values attaching to traditional forms of family hospitality were particularly strong among South Asians, persisting among the British-born in a way not found among Italians (Bush *et al.* 1996). Correspondingly, these South Asian women were a more encapsulated group than the Italians in their linguistic and marriage patterns; but we found no evidence that this is caused by an experience of hostility, which in these data was no more evident in the lives of South Asians than of Italians or general population women, possibly because of the close protection of young South Asian mothers within the enclave. Other Glasgow data have in fact suggested a greater experience of mugging and assault among South Asian women (Williams, Bhopal and Hunt 1994), so this question remains open.

Similarly, information differences were more prominent in restricting the patterns of exercise than barriers to action such as the fear of going out. South Asians were much less likely than Italians or controls to ascribe exercise a role in heart disease, were much less aware of the exercise facilities available, and more likely to say that there was no barrier to their using the exercise facilities they knew.

In some ways, ethnic divisions were less evident than ethnic interchange; this was particularly apparent when we considered the hospitality meals of women from the Glasgow general population. Along with a tendency to choose easy meals for family hospitality ran a tendency, predominantly in the ethnic majority, to mix in exotic items such as pizza, lasagne or curry (Bush *et al.* 1996). It is not for nothing that postmodern life has been described in terms of an 'ethnic pick 'n' mix' (Keith and Cross 1993).

However, this apparently harmonious picture should be treated with due caution in future studies, considering the evidence from both Glasgow and elsewhere that racism continues to be active.

Influence of religion and gender on food choice

A relatively segregated gender division of labour is often characteristic of peasant societies, and may be sustained by religious values, quite apart from the constraints we discussed earlier deriving from the breadwinner's occupational insecurities. In the 'new' Italian communities of the postwar era, migrant women tended to take up paid employment (Colpi 1991) but despite full-time work in factories, often with overtime, these women ran their homes and cared for their children without assistance from their partners since this was against the traditional value system. All meals were said to be prepared from fresh ingredients and 'fast foods' were never considered, with women sometimes rising early to make some preparation for the evening meal before going out to work.

In some cultures a woman's character is categorised by the amount of time she spends on cooking. In France, for example, according to Bourdieu (1984: 187) a housewife is known as a *'pot-au-feu'* since the time and dedication required to produce such a dish are only at the disposal of women who fill their traditional role in the gender division of labour. A woman's mode of cooking may reveal even the extent of her virtue: among Asia Minor refugees in urban Greece, real culinary skill involves complex dishes requiring many hours of work, but grilled food and other quickly prepared meals are called 'prostitute's food' (Hirschon 1989: 150). For Italian Catholics 'the female is the guardian of the family nucleus and the concept of the mother is the symbol of what is most sacred within a family' (Colpi 1991: 216). A mother is controlled by strict rules of behaviour, to deviate from which damages her family's reputation as well as her own. In both these cultures the reputation of the family depended on the mother's behaviour, especially with regard to cooking and food preparation.

Muslim values relating to motherhood are similar to those of Italian Catholics:

> She is sacred and respected in her capacity to perpetuate the group (i.e. as a mother) because children are highly valued for religious and economic reasons. This capacity is, however, often interpreted as a danger. She has the power to defile the 'pure' blood of the group, and this is often used to legitimate the strict control over her movements. (Saifullah-Khan 1976: 236)

In Muslim countries the social control of gender is achieved through *purdah*, although a 'strongly patrilineal and virilocal society', rather than a particular religious ideology, is the prerequisite of this system. Saifullah-Khan presents a detailed analysis of *purdah* as it exists in Punjabi culture in Pakistan and in Britain, but we concentrate here on one of its four basic rules: the division of labour by sex which begins at puberty.

In Pakistan, the observation of *purdah* varies with socioeconomic status, because to practise the system in its ideal form requires a standard of living which only the wealthy few can attain. The majority of Pakistan's population follow a village-based subsistence economy, but although some aspects of *purdah* have to be relaxed as a consequence, the basic rules remain: woman's work is home-based, involving housework and caring for her children, her husband and their animals. Men work in the public sphere outside the house, on the land or at a craft.

In an earlier study of migrant Pakistanis in Bristol, Jeffery found a fairly traditional reinterpretation of this way of family life (Jeffery 1976). At about the same time, Saifullah-Khan (1976) actually found that, for a number of reasons, women who migrated to Bradford from rural Mirpur experienced a stricter form of *purdah* than they did in their home villages. Over a decade later, Werbner (1990), while agreeing that some of the women she studied in Manchester were physically isolated, proposed that in most cases this is a stage of early migration which passes. Where a family is involved in competition for status with others through gift-giving, the wife will often work to assist in the maintenance of a munificent lifestyle. The outcome is generally a more equal relationship between men and women and 'often a more flexible domestic division of labour'.

In her study of Sikh women, Bhachu (1988) (herself a Sikh) sees the fact that they are not in *purdah* as one of the keys to their greater independence and ability to control their earnings. Bhachu proposes that while men still dominate the community, the combination of Sikh religious ideology and the customs of the community influences ideas about the roles of men and women, and helps to temper this dominance.

The participation of Sikh women in paid work outside the home has also caused changes within the household and in the organisation of the Sikh community. Households are increasingly nuclear which has meant that gender roles have been redefined, particularly for younger couples. Men are much more involved with child care and housework than before because of female employment; even when older female relatives are to hand they are also often in paid work so not available to take care of children, necessitating male participation (Bhachu 1988).

Nevertheless, Bhachu notes that traditional cultural values have not been lost as a result of these changes within Sikh society. The dowry system has expanded and there has been an increase in religious rituals and wedding ceremonials, which are almost completely female in the case of older women, and may be paid for by them entirely. Significantly, food is an integral part of religious functions (Bhachu 1988), and the wedding celebrations of East African Sikh migrants may last almost two weeks and involve extensive food consumption (Bhachu 1985).

Each of the studies drawn on in this section is concerned primarily with a single religious group without comparative data, which means that the contrasts between Sikhs and Muslims may be overdrawn. Nevertheless we can see how the gender division of labour may be deeply embedded in a minority's culture and its religious values, though it also undergoes change and renegotiation in the British context. Because of this gender division of labour, the initial migrants place an emphasis on home-prepared meals, but whether this remains part of the stable pattern or forms an element in the changes is an issue for research.

The Glasgow study

In Glasgow, for family hospitality at any rate, traditional forms of food preparation are more characteristic of British-born South Asians (in this case mainly Muslims) than of British-born Italians (Bush *et al.* 1996). We noted earlier, in the section on social class and occupation, that the division of labour in the household is correspondingly more segregated among the South Asians than the Italians, and the association of men with the public and women with the private sphere more pronounced. Since this is not because of the pattern of self-employment, which both groups have in common, the case for religious influence is reinforced. Certainly conservative values are involved: asked whether they thought a woman should go out to work if she wanted to, even if she was well provided for by her husband, 24 per cent of migrant and 13 per cent of British-born South Asians said no, compared with 3–6 per cent of Italians and controls.

Whatever the feminist issues here, the nutritional consequences may well be important; for the traditional home-prepared South Asian cuisine has many health benefits (McKeigue and Chaturvedi 1996).

Conclusion

There remains the question whether, and in what sense, our Glasgow study has documented the processes of choice. We have considered the alternative possibility that variation in the diet and exercise patterns of the two minorities studied here were the product of coercive circumstances: low income and racist hostility. Our evidence does not support this possibility, though the extent to which low income reduced choice is still an open question. Low income certainly did not produce the single undifferentiated outcome that coercion implies. Racism was not a factor in our study, though evidence for it continues elsewhere. Thus choice in some sense was an essential element. However, it was a choice closely linked with cultural values – a health value given to large body size, a traditional home-prepared cuisine, obligations of hospitality, little concept of leisure exercise, a conservative gender division of labour. These things may well be linked with past experience of food scarcity and of a peasant-based food economy, but again not in the undifferentiated way implied by coercion. Rather, they are the product of choices made by sharing understandings and values collectively over a long period, and the results among South Asians and Italians are both similar and different. In Britain, the expansion of individual choice does not mean that members of ethnic minorities wish to throw over these cultural inheritances; rather, they seek to build them in to their strategies for living in varied ways. The benefits to be gained by this are apparent: it is these cultures, after all, that invented the low fat/high carbohydrate diets now considered ideal for health, whose recipes are highly marketable for Glasgow family dinners. In the process of maintaining or recovering these diets, or (in the case of the general population) acquiring them, a subtle and complex balance of individual and collective choice is involved; and for health professionals or food producers interested in assisting the process, a sociological sensitivity will be essential.

Acknowledgments

Many thanks to our respondents, and to our interviewers and dieticians for their help in this study; to the Registrar-General's Office in Edinburgh, and the staff of the Greater Glasgow, Lanarkshire and Argyll and Clyde Health Boards for help with the sampling; to numerous other members of our unit and department who helped with training, quality control, coding, typing and statistical analysis; and to Sally Macintyre and Anne Murcott who commented on earlier drafts.

Part Three

Social Sciences and Food Choice
Additional Perspectives

Part Three

Overview to Part Three

Part Three represents a departure from the rest of the book. The chapters here are based on work of much shorter duration and more limited scope than that reported in Parts One and Two. Each is a revised version of three separate literature reviews commissioned by the Steering Committee. Work in social history and in a specialist branch of social policy analysis is thereby introduced, along with an early step on a possible path between academic and market research in food and food choice. While all three chapters address demand rather more than supply, they none the less contribute to extending the Programme's diversity still further.

Chapter 17 introduces a topic that, in the event, is included nowhere else in the Programme's projects. It examines the influence of formal and informal welfare provision on dietary choice. More accurately, Diana Leat finds she has to deal with a surprising dearth on this topic. It would seem that neither those concerned to debate and formulate policy nor those with a research responsibility have paid much more than passing attention to the matter. Given so little material, whether, in what manner, or how far, welfare provision influences dietary choice is largely unknown. All that is possible in such circumstances is to work at identifying questions that deserve investigation. For instance: in what fashion and to what extent is concern with diet and healthy eating part of policy and practice among agencies providing residential or day care for vulnerable members of the population? Are dieticians employed or professional nutritional advice sought? How far is the provision of food reckoned to be part of social care, or is it considered closer to domestic service? Without developing some answers to these and a good many other questions Leat uncovers, the forces shaping the dietary intake of disadvantaged sectors of the nation will remain insufficiently documented.

Shifting to the sphere of the majority with money to spend, Chapter 18 is least like any other in the whole book. It is aimed primarily at academic social scientists, and attempts to counteract their seeming profound ignorance of commercial applications in market- and marketing-research – at least as witnessed among those involved in studying food and food choice. As the chapter illustrates, there are excellent commercial grounds for the great distance in mutual understanding between market researchers and academics. The purposes of the two do not merely differ, they positively require each stands pretty much in opposition to the other. All the same, there may still be grounds for some *rapprochement*, some judicious mutual exchange of data or reanalyses, if only to reduce research costs. Recognising the width of the gulf between them the Steering Committee sought to make a modest start on discovering the feasibility of building bridges by commissioning a preliminary review from Leslie Gofton. Chapter 18 is a revision based on that review.

Chapter 19 provides a social history of the shifting relationship between nutrition science and moves to effect change in the nation's diet. Over the last 70 years or so, some nutrition scientists sought actively to influence government policy, others refrained: some argued that achieving dietary change needed no more than public nutrition education, others that it was not so straightforward. At times, this included calls for attention to what nutrition scientists called the 'psychological and sociological' aspects of food habits, and collaboration with social scientists was promoted. Continuity as well as contrast is evident in the debates David Smith documents, and his chapter provides some introduction to selected historical antecedent to 'The Nation's Diet' Programme itself. Thus coming full circle, Smith's discussion paves the way for future social historians to examine the relationship between the nations' eating habits; nutrition science; governments' attitudes to science policy, to wealth creation and to quality of life; and diversity in the social sciences.

CHAPTER 17

Food choice and the British system of formal and informal welfare provision: questions for research

Diana Leat

Introduction

Formal policy intervention in diet and food choice may be designed to influence the supply of food or demand for food. Interventions on the supply side generally belong within the realm of agricultural and economic policies. Social welfare policies are more likely to be concerned with influencing the demand for food.

The focus of this chapter is not state intervention and influence on the national diet but more narrowly the way in which diet and food choice is influenced by formal and informal welfare provision. Given the lack of research in this area, the chapter cannot be a review of the literature; it rather attempts to identify areas for future research.

Given the widespread acknowledgement of and current emphasis on the role of diet in promoting health and welfare, it is surprising how little attention has been paid to welfare policy in relation to food choice. Social policy analysts have been concerned with the history and structure of services, policies and provisions for particular groups, such as children and the elderly, and policies relating to 'social problems'. More recently, analysts have been interested in the policy process and, most recently, in the ways in which formal and informal welfare systems do or do not work together. In general, the study of welfare provision has been dominated by the myth of the all-encompassing welfare state; provision within, and policies directly or indirectly impinging on, the informal, voluntary and private sectors have begun to receive attention only in the last five to ten years.

There are some exceptions to the surprising dearth of attention to food and social welfare. There are odd references to food choice, or more particularly the constraints on food choice, in the literature on poverty and on unemployment (Marsden and Duff 1975; Townsend 1979). In the 'new' literature on the informal and voluntary sectors (there is, as yet, very little on the private sector) there are passing references to food and the provision of meals, but these are as likely to be mentioned informally between researchers as to be written up in any report. Explicit attention to the place of food in social policy is rare, but again there are exceptions. For example, Wilson in one of the very few articles on food and social policy, points out that both the NACNE and COMA reports of the early 1980s 'arrived at clear recommendations for changes in diet but gave relatively little attention to the policy framework within which the changes could be brought about' (Wilson 1989: 170).

Modes of state intervention

Formal policy intervention may be direct or indirect. Thus:

1 the state may intervene directly by denying people some choices, or by rationing certain types, or all, food
2 the state may intervene directly by providing or requiring provision of certain types of food, or food to certain groups, such as orange juice and cod-liver oil to infants, school meals and milk
3 the state may intervene directly by providing sums of money or vouchers (or goods) tied to purchase of certain items.

Alternatively, or additionally, state intervention may be indirect. Thus:

1 the state may intervene indirectly by providing monetary benefits/ income maintenance which are in some way, explicitly or implicitly, related to the cost/purchase of food or to notions of a 'healthy diet', but are not tied to food purchase or choice (i.e. and may therefore be spent in other ways)
2 the state may intervene indirectly by funding or in other ways encouraging others to provide food and/or certain types of food to certain groups, such as local authority provision of meals-on-wheels for housebound people, the funding of lunch clubs catering for ethnic minority elderly people
3 the state may intervene indirectly by attempting to influence people's food choices via, for example, health-education programmes.

This swift sketch of various modes of intervention raises a series of questions about formal policy intervention/influence over food choice. Under what circumstances do governments choose to intervene in each way? What is the logic of such intervention and how is it legitimated? Under what circumstances and on what grounds do governments withdraw from different forms of intervention, such as the withdrawal in Britain of free school milk or meals? How is such withdrawal legitimated? Do the answers to these questions differ cross-nationally? Do they change over time? Why is one type of intervention chosen rather than another? What factors inhibit government choice of different modes of intervention, and do these differ cross-nationally? Cross-national studies, within the European Community, for example, would be especially interesting but fraught with difficulty given the different systems and balance of financial and direct welfare provision as well as different monitoring procedures and non-comparable official statistics.

A second set of questions concerns the policy process. How are choices between forms of intervention made? Who is involved? What sorts of pressure groups favour which types of intervention and why? A third set of questions concerns the effects and effectiveness of different forms of intervention. Historical and cross-national case studies of particular policy interventions would undoubtedly shed some light on these questions.

For instance, the history of the introduction of family allowances in Britain provides an important – and fascinating – case study of the role of diet-related considerations in the case for provision of child benefits by the state. It also highlights the anxieties about state intervention in domestic 'family responsibilities' and the subtle distinctions, related to location (see below) about the social acceptability of state intervention in the provision of food and food choice. In its early stages the campaign for family allowances was explicitly related to 'physical deterioration of the industrial population' as a 'grave national danger'. Despite the introduction of free school meals, Ramsay MacDonald and Mrs Pankhurst, among others, were opposed to any extension of state maintenance of children on the grounds that this would weaken the family as a social institution. School meals were acceptable because 'the common meal will be regarded as a ceremony of greatest educational value' (quoted in Hall *et al*. 1975: 159). An alternative explanation of this distinction between intervention in school and within the family might be that state intervention in food choice is acceptable in public institutions but not within the home (and see Burgess and Morrison's Chapter 13 in this book).

As the campaign progressed, it became associated with a whole range of other themes:

> Family allowances could be approached from so many directions with such an infinite variety of emphasis and application. It could be handled as a problem of vital statistics, housing administration, minimum wage legislation, child nutrition, national insurance, teachers' salary scales, coal-mining economics, feminism social philosophy or pure finance. (Stocks quoted in Hall *et al*. 1975: 165).

During the 1920s and 1930s the campaign for family allowances became associated with, among other things, fears of the effects of a falling birthrate. However, towards the end of the 1930s nutrition assumed prominence once more. Rowntree's second study of poverty in 1936 exposed the extent of poverty and malnutrition, and the link between them.

291

Although definitions of 'poverty' and adequate nutrition were (and are) debatable, the accumulation of these findings did make an impression and convinced more people of the need for family allowances, particularly when viewed against the background of a declining population at home and the pro-natalist policies of our competitors abroad. (Hall *et al.* 1975: 174)

With fears of war looming, Leo Amery supported family allowances on the grounds that: 'when we are faced with the competition of a people who lay stress on the healthy development of their young manhood and womanhood, how can we afford a situation in which something like 25 per cent of the children of our country are growing up undernourished?' (Hall *et al.* 1975). Support from the Conservative benches increased and outside Parliament an all-party Children's Minimum Campaign Committee was formed 'to ensure that no child shall by reason of the povery of its parents be deprived of at least the minimum food and other requirements for full health' (Hall *et al.* 1975: 174–5). Free school meals were increasingly regarded as inadequate alone to ensure child health and, interestingly, were arousing some controversy on the grounds that school-feeding was a public health measure and should not therefore be the responsibility of the Education Department.

Thus the campaign for family allowances highlights the way in which the significance of diet and food choice ebbed and flowed over time in the campaign, the resistance to state intervention in diet and food choice and the reluctance by government and by government departments to accept responsibility for the provision of food. It also highlights the manner in which diet-related considerations alone were insufficient to provide adequate legitimation for such a policy. Other case studies (in Britain and elsewhere) are needed in order to understand better the considerations, alliances and obstacles related to state responsibility for and intervention in food provision and choice.

Direct state intervention in food choice

The history of British social policy suggests that direct state intervention in food choices is neither a first nor easy policy option. Notions of personal privacy and freedom, family responsibility and an individualist, rather than collectivist, approach to the state militate against such intervention. In Britain direct state intervention in food choice has generally been obvious only in periods of perceived national emergency, usually related to war. In the early years of this century concern for the health of children as future recruits to a fighting-fit army had a direct influence on welfare provision in the introduction of free school meals and milk. In the light of much more recent welfare preoccupations, the provision of school meals and milk is especially noteworthy. These measures were direct state interventions in food provision and choice, targeted at a particular group, providing goods not money (therefore reducing choice) and restricted to a non-domiciliary setting thus, presumably, avoiding objections on the grounds of interference with parental freedom and responsibilities. And, as noted above, those who objected to the introduction of family allowances on the grounds that this would weaken the family as a social institution accepted the provision of free school meals because the common meal was held to be an educationally valuable experience.

During the Seond World War, the state intervened on an unprecedented level in food supply, choice and preparation. More detailed study of policy formation and implementation remains to be undertaken. On what grounds was such intervention legitimated? As Burnett (1968), has indicated, it would appear from contemporary accounts that economic considerations, health concerns, military efficiency and issues of social justice were all brought into play (and see Smith's Chapter 19 in this book for a discussion of the role of nutritional scientific knowledge). But different types of consideration may have influenced different aspects of policy. For example, it was presumably concern about health and population renewal which led to special provisions for pregnant women and children. Were other groups singled out as requiring special treatment and, if so, on what grounds?

Income maintenance benefits and food choice

Historically, concern over the nation's diet was raised not by medical professionals but by social welfare reformers such as Booth and Rowntree, and nutritionists such as Boyd-Orr (1936). Concern with food, especially for the poor, was based on nutrition/health considerations but because of the perceived direct link between diet and income, food was cast as a matter of welfare reform rather than solely of health education.

As Wilson (1989) suggests (health-dominated) approaches to food choice of the 1980s were based on personal responsibility and assume that income is not a limiting factor. Evidence from a small study in inner London suggested that:

> (E)xpenditure on food was not a problem over a wide range of household incomes and financial limitations on dietary change were small or non-existent. *There were, however, two important exceptions to this rule.* The first was low income households. The second was households where the method of financial organisation left little money for food. (Wilson 1989: 172–3; emphasis added)

These two exceptions are, one might argue, the very groups with whom social policy is most concerned. The historical link between diet,

293

food choice and income maintenance raises some significant areas for research which extend beyond concern about the consequences of low income. One broad question concerns the apparent erosion of the link between nutrition and income-maintenance benefits: has concern with diet and food choice dropped off the social policy agenda as a corollary of increasingly being seen to belong to the domain of health education? When and why did this happen? Has it happened in other European nations?

Other more specific areas for research both in Britain and cross-nationally include:

1 The relationship between the introduction of income maintenance benefits and concern with nutrition and food choice.
2 The history of the British benefit system is widely acknowledged to be one of *ad hoccery* and many benefits may have lost sight of their original intentions. What explicit or implicit role does food choice and diet-related considerations currently play in income maintenance benefits?
3 The relationship between the calculation of the level of benefit and the assumed cost of a 'healthy' diet. For example, in Britain today many benefits are, in theory at least, uprated annually in line with rises in the cost of living; the cost-of-living index includes a shopping basket – what is in this basket, who decides its contents and by what criteria? Is the basket – and thus the assumed rise in the cost of food – the same for all groups/benefits?
4 Do benefits designed to cover the cost of, for example, special needs associated with disability include any explicit or implicit recognition of special dietary needs? There is, incidentally, evidence that benefits designed to assist with the costs of care – such as Attendance Allowance – are actually spent on heating and extra/special food rather than the purchase of care (Horton and Berthoud 1990).
5 What implications, if any, does the choice of benefit recipient have for expenditure on food and food choices? For example, family allowances have always been paid to the mother; Attendance Allowance (now Disability Living Allowance for those under 65) is paid not to the person providing care but to the person requiring care. To what extent does the choice of benefit recipient rest on assumptions about who is, or should be, in control of welfare – and food – provision? This issue may be particularly important given the points noted above about the limitations on food choice created by particular forms of household financial organisation (Pahl 1990). Benefit recipients, the provision of care and household financial organisation raise the fundamental, wider issue of power and control over money and food choice (see Kemmer, Anderson and Marshall's Chapter 12 and Henson *et al.*'s Chapter 11 in this book). In many informal care relationships the previous balance of power may be disturbed if not reversed: an elderly mother or father becomes the equivalent of a dependent child and the son/daughter

becomes mother. Discussions with carers suggest that this transformation is difficult and painful for both parties and may constitute a daily source of tension. How does this affect control over food choice? How, if at all, is this related to control over income – for example, via the benefit system's nomination of benefit recipient?

6 In Britain the amount of residential care benefits varies between groups. In what ways, if at all, does this variation rest on assumptions about different dietary needs?

7 The case of residential care benefits in Britain raises another more fundamental issue central to current social policy: what is social care? As Hurst (1990) has put it, care has become the chewing-gum of social policy; but is provision of food part of social care? Commonsense understandings suggest that the provision and preparation of food is a major part of social care; indeed women are encouraged to believe that preparing meals is a way of showing how much they care. But, at the same time, various wider social changes are encouraging the professionalisation of care. Care is increasingly presented as set apart from domestic service (cf. Leat 1990). Where does food provision and preparation now fit: in care provision or in domestic service?

In the 1980s, in an attempt to stem escalating expenditure on residential care benefits, a distinction was introduced between the benefits for provision of 'board and lodging' and for 'care'. Presumably the provision of food would come under the former heading, thus implicitly excluding food from the definition of care. Care appears, in this case, to be to do with the provision of help with bodily functions other than the provision of food. The professionalisation of care is occurring in other European states. How is care defined in different states and where does food provision and preparation fit on the care-domestic service continuum?

8 There is a growing number of areas in which the state provides, directly or indirectly, payments for care. For example, in Britain foster parents receive allowances in return for care of children. The history of the payment of allowances for child-fostering is complex and fraught with moral assumptions about the relationship between love and money. But part of the legitimation has always been to cover some of the direct costs, such as the provision of food, and to enable people to become foster parents without excessive financial loss (Southon 1986; Leat and Gay 1987; Leat 1990). At the time of writing, fostering allowances (as opposed to payments on top of assumed costs) are paid by most local authorities under a variable and complex set of expenditure headings and weighted according to the child's age. What significance is attached to the assumed cost of food in these calculations? What food items are assumed to be necessary and desirable? Do these differ according to age (and gender)? How is the amount allowed for food calculated? A study of foster parents (and other paid carers) found that, for carers themselves, the cost of

food and the provision of a 'healthy' diet were issues of some importance (Leat 1990).

Food choice as a health issue

Despite the historical link between nutrition and income-maintenance benefits, in the last decade food choice has been constructed primarily as a matter for public health, health promotion and health education rather than one for income-maintenance/welfare rights/social care. Diet seems increasingly to be seen as a matter of personal responsibility and choice rather than money. Some issues about the possible effects on welfare policy of the (re)construction of food choice as a health-education matter have already been raised, as have some queries about the role of food choice and preparation in the definition of social care. But there is a range of other questions.

For example, in what ways and to what extent do social care (as distinct from health care) agencies display institutionalised concern with diet and food choice? Given social services departments' involvement in food provision in residential and day care for vulnerable groups, how many employ nutritionists? If nutritionists are employed when, why and where were they first employed in social services departments? How many care homes employ or consult nutritionists in constructing menus? Will the now emerging contracts for provision of residential and domiciliary care include requirements concerning diet, for which groups, in what settings? Will residential care contracts include dietary requirements while domiciliary care contracts exclude them on the grounds that in their own homes people should be allowed to eat what they like? What considerations – for example, both price and transaction costs – will enter into the inclusion or exclusion of dietary requirements in contracts? In so far as menus are excluded from specification for social care contracts, this could be construed as further evidence for the exclusion of food choice from the domain of social care provision. These questions about food choice in residential (and domiciliary) settings are just some of those which might be asked in the wider investigation of food choice in total institutions – a subject which, as Mennell, Murcott and van Otterloo (1992) have pointed out, has attracted virtually no research interest.

Formal and informal welfare provision and food choice – the role of the voluntary sector

There are several reasons for suggesting that consideration of the role of the voluntary sector, though supposedly independent of the state, may be especially important in examining formal and informal welfare provision and food choice. First, as has often occurred in the history of British welfare provision, those issues which fall outside the concern of the state or which straddle departmental policy boundaries (such as between health and social care) may be taken up by the voluntary sector. Second, one function of the voluntary sector is to work in those areas for which neither the state nor the market adequately or equitably provide. Third, some also suggest that one role of the voluntary sector is to substitute for or enable indirect state intervention in politically controversial areas. In practice the voluntary sector in Britain has played various different roles in influencing or attempting to influence food choice.

Campaigning and policy influence

The role of the voluntary sector in influencing policies relating to food choice has been neglected by researchers in Britain. There is, however, little doubt that the voluntary sector has been active in this field via various organisations concerned with health, education, consumer rights and representation, women's organisations, as well as organisations concerned with poverty, children, the elderly and with family welfare. What sorts of organisations have seen policies relating to food choice as within their domain? What sorts of organisations have attempted to influence policies relating to food, how have they gone about this, why and with what effect? How does the role of British voluntary organisations in influencing policies relating to food compare with the role and activities of voluntary organisations in other countries?

Case studies of larger selected national voluntary organisations with a known interest in issues to do with food choice would provide a valuable starting point in such research. The National Federation of Women's Institutes, for example, has a wide national network, a known interest and campaigning role in relation to food and welfare and has in the past been used as a sounding-board by, and as an 'agent' of, government on food matters (Goodenough 1977). Similarly, it would be worth exploring what, for example, the Child Poverty Action Group and/or Citizens Advice Bureaux and/or Rural Community Councils have had to say about policies relating to food and social welfare.

In turn, it would also be worth exploring the impact of policies relating to food on voluntary organisations and their activities, and their responses. The Food Safety Act 1990, for example, has had a striking effect on voluntary organisations' costs and activities. Organisations ranging in size and income from village halls to playgroups, day centres to large national organisations have required new equipment, procedures and training as a result of the Act. The Act may, ironically, have a doubly damaging effect on organisations raising their costs and at the same time damaging their fundraising capacity if food preparation is involved.

Public education about food choice

The role of voluntary organisations – at national and local level – in providing public education about food choice is also largely uncharted water. Again the National Federation of Women's Institutes is one example of a nationwide organisation with a known and obvious role in educating its almost half-a-million members, as well as the wider public via its publications and demonstrations, about nutrition and food choice. Other organisations, such as the British Heart Foundation, have undoubtedly played a major role in health-education campaigns relating to diet. Voluntary organisations may be particularly important in reaching targeted, high-risk groups likely to be members or supporters. At the local level voluntary organisations may play an important part in reaching those less likely to be touched via other channels, such as groups of Asian women. Voluntary organisations have also provided back-up and local contacts for several media campaigns relating to diet and health education (Parker 1988).

Though the role of voluntary organisations in public nutrition education is widely acknowledged in the Third World, it remains unnoticed and in need of research in Britain and other European states. Who does what in providing public education about food choice, how, at what cost, funded by whom and with what effect? To what extent and why is the voluntary sector deliberately used (and funded) by government as a channel for influence about food choice for example, in order to sidestep philosophical and political controversies surrounding direct state intervention in food choice.

Voluntary organisations and food provision

For many of the most vulnerable groups in society – those with whom social policy is especially concerned – voluntary organisations play an important role in providing food. Good neighbours' groups providing meals for elderly and disabled people, organisations running playgroups, nurseries, lunch clubs, day centres, as well as those providing long– and short-term residential care facilities are all engaged in choosing and preparing food for others.

In relation to the direct provision of food the voluntary sector in Britain is probably most famous for its pioneering of meals-on-wheels. In some areas this service has been taken over by the local authority; in others it is contracted out to voluntary organisations such as WRVS. But in Britain it was the voluntary sector which through its direct provision gained acceptance that providing one hot meal per day to housebound people was a proper modern concern of state social welfare agencies. However, Johnson, Di Gregario and Harrison's (1981) findings regarding the provision of meals-on-wheels today raise questions about the purpose of meals' provision by the state and by voluntary organisations. Is provision concerned with the prevention of malnutrition and the promotion of health? If so, Johnson's findings suggest that the service is of questionable effectiveness. Few of those receiving meals were considered to be in need of nutritional supplement and few had been properly identified as being at nutritional risk (Johnson, Di Gregario and Harrison 1981; Audit Commission 1985; Sinclair *et al.* 1990). If meals-on-wheels is not primarily concerned with nutrition, does it have some other purpose such as support and monitoring, the provision of social contact or the tangible expression of care and concern? More practically, how does the purpose of provision affect the choice of recipients, food choices and menu-construction by providers?

Specific questions abound. Do similar arrangements exist for the provision of meals to the housebound in other European states? If so, how are these funded and regulated? What are the minimum and maximum requirements laid on such provision? What role does the voluntary sector play in such provision/delivery? Why is the voluntary sector used rather than direct state provision? How does this type of provision relate to wider philosophical objections to direct state intervention in food provision and choice? If there are no formal arrangements for the provision of meals to the housebound, how is the problem of feeding such vulnerable groups dealt with?

More general questions for research arise wherever food is chosen and prepared by voluntary (i.e. semi-public) organisations for others. What factors enter into decisons about food choice, for example, cost, convenience, notions of nutrition and a 'healthy/balanced' diet, consumer preferences and available facilities? In the for-profit commercial sector equivalent – restaurants, hotels – it might be expected that cost/profit and, closely related, consumer preferences would dominate menu construction. But voluntary organisations might be expected to display different considerations:

1 Recipients do not typically pay for meals, and costs therefore cannot be recovered in the same way. Furthermore, costs/ expenditure may be set by a third-party funder, such as the local authority.
2 Voluntary organisations are not typically concerned with the provision of food *per se* but with the welfare and health of those they serve. They might therefore be expected to put the provision of a 'healthy' diet higher on their list of priorities than a for-profit enterprise with no welfare or health mission. If, however, the provision of food is seen by voluntary organisations as serving purposes other than nutrition, such as social contact, a 'healthy' diet may be less immediately relevant in food choice by such organisations.
3 Most, especially smaller, voluntary organisations are probably unable to offer menu alternatives. For this reason the preferences of the majority may be a more important consideration than in a for-profit outlet able to cater for a range of preferences.
4 The notion that voluntary organisations are not concerned with profit is, as a general assumption, increasingly outdated (Leat 1993). The provision of food may be one area in which voluntary organisations may have sufficient leeway to contain costs, if not to

generate small surpluses to subsidise other activities which may, within the organisation's mission, be seen as more important.

There is another way in which the voluntary sector provides food for individuals and families. Some voluntary organisations still fund, organise or deliver food parcels/hampers or other foodstuffs, such as Easter eggs, to those deemed in need. In some cases voluntary organisations purchase food from their own funds; in other cases deliveries are done in conjunction with or on behalf of other commercial – and, less often, statutory – organisations such as super-markets and local radio stations. Voluntary organisations may also be responsible for the distribution of the produce from harvest festival services in schools and churches.

The impression – which, in the absence of research evidence is all there is to go on – is that this practice is dying out. If so, this is possibly on a combination of nutritional grounds and a view that giving people food rather than money is both demeaning and inconsistent with ideologies of self-determination and consumer choice. At the same time in other spheres voluntary organisations' involvement in food provision and distribution may be increasing. Voluntary organisations, especially in the major cities, distribute food, often donated by others (including retailers) to the homeless. Some national voluntary and commercial organisations ensure that all food left over from corporate entertainment is distributed in this way – though just possibly the smoked salmon canapés and quails eggs they are given may not be the first choice of the homeless.

To whom do voluntary organisations consider it appropriate to distribute food? What considerations enter into the distribution of what sort of food, to which groups and under what circumstances? To what extent have voluntary organisations' practices in this respect been influenced by current ideologies about nutrition and 'healthy' food stuffs? Are objections to voluntary organisations' distribution of food similar to the objections raised in relation to direct state intervention in food choices?

The voluntary sector and income maintenance

Finally, the voluntary sector, especially grant-giving trusts and foundations, may play some continuing role today in providing financial benefits to those on low incomes or for other reasons deemed to be in need. In general, trusts and foundations are careful to emphasis that they do not fund those things which are statutory responsibilities: but where does this leave food? Do trusts and foundations provide funding for purchase of food and, if so, under what circumstances, to which groups and for what reasons? It is likely, for example, that some trusts provide funding for the provision of 'special diets' – but what is to count as a special diet? Are special diets medically defined and legitimated? If so, does this again suggest that food has become a health rather than a social care or welfare rights issue?

The role of the voluntary sector in both the provision of food, especially to the homeless, and in income maintenance and provision for those with special dietary needs may be seen as a means of providing for such groups without the need for direct state intervention. Provision via the voluntary sector avoids precedent-setting and political controversy.

Conclusion

This chapter has had to be a very preliminary excursion into the field. But the basic exercise of juxtaposing reflections on food choice with an element of familiarity with British systems of formal and informal welfare provision, has yielded an unexpected collection of questions. A near enough unknowable number of British citizens are caught up in these systems. Growing socioeconomic disparities of the 1980s and 1990s would suggest, however, that even if this number does not increase, it will be slow to decline. With implications for their health and welfare, the workings of these systems may have far-reaching effects on the diet of the citizens concerned. Without research to tackle some of the questions raised here, however, what these effects might be will remain obscure.

CHAPTER 18

British market-research data on food: a note on their use for the academic study of food choice

Leslie Gofton

Introduction

Despite their apparent similarities, the differences between market research and social scientific data are marked. Research in the two provinces is undertaken in quite different circumstances, and wholly separate criteria are applied in determining what needs to be done, how and why. Are, then the data on food consumption produced by market research usable by social scientists interested in food choice? After all, since they have been produced at considerable cost it seems sensible to draw on them (especially in straitened times) rather than incur the expense and effort of undertaking further primary research. This chapter considers the question, showing that, ironically perhaps, the matter turns on the manner in which marketing research must stand in sharp contrast to academic research. It is written as a note for the uninitiated among academic social scientists.

The discussion begins with an obvious, but important, preliminary. The academic approach to market-research data has to be contemplated in exactly the same way as is the conduct of any other secondary analysis. First, this means recognising that the data in-volved are diverse, and cannot easily be lumped together. Thereafter, the usual considerations when approaching secondary materials must be remembered (Dale, Arber and Proctor 1988). Among the questions to be asked are: What were the purposes of the original study? What information was collected, and how did this relate to the definition of the key variables which are being used in the present study? What sample was aimed for, and what was achieved? What evidence for the data's validity and reliability is there and can it be trusted? How old are the data, and how representative are they? With these questions in mind, the chapter turns to note the nature of marketing research, the distinctiveness of the data and the market for marketing research.

The nature of marketing research

Marketing research is an aid to commercial decision-making. It is:

the function that links an organisation to its market through information. This information is used to identify and define marketing opportunities and problems; generate, refine and evaluate marketing actions; monitor marketing performance and improve understanding of marketing as a process . . . Marketing research specifies the information required to address these issues; designs the method for collecting information; manages and implements the data-collection process; interprets the results and communicates their findings and implications. (American Marketing Association 1987: 21)

Since marketing activities and the needs of decision-makers differ markedly, a wide range of decisions is involved needing a variety of data and methods. Thus marketing research may be used to describe a market (gathering and presenting data which are 'market facts'); to diagnose (what if the marketing mix is changed?); to identify the factors which are relevant to a particular state of a market or to consumers' decision-making. It may also be used to predict the outcomes of one or other marketing mix combination (Gates and McDaniel 1992).

So market research is only undertaken to provide information which can be used to inform commercial decisionmaking (Chisnall 1991; Tull and Hawkins 1992). As a result, this dictates what and how the data are gathered, the analysis to which they are typically subjected, and the forms in which they are submitted to those whose work requires their use.

At the same time, marketing researchers present their work as science. Its status as such is sufficiently important for it to have figured as a theme of Frank Bass' leader for the thirtieth anniversary issue of the *Journal of Marketing Research* reviewing the 'history of serious research on marketing topics applying advanced research methods' (Bass 1993: 1). For Bass, and the large number of market researchers to whose work he refers, market research is science, not merely commonsense organised and classified. It 'seeks to provide generalised explanatory statements about disparate types of phenomena and to provide critical tests for the relevance of the attempted explanations' (Bass 1993: 2). He refers to the generality of results, the degree of consistency of observation with theory, as well as the extension of theories to predict new observations, all of which he proposes are 'likely to be of increasing importance in advancing fundamental knowledge' (Bass 1993: 3). Those involved in marketing research, like other scientists, are to be guided by recognising their efforts in what he calls the 'greater scheme of things'. There remains, however, a self-evident tension between these claims and the highly distinctive nature of marketing research.

The distinctiveness of marketing research data

Marketing research is almost invariably conducted in response to a client's *particular* need for information, to solve a problem, or to inform strategic decision-making. Thus, for example, Birds Eye, the largest producer of fish products for the UK market, carries out market studies which reflect highly specific interests, and not simply 'the market for fish'. The company focuses on consumer preferences in mass markets, for example, for frozen products based on white fish, and has less interest in, for example, markets for fresh fish, or little-used species (Gofton and Marshall 1992).

Clients require the marketing researcher to produce only information which is directly relevant to their specific needs, and to render it into a form which can be understood and used by the (non-specialist) individuals concerned. For their part, market researchers must 'translate' the client's problem into a suitable and viable research programme. The client's problem cannot usually be directly researched, because clients rarely have a clear idea of the kinds of information they need, the type of data which can be gathered, or how they can be interpreted. But the research still has to be highly focused. Even specialists in academic marketing departments, or in marketing research agencies or sections, have little autonomy in the way they carry out research, since the main criterion for successful and profitable research is customer usability. Marketing research only exists in order to produce information which can be of use to clients. Outside a very small part of the academic world of marketing teaching and research, marketing research is never done 'for its own sake' or simply to address the question of why consumers behave in the way they do.

The highly specific nature of the information required, and the generally very firm time limits within which it is needed, are reflected in the resources available for marketing research. The research appropriation is determined by the value of the information it is to yield, or rather by the potential profit to be generated by the decision(s) which it informs. A Bayesian or rational decision analysis may be carried out to assess the cost-effectiveness of undertaking the research. Information has to be relevant, timely, and also 'actionable', i.e. it should refer either to things about the product or market which can be acted on, or to defining the limits of action. Hence it must be completely case-specific. Anything more is surplus information representing unnecessary, unjustifiable time and cost.

By definition, good primary marketing research should not produce generalities. Primary market-research data are gathered, in the vast majority of cases, for the specific needs of particular clients. The final product, the findings and the report, are fitted to the clients and their organisational needs. There would simply be no commercial sense in producing data which were too complex to be grasped or easily absorbed by the client, or buttressed by 'superfluous' information. The best market research, like bespoke tailoring, should fit the client perfectly, but no one else. As a result, work for a named client is commercially confidential or, more accurately, it remains so for the period when it counts as still completely up-to-date. Apart from a small group of (competitive) businesses, the wider relevance or value of such information is hard to see. The *better* the marketing research – i.e. the more precisely it is targeted at the requirements of a particular client – the less generalisable are its findings and the *less use* it is likely to be to anyone else – including academics.

Not all market researchers' output is produced for a commissioning client, but this does not, however, make it any the less distinctive. Some is made available for sale on the open market, in which case it must be couched in terms which give it 'mass appeal': it should be easily digested and understood by a non-specialist business audience. To this end it is based on assumptions about what non-specialist decision-makers would be able to use – assumptions that reflect the characteristics of the 'typical client'. For instance, sociodemographic data are presented in terms of customer profiles, as 'actionable' characteristics such as patterns of media consumption or disposable income, residence or product usage, rather than in terms of age, occupation, educational level or the Registrar General's classification of social class.

The popularity of such 'psychographics' resides in the fact that they promise to describe key aspects of the ways in which different groups of existing customers think, feel and act, the kinds of activities they enjoy, or which newspapers and TV they see – in short, a description of their 'lifestyle' (a term, it should be noted, used in a colloquial rather than a social scientific sense). In this fashion they should enable the marketer to see where the product could be fitted in, and therefore how it should be 'conceptualised' and best communicated to the consumer. The dimensions included in profiles are usually selective, chosen on the basis of the typical client's likely interests. Caricatures such as 'grabit and runs', the 'traditionalists' or 'green consumers' are commonly used to describe the segments into which a market can be divided.

Market-research methods

The popular impression that market-research data are mostly derived from interviewing dozens of passers-by, or from large numbers of long questionnaires sent through the post is inaccurate. Whenever possible, secondary materials, such as official statistics in the *National Food Survey*, or figures compiled by bodies such as the Meat and Livestock Commission are used instead, or else, if primary research is undertaken, small-scale qualitative studies are substituted. In a way that will be entirely familiar to academic social scientists, market researchers commonly distinguish two main types of primary data-collection: qualitative and quantitative. Only some of the key differences in market-research methods of which academic researchers ought to be aware are noted here.

Secondary analysis – a brief aside

In contrast to the majority of academics, however, market researchers make particular use of data internal to a company. The widespread use of information technology has increased the range and application of such data, giving rise to uses possibly less well known among academic social scientists. The advent of Electronic Point of Sale (EPOS) systems, using optical-scanning equipment recording customer purchase data, has had a dramatic effect in making the collection of such information very much simpler. Cheap and accessible means of storing, handling and processing the immense volume of data they generate is revolutionising marketing research – as well as management-information systems. The extent, accuracy and immediacy of the information they offer about stock levels, ordering patterns, product distribution and customer profiles is readily apparent and widely used by business.

Database marketing has grown out of this new development. Identified as 'interactive', using individually 'addressable' means of communication, database marketing is to 'extend help to a company's target audience, stimulate their demand' and 'stay close to them by recording and keeping an electronic database memory of customer, prospect and all communications and commercial contacts, to help improve all future contacts' (after Fletcher, Wheeler and Wright 1990). It is suggested that these new developments are, to a degree, de-skilling market research and analysis, by making it possible for non-specialists to use and manipulate data very quickly, and at very low cost. The latest development in this direction is 'datamining'. A number of companies now offer to 'mine' information to order from the extensive databanks that are being accumulated.

Qualitative market research

Qualitative research has had a limited role in marketing research. It has largely been confined to the generation of hypotheses, the development of attitude measure or scales, the design of questionnaires about use or behaviour, and geared to gaining insight into the meanings of a product for consumers or to gauging consumer reactions to changes in the marketing mix.

Both depth interviews (with a single respondent) and focus groups (with between eight and 12) are used. Data are gathered and analysed in much the same way in each. Focus groups have recently become very widely known. Originating in the US, some credit market and opinion-researchers of the 1920s with their invention. Others ascribe it to the American sociologist Robert Merton who, with colleagues, used them in his 1940s investigation of the impact of wartime propaganda (Merton and Kendall 1946; Merton 1987). Merton's work on the method was not pursued by academic social scientists until very recently with its adoption in selected academic research. The style of questioning aims to 'focus' discussion on whatever topic is of interest. It owes much to the procedures of practitioners in their professional relationships with patients or clients, such as those in clinical psychology, counselling or health education (Basch 1987; Stewart and Shamdasani 1990; Lengua *et al.* 1992).

The re-emergence of the focus group in marketing research may, in part, be due to the availability of cheap and manageable audio- and video-recording. The supposed 'softness' of the data has long been a source of suspicion and one of the reasons for neglecting the method. A permanent record of 'what happened' is held to provide 'harder' data. Discussions can be transcribed, and new software allows quantitative analysis – for example, the generation of word counts, or lists of phrases or terms used to describe a particular product – in addition to the qualitative identification of concepts and ideas. Video-recording can be particularly useful when products are being tested to examine the way consumers may hold or use them.

Quantitative market research

Experiments such as 'sensory testing' or 'taste testing' in either a food laboratory or as a 'hall' test in a public place such as a supermarket, observational studies, such as watching and classifying shopping behaviour or eating, conducted under natural or contrived conditions, are used in addition to surveys using either (self-complete) questionnaires or interviews. Although superficially similar to their academic use, the use of surveys in marketing research has a number of distinctive features. For instance, they commonly involve incentive payments or the offer of gifts or other material inducements to obtain respondents' cooperation. This may well make securing a suitable response rate somewhat easier. But it raises difficult questions about the nature and quality of the data and the representativeness of the sample. Or again, since marketers are seldom concerned with the whole population and mostly interested in quite precisely defined respondents (e.g. consumers of one brand) or market segments, they often use quota, stratified, or even skewed samples.

Quantitative data are most important for marketers. They indicate the total size of the market (volume, value); the segmentation of the market (different usage on different occasions or in different settings); market share (by brands); and the use of a product (when it is eaten, in what combinations, how it is cooked). These data offer information on markets, on consumer behaviour, 'lifestyles' and attitudes which are simply not available elsewhere. A very good example is the use of panels to gather information about changes in consumer purchase and use of products

The market for market-research

Marketing information, on food consumption as on anything else, is itself marketed: it is formulated, made available and promoted as a product and service which will satisfy the needs of consumers: business decision-makers. Market-research companies (the small, local examples as well the large, well-known ones such as Neilsen, National Opinion Polls, the British Market Research Bureau, or Marketing Intelligence) and, in addition, some college/university marketing departments and business schools, are in the business of selling their services to clients in the food industries. Marketing research data are sold on the basis of representing up-to-date information which is relevant and understandable. The claim to be scientific is essential when seeking to sell its products and services.

The authority of 'science' provides 'value added' as an important assurance to the customers for marketing research information. But market research which actually pursued scientific aims and methods would be neither cost-effective nor, expressed in scientific and technical terms at least, understandable by, or relevant to, the client. Claims to produce 'general laws' or 'generalisable findings' cannot be anything other than a by-product of the main marketing research objective. Bass (1993) rightly recognises that testability is only an issue when the generalisation derived from specific findings is taken outside the setting in which the original findings were generated. But that cannot be any concern of marketing research itself, since its *raison d'être* is to satisfy the need for specific and highly contextualised information – the opposite of the production or testing of general laws. Only the specialist academics involved in teaching marketing research would be likely to find such general laws of any value.

The use of market-research data for academic study

As the above implies there is, then, a number of factors limiting the value of market-research data for academic investigation. Equally, their strategic use can augment academic investigation in a manner that has inadequately and/or infrequently been attempted.

Over and above the usual precautions required in secondary analysis, there is a series of quite significant drawbacks. First, the availability of primary market-research data is highly likely to be restricted. Reports are often commercially sensitive. If they are made available to anyone other than the client, they may be either extremely expensive, or only offered for sale some time after they have been produced. Furthermore, data are typically presented 'ready-interpreted'. As noted earlier, they need to be presented in terms that suit the client, but which correspondingly convey much less for more general or other purposes. Inevitably, too, many marketing studies (especially observational work) tend to interpret the results in terms of individual behaviour and as the outcome of physiological or psychological processes, rather than as evidence of complexities of culture, economic factors or the social structure. It is these latter which are likely to be of more central interest to many academic social scientists. But obtaining 'raw' data is very difficult, thus severely restricting the opportunity for reanalysis.

The quality of the data can also be highly variable. This chapter has indicated that what is needed to answer commercial questions – including inducements for respondents, unrepresentative sampling, the use of non-social scientific styles of questioning – does not neatly correspond with what is required for academic social scientific investigation. Street interviews, for instance, using a 'convenience' sample and a short, simple questionnaire, can often yield very interesting material. But, for academic purposes, it may also be highly unreliable and should only be used with extreme caution.

There are, however, potential benefits to be gained from the judicious use of market-research data which have been neglected by academics. Marketing research focuses on behaviour, actions, choices and ideas relevant to the world of commerce. As a result it concentrates on brands of products, retailers and their activities, and advertising which is often by-passed by academic social scientific research. In other words, it provides information on details of consumer behaviour which are infrequently, if at all, apparent in official statistics, other social research, or academic social scientific investigation. Yet consumer activities are facts of social life and can obviously be extremely important, especially in the nature and place of food choice in modern society.

For instance, in looking at changes in the use of drugs and in drinking behaviour over 20 years, it was found that it was the shifts between different brands and types of drink (along with the meanings attached to them), rather than changes in gross consumption which turn out to have been important (Gofton 1983, 1986, 1990). It would not have been possible to address many central questions of that research without recourse to marketing research data on, for instance, profiles of the 'market segments' for different products; information on patterns of public-house usage, and traffic flows within the main drinking areas of city centres; evaluation criteria which drinkers used, perceptions of various products and brands relative to each other and, in some cases, 'competitive products' such as illegal drugs. In principle, this kind of information could be gathered by social scientists, but in practice it almost never is. This highlights the particularly important potential for academic study, of market researchers' consumer panels in providing trend data that are, it seems, simply unavailable anywhere else.

Conclusion

Academic social scientists using market-research data should first and last regard them as a secondary source. Whenever they are used, it is essential that the objectives of the market researchers, the context in which the work was conducted – including the methods employed, the constraints involved and the clients for whom the data were gathered – should be taken into account throughout. Methodological differences are the key to understanding the value and limitations of marketing research data. Market research is bound to differ from academic research because quite simply, it is intended to serve very specific purposes for a limited audience. For this reason, the data themselves represent a research problem for academics, and not simply a resource to be added to those already available. Used circumspectly, in strategic conjunction with other materials, marketing research findings may well supply invaluable information in addressing academic social scientific problems in the study of food choice.

CHAPTER 19

The discourse of scientific knowledge of nutrition and dietary change in the twentieth century

David Smith

Introduction

For several decades before the First World War scientists had been discontented with the lack of governmental support for their activities, and the war offered an opportunity for them to display the utility of their knowledge (Turner 1980). The Royal Society helped to press the claim that scientists could play special roles in the pursuit of the war, and quickly became involved in initiatives concerned with munitions' research and development. In March 1916, however, the Royal Society set up a committee to consider food problems, at a time when the government was still reluctant to undertake any substantial intervention in the food system (Barnett 1985).

Soon after the formation of what became known as the Food (War) Committee, its secretary, W. B. Hardy, informed an official of the Board of Trade that the Board of Agriculture operated a scheme involving the collection of data on the availability and prices of animal foodstuffs. A professor of agriculture then applied 'physiological corrections' and drew up 'definite advice to farmers' which was embodied in leaflets, distributed monthly. The rations of animals could thereby be modified according to the combination of raw materials providing the nutrients required most economically. If appropriate information about human food was made available, Hardy suggested that a similar service could be provided for the guidance of the public.[1]

Hardy's vision of how the Committee would operate implied a direct connection between nutrition experts, the population and food habits. However, as it became clear that active management of food supply by government was required, he adopted a different model for the work of the Committee. The expected role became that of providing the scientific knowledge on which the government would base its policies. With this in mind, Hardy told a colleague that they should act as 'a body of specialists to fix the fundamental scientific data' and cautioned him not to allow differences of opinion to appear in memoranda because 'It is so important that the prestige of the scientific man should not suffer at this juncture in Government circles'.[2] In late 1916 a Ministry of Food was established and the Food (War) Committee achieved a degree of recognition as an advisory body, but found itself engaged in a more or less continuous struggle to maintain some influence (Smith 1997).

In this chapter, it will be shown through a series of glimpses at episodes in the history of nutrition science between the First World War and the 1960s that a range of views have been expressed by nutrition scientists, scientific and medical adminstrators and others, about the actual and desirable connections between nutrition science and dietary habits. Some scientists and administrators wished to influence government policies; others held no such ambitions. Some believed changes in dietary habits will simply follow the dissemination of nutritional knowledge; others emphasised the great complexities involved in bringing about dietary change. Some have changed their views dramatically in response to changing circumstances. These varying perspectives will be interpreted in terms of the individual or collective professional interests involved, in particular historical contexts. It will also be seen that, on several occasions during the twentieth century, there have been explicit calls for the development of social scientific approaches to food. Part of the purpose of this chapter is therefore to provide an account of some of the historical antecedents of the ESRC's 'Nation's Diet' programme.

Science, scientists and dietary habits in the interwar period

The work of the Food (War) Committee consisted mostly of the preparation of memoranda and reports which made specific recommendations based on existing knowledge. However, at the end of 1918 the Committee argued for the establishment of a 'Human Nutrition Research Board' and 'National Laboratory for Research in Nutrition'. Some bold claims were now made. It was asserted that new calorimetric studies could not only prevent the 'imperfect nutrition of the working classes' being 'a hindrance and danger to the state' but that they would also be 'of immense value in dealing with the labour problem in tropical and sub-tropical climates' and would 'assist the solution of the vexed question of equal pay for equal work irrespective of sex'.[3]

Support for the Board and Laboratory soon dissipated and the Committee formed to pursue the project ceased to meet long before the Ministry of Food was dismantled in 1921. The proposals cut across the interests of a range of new institutions, including the Medical Research Council (MRC). Walter Fletcher, Secretary of the MRC, regarded nutrition science as the prerogative of his organisation and without the

MRC's enthusiastic support, a Human Nutrition Research Board would not be viable. Fletcher regarded research on nutrition, and on vitamins in particular, as a 'showcase' for the value of medical research, which could help protect MRC funding (Petty 1989).

The Ministry of Health, established in 1918, soon became the main government department towards which scientists concerned about the application of nutritional knowledge usually directed their attention. Fletcher proposed that while the MRC would be responsible for basic research, the Ministry's Food Department would undertake 'investigations necessary for converting new theoretical knowledge of foods into terms applicable in administrative practice'.[4] This presupposed that the Ministry would make vigorous efforts to apply nutritional knowledge and in this respect Fletcher was soon disappointed. In 1921, when commenting on a memorandum on nutrition produced by the Food Department, Fletcher remarked that while the document summarised recent work for 'the intelligent doctor', it did not give 'strong and clear guidance' to the public. There was 'not much . . . help given, to the mother of a family, to tell her what to buy, and what not to do in the kitchen'. Fletcher thought the Ministry ought to disseminate such knowledge 'as from the housetop'.[5]

The MRC's work on vitamins was supervised by the Accessory Food Factors Committee, chaired by F. G. Hopkins, pioneer vitamin researcher. In 1922 a Committee on Quantitative Problems on Human Nutrition was also formed, at the suggestion of Major Greenwood, a medical statistician employed by the Ministry, who also worked closely with the MRC.[6] In view of allegations that there was 'actual starvation' in mining districts because of the unemployment and pay cuts, the Committee embarked on a study of the diets of miners and their families, leading to an MRC *Special Report* (Cathcart, Paton and Greenwood 1924). E. P. Cathcart and D. N. Paton were, respectively, Professor of Physiological Chemistry and Regius Professor of Physiology at Glasgow University. A total of 140 families was studied in five areas. Little evidence of a direct relationship between the weight of children and calories consumed could be found and the differences between the miners' and other local children were small. While there was a correlation between income and calories there was great variation in the yield of calories per penny spent and it was possibilities suggested by this observation which received greatest attention:

> quite apart from differences of income there are variations of diet . . . which suggest that housewives could be helped to secure a more adequate return for their expenditure by a better dissemination of knowledge both of the economic and hygienic aspects of diet. (Cathcart, Paton and Greenwood 1924: 47)

In June 1924, in a letter to George Newman, Chief Medical Officer of the Ministry, Fletcher cited these findings as evidence of the need for a nutrition-education campaign.[7] Fletcher's expectations of the Ministry eventually became a serious bone of contention which came to a head in October 1931.

Newman remarked in his annual report for 1930 that the 'adequate nutrition of the child' was 'one of the primary functions of the home', that the 'appropriate nutrition . . . of the pregnant woman', was a matter of 'common sense' and that there was 'no royal road to national health and sound nutrition' (Newman 1931: 163). Fletcher told Newman that he had received a 'great shock' when he had read these views. Fletcher thought nutrition had given 'greater practical results' than any other field of medicine during the past twelve years. He referred to the importance of vitamins in the diets of pregnant women and declared: 'There *is* a royal road, which is along the advancing line of scientific progress. This is steadily and very rapidly replacing ignorance and rule of thumb and "common sense", by precise and available knowledge.'[8]

Newman enquired evasively 'In what way do you suggest that we can do more than we are doing in the matter?' adding: 'As you know, we possess no proven powers of compulsion as to the selection, purchase or consumption of dietaries.'[9] Fletcher's complaints were referred to the Ministry's Advisory Committee on Nutrition which had been set up at the beginning of the year, which included the leading MRC nutrition researchers, resulting in a circular to local authorities which advised on the prevention of anaemia, rickets and dental disease, and the value of milk for growing children (Ministry of Health 1932). The application of this advice, like the provision of welfare foods, school-feeding and nutrition education, depended greatly on the initiative of individual Medical Officers and Councils, and other local conditions. The measures taken certainly failed to satisfy those who thought the Ministry slow to take note of and act on new nutritional knowledge. Nutrition became a subject for public debate as a series of claims and counter-claims were made about the effect of the economic depression on the incidence of malnutrition (Webster 1982).

Fletcher's use of the report on miners masked a diversity of opinion among the MRC-supported scientists. During the late 1910s and early 1920s the Glaswegian physiologists had opposed Edward Mellanby's theory of rickets as a vitamin deficiency, and Cathcart, chair of the Committee on Quantitative Problems in Human Nutrition, was sceptical about the practical importance of vitamins in human diets (Smith and Nicolson 1989). Cathcart supervised a series of MRC surveys concerned with other aspects of nutrition. A man of strong religious convictions, Cathcart's research was closely linked to a moral perspective on the determinants of food habits. His surveys aimed to provide analyses of diets in terms of calories, carbohydrates, fats and proteins, and to correlate the condition of children with 'maternal efficiency' (Cathcart and Murray 1931). His remarks during a talk at the Domestic Science College in Glasgow were typical:

> Improved education is badly required; education in budgeting marketing and cooking. But it must be education of a type suited to the needs, skill and intelligence of those who require assistance . . . the problem is not an easy one because good marketing and cooking

demands knowledge, time, interest and enthusiasm. It will mean, in many instances, a development of character, a change of heart, a conversion . . . the stimulus will not be achieved by such impersonal propaganda as lectures and leaflets.[10]

According to Cathcart, dietary problems were best tackled by voluntary organisations, and Newman adhered to similar views. Fletcher's charge that the Ministry was not involved in nutrition education was not entirely valid – a substantial, if fragmented, educational programme was undertaken by voluntary organisations and local health departments, helped and encouraged by the Ministry (Newman 1924).

Researchers such as Mellanby were aware, however, that the messages delivered by voluntary organisations were not necessarily in line with their own positions. Mellanby regarded rickets as a disease caused by an excess of cereals as well as a vitamin deficiency, and was particularly harsh in his condemnation of oatmeal. His views were attacked by organisations that praised the nutritional qualities of oatmeal and other cereals as part of their programme of dietary reform.[11]

Mellanby became Fletcher's successor as Secretary of the MRC in 1933 and in early 1934 he and Greenwood, now Professor of Epidemiology and Vital Statistics at the London School of Hygiene and Tropical Medicine, exchanged views about the future work of the Advisory Committee on Nutrition, of which Greenwood was chair and Mellanby a member. Since its formation, the Committee had achieved little, partly because Cathcart, who was also a member, often blocked consensus on key issues (Smith 1987: ch. 3). Most recently, the Committee had become embroiled in controversy, after a report of the British Medical Association (BMA) contradicted the Advisory Committee's figures for calorie and protein requirements (Smith 1995).

Greenwood had been in discussion with Arthur Robinson, Permanent Secretary at the Ministry, about the future activities of the Advisory Committee. Robinson, apparently, had 'long lamented that the Ministry has no food policy' and suggested that such a policy could be based on a study of food habits:

If one takes different industrial areas . . . for example, the cotton towns and the centres of heavy industries, the eating habits . . . are different. Indeed, the ordinary tourist can notice the greater frequency of shops selling black puddings and pork products in Staffordshire as compared with cotton towns. Robinson's idea is that a careful comparison should be made between the food habits of wholly different industrial places and that consideration should be given as to whether the differences correspond to real needs and to how far the necessary conditions are satisfied. In this way he suggests a scientific foundation might be obtained for a ministerial food policy.[12]

Mellanby could not see where such inquiries could lead. His own sympathies were with 'nutritional research of an experimental type' and since animal experiments had established facts 'likely to be beneficial to mankind' he could not see why 'an attempt should not be made to apply such facts to human beings at once'. Mellanby asked why it should not be possible to

> take some . . . area where the general health is notoriously bad . . . and introduce some feeding system . . . so as to ensure in the first place that every pregnant woman can get an abundance of milk, butter, eggs and green vegetables. This should continue through-out lactation, and after this stage the infant should receive a diet which is considered to be the best possible on the basis of present knowledge.[13]

Mellanby thought this scheme would clearly demonstrate the value of good feeding and that the health authorities might then 'place facilities for proper feeding on the same basis as the existing facilities for proper housing and proper water supply'.

Neither the Robinson/Greenwood proposals nor Mellanby's plan made much headway as the Committee was preoccupied with the controversy with the BMA. Greenwood resigned in July 1934 and the Committee was discharged and reconstituted on a different basis following discussions in November of a report of the Economic Advisory Council Committee on Scientific Research, on 'The Need for Improved Nutrition of the People of Great Britain'.[14] This document had been prepared by Hopkins and Mellanby. However, the new Committee, which first met in June 1935, adopted a programme of work much closer to the Robinson/Greenwood proposals than Mellanby's. Before the first meeting Robinson advised the new chair that the Minister wanted the Committee to 'find out what are the principle articles of food that are being consumed' and to advise whether changes are desirable and how any conclusions might be 'got across to the general population'.[15] These investigations were still on-going at the beginning of the Second World War and were never completed. In the context of the continued political agitation around nutrition, which became better organised during the later 1930s, the second Advisory Committee on Nutrition mainly served in the cause of governmental prevarication over the issue (Smith 1987: 168–84).

Mellanby's was not the only voice which placed little emphasis on education and food habits. G. C. M. M'Gonigle, co-author of *Poverty and Public Health* (M'Gonigle and Kirby 1936), resolutely opposed the 'ignorance' argument, remarking in the film *Enough to Eat?*, first screened in October 1936, that

> the average working class housewife by rule of thumb methods knows pretty well which foodstuffs to buy to feed her family . . . as her income increases she approaches more and more nearly to a really satisfactory diet. But there are hundreds of thousands of housewives who cannot afford to buy enough of the high-grade protective foods.[16]

Enough to Eat? was directed by Edgar Anstey, and was celebrated as one of the finest examples of the potential of film for informing the public about major social issues (Rotha 1973: 158, 274). The film presented data compiled by John Boyd-Orr, Director of the Rowett Research Institute in Aberdeen, and published in *Food, Health and Income* earlier in 1936. Boyd-Orr claimed that the adequacy of diets depended largely on income, and that the diet of about half the population was deficient in some respect. He called for measures which could solve the problems of both nutritional under-consumption and chronic agricultural over-production.

More radical voices were also represented by two pressure groups, the 'Committee Against Malnutrition' and the 'Children's Minimum Council'. Both organisations de-emphasised the importance of individual food habits, emphasising such measures as improving unemployment benefits, free school milk and the compulsory provision of school meals. Despite this pressure, in some areas progress was very slow. The number of solid school meals served during the interwar period, for example, rarely covered more than 2–3 per cent of the school population. However, school milk expanded substantially, encouraged by the National Milk Publicity Council and the Milk Marketing Board, which were anxious to dispose of surplus milk. By 1939 more than 85 per cent of local education departments in England and Wales participated in the Milk Marketing Board Scheme, in which areas over 55 per cent of children received school milk (Harris 1995: 125; Petty 1987: ch. 5). The nutritional value of milk was also one area in which a broad scientific consensus existed which also helped to stimulate commercial attempts to popularise milk through the milk bars which opened in many cities during the 1930s (McKee 1997).

During the interwar period, as has been seen, there were a variety of positions on the connections between scientific nutritional knowledge and the food habits of the population. Fletcher, who was interested in the development and protection of the MRC's research programme, presented the results of MRC nutrition research as more unified than they were, celebrated the importance of vitamins, and placed the responsibility for application on the Ministry of Health. He assumed that changes in dietary behaviour would automatically follow the dissemination of nutritional knowledge.

Newman's view that the selection of an adequate diet was largely a matter of commonsense, and that nutrition education was the responsibility of voluntary organisations, protected the Ministry both from the charge that it was neglecting its duties, and from potentially great expenditure. Cathcart's interest in dietary habits and his emphasis on educational and moral factors sprang from his long-term adherence to philosophical and political positions which regarded simplistic approaches to social problems in general, and nutritional problems in particular, as anathema.

Mellanby, whose theory of rickets had been attacked by rival scientists and voluntary organisations, took little interest in food habits and rather sought solutions which would by-pass the need for nutrition education. The broad trend in opinion of the late 1930s which

317

de-emphasised individual food choice in favour of economic factors, illustrated by the views of Boyd-Orr, M'Gonigle and the campaigning organisations, represents a complex alliance of professional and political opinion, characteristic of the popular front politics of the period.

The Second World War and the impulse towards social scientific approaches to nutrition

With the outbreak of the Second World War, intervention by the government in the production and distribution of food started immediately and soon became extensive. A Ministry of Food was established within days, and policies were steadily introduced which effectively combined the competing approaches to the improvement of diets advocated during the 1930s. Once the wartime food machinery was established, its existence effectively shelved the question of how scientific knowledge was to influence dietary habits – scientific knowledge could now guide the system of controls over production and distribution and the messages delivered by government propaganda.

Precisely what advice should inform the operation of the system, and exactly how it should be provided remained controversial. Mellanby successfully manoeuvred himself into a powerful position which he subsequently jealously guarded from rivals. In December 1941 he became the main nutrition expert on an interdepartmental committee established by Wilson Jameson, Chief Medical Officer of the Ministry of Health. This become known as the Standing Committee on Medical and Nutritional Problems or the Jameson Committee.

Wartime conditions also provided a stimulus towards the broader professionalisation of nutrition, as shown by the establishment of a new scientific society, the Nutrition Society, which was formed as a result of the activities of a group of junior scientists who felt that their skills were not fully deployed. These scientists began to hold monthly 'Informal Conferences of Nutrition Workers' from the autumn of 1940, preparing reports and recommendations which were sent to government departments. The reaction of Mellanby to this movement, and the intervention of Boyd-Orr, led to the formation of the new formally constituted organisation, which held its first meeting in October 1941. Each of the early meetings of the Nutrition Society addressed a policy-orientated theme, but there was never any attempt to arrive at and issue recommendations, although one current of opinion within the Society favoured such a procedure (Smith 1992a).

Discontent with the policy-making process is also indicated by an article in *The Times* written anonymously by John Yudkin, a researcher at the MRC's Dunn Nutrition Laboratory in Cambridge. Yudkin argued that currently policy was fragmented because of the wide range of government departments involved. He suggested that a 'Nutrition

Council' should be formed to organise surveys and to coordinate policies. The surveys would use new methods for the 'detection of very early signs of nutritional deficiency' which, Yudkin claimed, made it possible to 'diagnose deficiency which may not lead to any obvious symptoms . . . [and to] advise the authorities . . . on the relative merits of food policies' (*The Times* 1942). These proposals were debated in the letters column of the newspaper for five weeks, soon after which Jameson invited the Nutrition Society to establish a 'Bureau of Nutrition Surveys' to standardise survey methods – a development which was not well-received by Mellanby (Smith 1992a).

The wartime arrangements for the production and distribution of food reduced the role of individual decision-making by members of the public as a determinant of dietary habits, and in general food propaganda aimed simply to persuade people to make the best of what was available. Nevertheless, one activist began to argue that once the food controls were dismantled, a new understanding of the social determinants of food habits would be required, if the population was to be persuaded to choose diets favoured by scientists. This perspective was developed not by officials or established scientists, but by one who operated on the fringes of the food system: the left-wing, blind and disabled founder member of the Committee Against Malnutrition, Frederick le Gros Clark. At the beginning of the war Clark had become Secretary of the Children's Nutrition Council (CNC) formed by merger of the Committee Against Malnutrition and the Children's Minimum Council.

In the 1930s the nutrition campaigns consistently criticised the government, but the CNC increasingly supported wartime food policies. Reforms that the movement had long advocated seemed within sight of being realised and in 1943, the CNC congratulated itself:

> the scientific and medical point of view is beginning to influence administrative decisions now to a greater and greater extent: and this is particularly clear in matters of nutrition. The CNC has from its inception played no inconsiderable part in the changed attitudes of the authorities. (*Wartime Nutrition Bulletin* 1943)

The CNC not only welcomed the expansion of welfare foods, school-feeding and other communal feeding schemes, but also warmly approved of the food-advice schemes. While the Committee Against Malnutrition had regarded the 'ignorance and education' argument as a diversion, the CNC's *Wartime Nutrition Bulletin* now urged its branches to 'expand the principles of sound diet to all organisations by means of lectures, public meetings, exhibitions, literature' (*Wartime Nutrition Bulletin*, 1941). In this way the CNC began to assist the government's food-advice organisation. Clark even became a member of the Ministry of Food's speakers' panel.

The promise of the plans for postwar reconstruction created an assumption that, after a period of transition, employment would be full, wages adequate and food supplies abundant and varied. In the fairer, postwar society, it seemed that there would be little necessity for the movement to return to its prewar agitational role and the question of the future of the movement therefore arose. In 1936, Clark had remarked that

> a community that is conscious of a growing variety and cheapness in its food supplies can easily be induced to study the rules of correct nutrition . . . even the more abstract problems . . . are well within the comprehension of simple folk. (Clark and Brinton 1936: 159)

However, as the CNC aligned itself with the government's efforts to safeguard the nation's diet, along with this came the acceptance of the idea that the population could not always be relied on to enthusiastically embrace the provisions made for it. In 1944 an article in the *Bulletin* began to argue that a new approach was needed:

> It still remains necessary for a pervasive and patient campaign to be carried on, especially among housewives, to effect a continuous improvement in the choice of food and the understanding of food values . . . If food is in adequate supply and wage levels sufficiently high, the old patterns of food habits will begin to reassert themselves. It is clearly the function of Food Advice to work patiently on a long-term programme for the steady improvement of these habits and the correction of traditional prejudices . . . Above all, it is necessary for the staff to understand intimately the mind of the public. (*Wartime Nutrition Bulletin* 1944)

Clark had great hopes for the future of the 'Food Leaders Scheme': a system whereby the Ministry of Food recruited a network of volunteers to work in conjunction with their local Food Advice Centres (Smith 1992b). In 1945 he commented:

> They are the true spirit of this campaign of enlightenment and through whatever modification of terms and usages the campaign will pass into a post-war world, it is on such spiritual rock as this that it will have to be built. (Clark 1945: 76)

But while the postwar food-advice programme was to rely on the 'spiritual rock' of volunteer food activists, their activities were to be guided by a new scientific understanding of food habits and how to change them. The *Wartime Nutrition Bulletin* advocated the development of a new 'field of science' called 'social nutrition' or 'food sociology':

> *Food Sociology* deals . . . with the actual manner in which human beings, under varying conditions of culture and custom, choose, prepare and consume their food . . . with the more or less fixed patterns of food habits and traditions, with prejudices and taboos, with the relations between domestic feeding and communal feeding.

Investigation of these matters could form the basis for effective application of nutritional knowledge:

We should doubtless like . . . [Man] to be a creature who does without question all that the dietetic expert advises . . . Few if any of us do that. We have therefore to study ourselves as food consumers and both accumulate knowledge about ourselves and apply it towards a steady and irreversible improvement in our nutritional levels. (*Wartime Nutrition Bulletin* 1945)

It is unnecessary to speculate whether Clark's choice of the term 'sociology' signalled any special theoretical position about the nature of food choice. Sociology's image of being a progressive academic discipline, which had, for example, recently been reinforced by the founding of the monograph series *International Library of Sociology and Social Reconstruction* by Karl Mannheim, and the increased use of social surveys for government purposes during the war, made it an attractive label for activists interested in the professionalisation of their field of work. Similarly, the use of the phrase 'consumers' should not be taken to indicate a commitment to modern consumerism. The term was used, for example, by the technocratic planning organisation 'Political and Economic Planning' during the 1930s, which appointed a Research Group on 'Consumer Research' and prepared a memorandum on the need for a national food policy.[17]

Clark's 'food sociology', he stated, could be divided into the study of food services 'already in operation and those which might theoretically be brought into existence' and the study of 'Food Customs and Traditions'. The *Bulletin* suggested that the new field could be a source of employment for at least some of the people who had been recruited to the Government's wartime food machinery:

many inquiries of this kind are well within the capacity of experienced persons whose training in chemistry, physiology or medicine may have been elementary. We shall have after the war a large body of canteen supervisors, hospital caterers, dietetic advisers and domestic science teachers . . . Many of these should be able to contribute useful observations . . . But emphatically the technique of research will have to be learned and mastered . . . Allowing for that, we may believe that here is a field of science open to numerous practitioners, that it is not only of theoretical interest but has a normal outcome in social amelioration. (*Wartime Nutrition Bulletin* 1945)

Early examples of 'food sociology' were Clark's studies for Hertfordshire County Council on school children's views on school meals and their taste in vegetables, based on analyses of pupils' essays on these subjects (Clark 1943a, 1943b).

During the early postwar years, Clark found a niche with the Central Council for Health Education (CCHE), the forerunner of the Health Education Council. This organisation took over the CNC *Bulletin* after October 1946, retaining Clark as editor. After May 1951 the *Bulletin* was incorporated into the *Health Education Journal*. Clark participated in the formulation and discussion of the CCHE's memorandum 'The

Improvement of the National Diet', published in *The Lancet* in May 1948, and organised courses for food operatives on behalf of CCHE.[18]

The introductory declaration in the first number of the CCHE's *Nutrition Bulletin* suggested that it would prove an outlet for 'food sociology'. The purpose of the publication would be to examine:

the growth of the public services, the response made to them and the influence they exert over our social customs, the techniques of instruction in food values, the nature and origin of food habits, the class differences in diet and the role of diet in the health of the community. (*Nutrition Bulletin* 1947a)

However, the 'food sociology' that appeared in the *Bulletin* consisted largely of programmatic essays and occasional reports of small-scale research projects. One example was a study of the National Milk Cocoa Scheme which provided subsidised cocoa for young factory workers. It was found that the scheme could be made more popular if the workers were allowed to make their own cocoa, take it between mealbreaks, and drink it at their machines (*Nutrition Bulletin* 1947b). Investigations of the diet of young people at work was taken up by a research group of the London Council of Social Service, directed by Clark. This group had already conducted a study of communal restaurants during the war, and in 1948 published a booklet called *Young Workers at Meal Time* (London Council of Social Service 1944, 1948).

Clark sought to promote the study of food habits of young people through his membership of the sub-committee on 'Psychological and Practical Aspects of Nutrition' of a BMA Nutrition Committee which was established in October 1947 to 'consider and report on the problem of nutrition in this country, including current nutritional standards' (Anon 1947). This Committee was formed against a background of agitation for an end to rationing at a time when rations had been reduced because of the need to release supplies for the relief of war-ravaged countries (Zweiniger-Bargielowska 1993). Clark prepared two memoranda,[19] which were included, virtually unchanged, in the final report, published in early 1950. One of the final recommendations, based on Clark's memoranda, advocated an inquiry 'into any fundamental changes in food habits which may have occurred among young people aged 15 to 25 as a result of the diet in recent years' (British Medical Association 1950: 100).

'Food sociology' formed part of an attempt by Clark to professionalise the activities of the nutrition movement, but despite his best efforts it did not become established as a recognised field of study and practice as he had envisaged. By the end of the 1940s the food advice and communal-feeding schemes, which he had seen as major objects of study for 'food sociology', and as important mechanisms through which the results of 'food sociology' would be applied, were subject to severe financial retrenchment. In this new situation Clark adopted a different approach to nutrition education: he began to place most emphasis on the task of dispelling food prejudices. In 1947 he argued:

we should concentrate less on commending various foods to the public than on working to remove from their minds the mistaken and outworn ideas that still survive . . . in the course of history men have attached to food an emotional significance, amounting in some cases to a religious taboo; and our own task is simply that of reversing the process and gradually purging the human mind of the accumulated dross of centuries. (Clark 1947: 137)

The shift in Clark's thought on the links between scientific knowledge and food habits, during and after the war, allowed a degree of political disengagement as he moved from the oppositional stance of the 1930s to a position in which he hoped to deploy a social–scientific approach to food choice and to participate in the progressive management of the population in the interests of their health. But while Clark failed to realise his ambitions with regard to nutrition and food sociology and soon moved on to the social problems faced by elderly workers as his central interest (Clark and Dunn 1955), John Yudkin, who adopted some similar positions to those of Clark in his own attempts to find a viable role in the postwar world, successfully developed a career in nutrition, and eventually revived interest in research in social aspects of nutrition during the early 1960s.

John Yudkin and nutrition at Queen Elizabeth College

As a medically qualified researcher at the Dunn Nutritional Laboratory, compared to Clark, Yudkin worked more within the mainstream of nutrition research during the 1930s. During the war, however, his identity as the proponent of a 'Nutrition Council' came to the notice of Mellanby, who was greatly offended, seeing it as an unjustified challenge to the leadership of the MRC in the field of nutrition.[20] Since Mellanby remained Secretary of the MRC until 1949, Yudkin's position became that of a relative outsider to the medical research establishment.

In 1945 Yudkin was appointed Professor of Physiology at King's College of Household and Social Science of the University of London, where he had to rely almost entirely on industrial funding for research and received no support from the MRC until 1959 (Queen Elizabeth College 1960: 21). As soon as he took up the appointment, however, he started campaigning for a further step in the professionalisation of nutrition: the institution of a BSc in the subject. This involved a difficult process of defining the nature of nutrition as a science, and the practices of graduate nutritionists, and of convincing London University that nutrition was a respectable degree subject. The new course was finally approved in 1951 and the first students started in 1953, in which year the College was renamed Queen Elizabeth College (QEC). Yudkin was made Professor of Nutrition in 1954.

As has been seen, in 1942 Yudkin boldly claimed that tests for monitoring nutritional status could be employed as a guide to food policy. Later in the war, he published several papers which addressed questions of nutrition, class and economics, in ways reminiscent of Boyd Orr's *Food, Health and Income* (Yudkin 1944a, 1944b). By 1952, however, Yudkin had arrived at a quite different position. In *The British Encyclopaedia of Medical Practice*, he observed

It is . . . becoming increasingly recognised that the methods for assessing dietary intakes, for the determination of dietary requirements with which those intakes can be compared, and for the assessment of nutritional status by clinical and laboratory means, are all fraught with considerable difficulty. (Yudkin 1952: 134)

The emphasis in Yudkin's writings became that of opposition to simplistic approaches to nutrition and the assertion of the complexity and difficulty of the subject. This was the import of a lecture on 'Fighting Food Faddism' given in 1953, in which he argued that:

there is so much which is unknown in nutritional science; and because there is still so much room for differing opinions based on what is known . . . it is imperative, for all of us, that we approach the many nutritional problems which beset us with enquiring minds and with humility, not emotion and not with prejudice. (Yudkin 1953a: 186)

Emphasising the unknown in nutrition science served a variety of purposes. First, it helped to counter any feeling that the apparent success of nutrition during the war showed that the field was 'worked out'. Immediately following the war there were several setbacks which have been attributed to such a view. When Harriette Chick, pioneer vitamin researcher at the Lister Institute retired in 1946, and it was decided to close the Institute's Nutrition Department, the Director told one of the remaining nutrition workers, 'there's no future in nutrition'.[21] According to H. M. Sinclair, who had established the Oxford Nutrition Survey with funding from the Rockefeller Foundation during the war, this feeling also played a role in Oxford University's decision to renege on a promise to establish a permanent department of nutrition.[22]

Emphasising the difficulties involved in the assessment of nutritional status also allowed a withdrawal from challenges to government administration of food and health. Several events during the early post-war period illustrate the pressures in this direction, and the desirability of joining the trend. When Boyd-Orr retired as Director of the Rowett Institute in 1945, an opportunity was taken to limit its activities with a ruling that the research conducted there was not to be concerned with human nutrition. His successor recalled that when he was appointed it was 'made fairly plain . . . that I was there to encourage the study of the nutrition of animals of agricultural importance'.[23] The implication was that the new Director was warned not to revive the kind of campaigning that Boyd-Orr had taken up during the 1930s.

324

The trend away from policy and politics may also be illustrated by the development of the Nutrition Society in the early post-war years. In March 1946, Mellanby referred to the Society disparagingly as 'mainly concerned with the political, social and economic aspects of nutrition' and 'never . . . distinguished for any great desire to hear and discuss new truths and new discoveries'.[24] However, the Society was already taking steps to acquire a more respectable image by embracing more of the attributes of a conventional scientific society. The decision to start holding 'Open Scientific Meetings' where short preliminary communications about research in progress would be given, was taken shortly after the war. The Society's journal also soon started accepting original articles for publication, and the Conferences began to move away from exclusively policy-orientated topics. The Society also quickly shed its limited wartime role in the coordination of nutrition research (Smith 1987: 234–58).

All these developments after the Second World War encouraged some research scientists who had been involved in nutrition either to move on to other fields, or into research on the purely biochemical or physiological aspects of nutrition. Yudkin, however, based as he was at a college which had been dedicated to developing scientific approaches to the problems of the home, could hardly devote himself exclusively to pure science (Blakestad 1997). Yudkin's definition of what 'nutrition' consisted of needed to encapsulate some sort of vision of how nutritional knowledge might be applied: he needed something to say about how the graduate nutritionists he aimed to train would apply nutritional knowledge.

Yudkin's initial solution to these problems involved a broad vision of nutrition science, including consideration of social aspects of food, and a reliance on conventional education as the means to influence food habits. In 'Fighting Food Faddism' he explained that the science of 'Nutrition' should be considered a 'new entity':

> Our first principle is that nutrition concerns every aspect of food, from its growth as plant or animal, through its harvesting, transportation, preparation and consumption, to the effect of that consumption on the health of the people. We must teach something of the soil and agricultural methods . . . food preservation and cookery, and the economic, psychological and sociological aspects of food . . . We must do all this teaching of biology, chemistry, physiology and a variety of other subjects, in such a way that our students do not think of themselves as specialists in any of these fields, but as persons who have built up the relevant parts of these subjects into a new entity, nutrition. (Yudkin 1953a: 186)

The potential of graduate nutritionists for placing nutrition education on a sound basis was discussed in Yudkin's address to the Nutrition Society's conference on 'Education in Nutrition', which was held at QEC. He remarked:

> The difficulty. . . is that at present those who teach nutrition are

themselves not sufficiently trained in the subject. There is thus, for example, a tendency for domestic science teachers to learn their nutrition from other domestic science teachers, so that there is inevitably a perpetuation of ill-founded, inaccurate and out-of-date information. (Yudkin 1953b: 198)

Yudkin went on to make further points about the teaching of nutrition to medical students, caterers and food technologists, and continued:

The obvious question arises, 'Who is to teach the teachers?' It seems clear that the need is for the training of nutritionists having, on the one hand, a sound academic background and, on the other, a full appreciation that nutrition is concerned with what people eat. As well as providing the source from which can be drawn the teachers in nutrition at all levels, the existence of trained nutritionists might well in time influence those with administrative responsibility to realise the significance of the science of nutrition. (Yudkin 1953b: 199)

The last quotation suggests that Yudkin had not altogether given up the hope of eventually influencing government policies, but the vague and tentative nature of his remarks emphasises the dramatic change from his position of only ten years earlier.

However useful stressing the complexity of nutrition science, and pointing out the pitfalls of simplistic approaches, might have been in the process of establishing degree-level nutrition science in the early 1950s, such an emphasis could not indefinitely justify the subject in the long term. Yudkin needed to participate in wider developments in the field, which during the late 1950s included the nutritional aetiology of the 'diseases of civilisation', slimming, and the nutritional problems of developing countries. During this period Yudkin began to formulate distinct positions on obesity and slimming and on the role of diet in coronary heart disease and other degenerative conditions. He argued that the most effective approach to slimming was to limit carbohydrate consumption, and published a popular book based on this view. He also developed a theory linking the putative increase in coronary heart disease with increases in sugar consumption, and challenged alternative theories which emphasised the role of dietary fat (Yudkin 1958, 1959).

Positively taking up such topics as slimming and the 'diseases of civilisation', and the interest in nutrition in the developing world, again placed the question of how the work of nutrition scientists was to be applied back on the agenda, and demanded a novel solution. The problems in both the Western and the underdeveloped countries became defined by Yudkin as problems of changing food habits, but now the inadequacy of ordinary education in bringing about such changes was emphasised. Changes in food habits, it was now suggested, could only be brought about on the basis of an understanding of the factors, particularly sociological and psychological factors, which determine food habits.

In the early years of the nutrition degree, social scientists visited

Queen Elizabeth College to teach the nutrition students, but in 1959 J. C. McKenzie, a graduate in economics, was appointed 'Research Fellow in the Sociology of Nutrition', a post which was funded by a grant from the Leverhulme Trust, and in 1960 R. H. J. Watson was appointed Research Psychologist, funded by the Department of Scientific and Industrial Research. A 'Social Nutrition Unit' was established which began to conduct its own teaching in sociology and psychology, and started a research programme on social aspects of nutrition. Accompanying these developments was a striking revision of opinion about the value of nutrition education. In 1963, McKenzie and Yudkin commented in the *New Scientist*:

> Nutritionists . . . have a touching faith in the efficacy of education in improving food habits. Many of us have spent a great deal of time and energy in telling what people should eat for health . . . We are, however, becoming increasingly sceptical of how much education in nutrition can overcome all other 'social' factors which can influence food choice. (McKenzie and Yudkin 1963: 281)

In September 1963 a conference on 'Changing Food Habits' was held at Queen Elizabeth College. Eight papers were presented including one each by Yudkin and McKenzie. Most of the other contributors, who were from industrial as well as academic settings, spoke from the perspectives of psychology, sociology or anthropology. In a 'Conspectus' included in the publication containing the papers discussed at the conference, Yudkin and McKenzie make further remarks on the lack of connection between nutritional knowledge and food choice:

> Our . . . observations suggest that nutritional knowledge – correct or incorrect – does not affect the choice of many people other than those unusually preoccupied with their health. Nutritional value is more commonly used as a rationalisation for a choice that has already been made; for example, that sweets and sugar are especially good sources of energy. (Yudkin and McKenzie 1964b: 136)

Yudkin and McKenzie pointed out that many people, including the United Nations agencies, still believed in the efficacy of scientific nutrition education but suggested, however, 'that the success of the efforts to change food habits which have been made for 15 years or more has been disappointingly limited'. In their view the time had come:

> to ask whether we should by now not have done better if we had spent time in assessing the effectiveness of these efforts, and more particularly in studying the fundamental determinants of food habits and their relative importance, and then in examining the ways in which one or more of these determinants could be used to promote change. (Yudkin and McKenzie 1964: 142)

This emphasis on the need to study the 'determinants of food habits' was characteristic of the QEC approach to nutritional problems during the rest of, and beyond, Yudkin's tenure of the Chair of Nutrition.

'Social aspects of nutrition' no longer simply constituted just another component of the course, but became a cornerstone of the practice of the QEC-trained graduate nutritionist. The greatest emphasis was placed on psychological and sociological factors in food choice, and economic factors were largely ignored, as is clear from this passage from a further contribution by Yudkin to *New Scientist* in 1964. According to Yudkin's article, the major problem to be solved in the 'impoverished countries' was:

> how to persuade people to eat what is good for them and how to prevent them from eating what is bad for them. In other words the first problem is to persuade people accustomed to eating a narrow range of nutritionally poor foods to widen their choice so as to include the nutritionally more desirable foods, especially those rich in protein. We will need, for this purpose, information about what determines food habits and how people can be influenced to eat unaccustomed foods. (Yudkin 1964: 273)

Ironically, this article was part of the *New Scientist*'s '1984 Series', because Yudkin seemed to suggest that, armed with social–scientific insights, the nutritionist, in collaboration with the food industry, would be able to act as 'big brother' and manipulate the diet in both undeveloped and developed countries, in the interests of their health. At the 'Changing Food Habits' conference, market researchers David Pickard and Ray Cori, speaking on 'The Role of the Sociologist in Inducing Changes in Food Choice' advised nutritionists: 'If you can introduce changes in food habits surreptitiously, without anyone knowing, if necessary by plain deceit, then – assuming you are certain you are justified – do so' (Pickard and Cori 1964: 72). Similarly, Arnold Bender, Head of Research and Development at Farley's Infant Food Ltd, speaking of 'The Nutritionist in Industry', argued that if a manufacturer's food chemist was (like himself) also a nutritionist ('one who studies the supply of nutrients to society, to the individual, and, ultimately, to the cell') then:

> he has the opportunity of at least mitigating the effects of his processing, of placing the degree of damage in its proper perspective or recommending methods of consumption that will obviate any nutritional losses. For example, if vitamins are lost they can be restored, or raw materials of higher vitamin content chosen; if a cereal has lost some of its already limited store of the amino acid, lysine, the product can be recommended to be consumed with milk which makes good the deficiency, or synthetic lysine may be added. (Bender 1964: 111)

Bender was appointed to a personal Chair of Nutrition at QEC in 1972, shortly after Yudkin had retired, and later became head of the Nutrition Department. Under Bender's leadership, emphasis on the lessons of the study of sociological and psychological aspects of nutrition continued to play a fundamental role in the professional identity of the QEC-trained nutritionist.

328

Strategically, the emphasis on the sociological and psychological aspects of nutrition during the 1960s served a similar purpose to the earlier emphasis on the complexity of nutrition and 'Fighting Food Faddism'. During the early 1950s the formulation of 'Fighting Food Faddism' and the emphasis on complexity helped to provide a rationale for the political disengagement of nutrition, and formed part of Yudkin's initial efforts to professionalise the field and establish nutrition as a respectable degree-level science. Nutrition would no longer be associated with lobbying the government for changes in food policies: instead, the main task would be to counter unscientific food prejudices through nutrition education. By the 1960s, when some more positive messages had been formulated, which implied a definite need for changes in nutrient intakes, the emphasis on the need for the systematic study of the 'sociological and psychological aspects' of nutrition as the basis for action, helped to ensure the continued political disengagement of the field. In contrast to Clark's initial conception of 'food sociology' which linked the new field very clearly with the active citizenship of 'Food Leaders' and other nutrition campaigners, the social nutrition programme at QEC emphasised the role and potential of nutrition scientists working through an enlightened food industry.

Discussion and conclusion

In this brief and schematic account of the thought of a few selected actors on the question of the connections between scientific knowledge and dietary habits, the focus has largely been on nutrition scientists and activists, and medical and scientific administrators. Nothing has been said of why, from time to time, social scientists have become involved in questions of food choice, but in recent years that interest has not only increased, but ESRC funding for research in this area has become available through 'The Nation's Diet' Programme. This volume is one of the products of this new and concerted research effort.

This chapter has shown that in the past, views on the potential of scientific knowledge of nutrition for altering the food habits of the population have varied, along with the particular goals of individuals and groups involved in· nutrition. At times the potential of the dissemination of nutritional knowledge to change food habits has been assumed; at other times it has been denied. No doubt the findings of 'The Nation's Diet' Programme will provide a range of messages which will also be pressed into the service of a range of interests within nutrition science.

The actual roles played by nutritional knowledge in dietary change still await detailed historical investigation. Such topics as the role that scientific consensus on the nutritional value of milk played in the popularisation of milk during the 1930s, and the apparant failure of scientific opinion to prevent the general switch to white bread when controls over milling ended in the 1950s, seem worthy of further study.

Other possibilities have been suggested by Arnold Bender who has observed that, with reference to more recent trends in bread consumption, 'sales of breads of all kinds fell steadily until the publication of the COMA [Committee on Medical Aspects of Food Policy of the Department of Health and Social Security] Report on Bread (1981) which encouraged bread consumption'. And on trends in sugar consumption he remarked: 'Sugar and sweet foods are continually under pressure [from health educators] and sales of packet sugar have fallen steadily since a peak in 1958.' However, Bender also observed that the upturn in bread sales coincided with technological changes which make wholemeal bread more palatable, and that the decrease in sales of packet sugar has been accompanied by an increase in sales of sugar confectionery (Bender in Hurren and Black 1991: 127, 130). It is clear that the investigation of such episodes will not reveal any simple mechanistic connection between nutritional advice and changes in food consumption.

In conclusion, it is the contention of this chapter that a mature and comprehensive social science of food choice must neither over-emphasise nor exclude scientific knowledge as a factor in dietary change. But in order to move beyond existing views on the connections between nutritional science and dietary change, that have been closely linked with the discourse of a continuously insecure scientific enterprise, concrete and detailed historical studies are required that analyse the role of scientific knowledge in specific contexts. Such studies may then help to encourage realistic strategic thinking and expectations.

Notes

1   Memorandum, W. B. Hardy to Mr Eddison, 29 March 1916, Royal Society Archive (hereafter RS) MS 505, file 'Board of Trade'.
2   W. B. Hardy to D. N. Paton, 10 August 1916, RS MS 505, File 'Paton, D. N.'.
3   W. B. Hardy, 'Human Nutrition Institute', September, 1918, and 'Report of the Food (War) Committee upon the organisation of state research in human nutrition', 18 January 1919, RS MS 528.
4   'Memorandum on the suggested relations between the Ministry of Health and Medical Research Committee in regard to scientific work upon food', 25 November 1919, Public Records Office (hereafter PRO) FD1/2382.
5   W. Fletcher to A. W. MacFadden 20 September 1921, PRO FD1/2382.
6   M. Greenwood to W. Fletcher, 30 October 1921, PRO FD1/4365.
7   W. Fletcher to G. Newman, 20 June 1924, PRO FD1/4366.
8   W. Fletcher to G. Newman, 22 October 1931, PRO FD1/1375.
9   G. Newman to W. Fletcher, 30 November 1931, PRO FD1/1375.
10 'Domestic Science, Glasgow 1936' (Typescript), E. P. Cathcart papers, Glasgow University Library, Department of Special Collections.
11 M. Yates, Bread and Food Reform League to W. Fletcher, 6 May 1924, PRO FD1/90.
12 M. Greenwood to E. Mellanby, 8 January 1934, PRO FD1/4428.

13 E. Mellanby to M. Greenwood, 15 January 1934, PRO FD1/4428.
14 Minutes of Conference of Ministers on Nutrition, 6 November 1934, PRO MH 79/342.
15 A. Robinson to Lord Luke, 5 July 1935, PRO MH 79/343.
16 *Enough to Eat?* is available from the British Film Institute, London.
17 See Medical Research Council file, 'PEP and Medical Research', PRO FD1/3532.
18 Central Council for Health Education, 'Report of a Conference on the National Diet', 4 November 1948, Wellcome Institute, London, Contemporary Medical Archives Centre (hereafter CMAC) SA/BMA/G48.
19 A. Macrea to F. Le Gros Clark, 19 January, Clark to Macrea, 23 January, 16 February 1948, CMAC SA/BMA/G58.
20 L. J. Harris to E. Mellanby, 11 October, Mellanby to Harris, 15 October 1943, PRO FD1/3813.
21 A. M. Copping, interview with D. F. Smith, 14 November 1979 (typescript available from author).
22 H. M. Sinclair, interview with D. F. Smith, 13 November 1979 (typescript available from author).
23 D. P. Cuthbertson, interview with D. F. Smith, 1 November 1979 (typescript available from author).
24 E. Mellanby to R. A. Peters, 7 March 1946, PRO FD1/4372.

References

ACHAYA, K. T. 1987. 'Fat Status of Indians – a Review.' *Journal of Scientific and Industrial Research* 46: 112–26

AHMAD, W. I. U. 1996. 'The Trouble with Culture' in D. Kelleher and S. Hillier (eds), *Researching Cultural Differences in Health*. London: Routledge.

AINSLIE, G. 1992. *Picoeconomics: the Strategic Interaction of Successive Motivational States within the Person*. Cambridge: Cambridge University Press.

AJZEN, I. 1991. 'The Theory of Planned Behavior', *Organizational Behavior and Human Decision Processes* 50:179–211.

AJZEN, I. 1996. 'The Directive Influence of Attitudes on Behavior', in P. Gollwitzer and J. A. Bargh (eds), *Psychology of Action*. New York: Guilford, pp. 385-403.

AJZEN, I. and FISHBEIN, M. 1980. *Understanding Attitudes and Predicting Social Behavior*. Englewood-Cliff, NJ: Prentice-Hall.

AMATO, P. R. and PARTRIDGE, S. A. 1989. *The New Vegetarians: Promoting Health and Preserving Life*. London: Plenum Press.

AMERICAN MARKETING ASSOCIATION 1987. 'New Marketing Research Definition Approved'. *Marketing News* 2 January: 21.

ANDERSON, A. S. and HUNT, K. 1992. 'Who are the Healthy Eaters?' *Health Education Journal* 51(1): 3–10.

ANDERSON, A. S. and LEAN, M., 1995. 'Healthy Change: Observations on a Decade of Dietary Change in Glaswegian South Asian migrants'. *Journal of Human Nutrition and Dietetics* 8: 129–36.

ANDERSON, A. S., LEAN, M., BUSH, H., BRADBY, H. and WILLIAMS, R. 1995. 'Macronutrient Intake in South Asian and Italian Women in the West of Scotland' (abstract). *Proceedings of the Nutrition Society* 54(3): 203A.

ANDERSON, C. A. 1983. 'Imagination and Expectation: The Effect of Imagining Behavioral Scripts on Personal Intentions'. *Journal of Personality and Social Psychology* 45: 293–305.

ANDERSON, D. (ed.) 1986. *A Diet of Reason – Sense and Nonsense in the Healthy Eating Debate*. London: The Social Affairs Unit.

ANDERSON, G. and BLUNDELL, R. 1982. 'Consumer Non-durables in the UK: A Dynamic Demand System'. *Economic Journal, Supplement* 94: 34–44.

ANON 1947. 'Standards of Nutrition'. *British Medical Journal* II: 740.

ANWAR M. 1979. *The Myth of Return: Pakistanis in Britain.* London: Heinemann.

ARCE, A. and MARSDEN, T. K. 1993. The Social Construction of International Food: a New Research Agenda. *Economic Geography* 69:293–311.

ATTAR, D. 1990. *Wasting Girls' Time: The History and Politics of Home Economics.* London: Virago Educational Series.

AUDIT COMMISSION, 1985. *Managing Social Services for the Elderly More Effectively.* London: HMSO.

BACK, L. 1996. *New Ethnicities and Urban Culture: Racisms and Multiculture in Young Lives.* London: University College London Press.

BAER, D. M. and DEGUCHI, H. 1985. 'Generalized imitation from a radical-behavioral viewpoint' in S. Reiss and R. R Bootzin (eds), *Theoretical issues in behavior therapy,* Orlando: Academic Press, pp. 179-217.

BAER, J. R., WILLIAMS, J. A., OSNES, P. G. and STOKES, T. F. 1985. 'Generalised Verbal Control and Correspondence Training', *Behavior Modification,* 9: 477–89.

BAER, R., BLOUNT, R., DETRICH, R. and STOKES, T. 1987. 'Using Intermittent Reinforcement to Program Maintenance of Verbal/nonverbal Correspondence': *Journal of Applied Behavior Analysis* 20: 179–84.

BAGOZZI, R. P. 1992. 'The Self-regulation of Attitudes, Intentions and Behavior'. *Social Psychology Quarterly* 55: 178–204.

BALL, S., BOWE, R. and GOLD, A. 1992. *Reforming Education and Changing Schools: Case Studies in Policy Sociology.* London: Routledge.

BANDURA, A. 1977. *Social learning Theory.* Englewood Cliffs, NJ: Prentice–Hall.

BANDURA, A. 1989. 'Social cognitive theory', *Annals of Child Development,* 6, 1–60.

BARGH, J. A., CHAIKEN, S., GOVENDER, R., and PRATTO, F. 1992. 'The Generality of the Automatic Attitude Activation Effect'. *Journal of Personality and Social Psychology* 62: 893–912.

BARNETT, M. 1985. *British Food Policy During the First World War* London: Allen & Unwin.

BASCH, C. 1987. 'Focus Group Interviews; an Underutilised Research Technique for Improving Theory and Practice in Health Education'. *Health Education Quarterly* 16: 389–96.

BASS, F. M. 1993. 'The Future of Research in Marketing: Marketing Science'. *Journal of Marketing Research* XXX: 1–6.

BAUMAN, Z. 1988. *Freedom.* Milton Keynes: Open University Press.

BDP PLANNING/OXIRM 1992. *The Effects of Major Out-of-town Retail Development: a Literature Review for the Department of the Environment.* BDP Planning/Oxford Institute of Retail Management, London: HMSO.

BEALE, D. A. and MANSTEAD, A. S. R. 1991. 'Predicting Mothers' Intentions to Limit Frequency of Infants' Sugar Intake: Testing the Theory of Planned Behavior'. *Journal of Applied Social Psychology* 21: 409–31.

BEARSDWORTH, A. and KEIL, T. 1997. *Sociology on the Menu*. London: Routledge.

BEAUCHAMP, G. K. 1987. 'The Human Preference for Excess Salt', *American Scientist*, 75: 27–33.

BECKER, G. 1965. 'A Theory of the Allocation of Time'. *The Economic Journal* LXXV: 493–517.

BELL, D. W., ESSES, V. M., and MAIO, G. R. 1996. 'The Utility of Open-ended Measures to Assess Intergroup Ambivalence'. *Canadian Journal of Behavioral Sciences* 28: 12–18.

BELLACK, A. S., HERSEN, M. and KAZDIN, A. E. 1985. *International Handbook of Behavior Modification and Therapy*, New York: Plenum Press.

BENDER, A. 1964. 'The Nutritionist in Industry', in J. Yudkin and J. C. McKenzie, 1964.

BENTLER, P. and SPECKART, G. 1979. 'Models of Attitude-behavior Relations'. *Psychological Review* 86: 452–64.

BERGER, P. 1963. *Invitation to Sociology*. Harmondsworth: Penguin Books.

BERGER, P. and KELLNER, H. 1974. 'Marriage and the Social Construction of Reality', in B. Berger (ed.) *Readings in Sociology*. New York: Basic Books, pp. 119–23.

BERGER, P. and LUCKMANN, T. 1966. *The Social Construction of Reality: a Treatise in the Sociology of Knowledge*. Harmondsworth: Penguin Books.

BERNAL, M. E. 1972. 'Behavioral Treatment of a Child's Eating Problem', *Journal of Behavior Therapy and Experimental Psychology*, 3, 43–50.

BERNSTEIN, D. J. 1990. 'Of Carrots and Sticks: A review of Deci and Ryan's Intrinsic Motivation and Self–Determination in Human Behaviour', *Journal of the Experimental Analysis of Behavior*, 54: 323–32.

BHACHU, P. 1985. *Twice Migrants: East African Sikh Settlers in Britain*. London: Tavistock.

BHACHU, P. 1988. 'Apni Marzi Kardhi Home and Work: Sikh Women in Britain', in S. Westwood and P. Bhachu (eds), *Enterprising Women: Ethnicity, Economy and Gender Relations*. London: Routledge, pp. 76–102.

BINGHAM, S. A., GILL, C., WELCH, A., DAY, K., CASSIDY, A. *et al.* 1994. 'Comparison of Dietary Assessment Methods in Nutritional Epidemiology: Weighed Records v. 24h Recalls, Food Frequency Questionnaires and Estimated Diet Records'. *British Journal of Nutrition* 72: 619–43.

BINNS, R., DAVIES, G. and PARRY, B. 1989. *A Taste of Wales: Good Food, Recipes . . . a Guide to Cooking and Travel*. Wales: Blas ar Gymru.

BJORNTORP, P. 1987. 'The Associations Between Obesity, Adipose Tissue Distribution and Disease'. *Acta Medica Scandinavica Supplement*. 723: 121–34.

BLAKESTAD, N. L. 1997. 'King's College of Household and Social Science and the Origins of Dietetic Education' in Smith, D. F. (ed.) 1997a.

BLAXTER, M. and PATERSON, E. 1983. 'The Goodness is Out of It: the Meaning of Food to Two Generations', in A. Murcott (ed.) 1983b.

BLAYLOCK, J. R. and SMALLWOOD, D. M. 1987. 'Intrahousehold Time Allocation: The Case of Grocery Shopping'. *The Journal of Consumer Affairs* 21(2): 183–201.

BLUNDELL, J. E. and ROGERS, P. J. 1991. 'Satiating Power of Food'. *Encyclopaedia of Human Biology* 6: 723–33.

BODY, R. 1982. *Agriculture: The Triumph and the Shame*. London: Temple Smith.

BODY, R. 1984. *Farming in the Clouds*. London: Temple Smith.

BODY, R. 1987. *Red or Green for Farmers (and the Rest of Us)*. Saffron Walden, Essex: Broad Leys Publishing.

BODY, R. 1991. *Our Food, Our Land*. London: Rider.

BOLESWORTH, S. and WALLER, D. 1997. 'The Secrecy that can Kill'. *Guardian* 15 March: 26.

BOLGER, N. and ECKENRODE, J. 1991. 'Social Relationships, Personality, and Anxiety during a Major Stressful Event'. *Journal of Personality & Social Psychology* 61: 440–49.

BOOTH, D. A. 1994. *Psychology of Nutrition*. London: Taylor & Francis.

BOOTH, D. A. and SHEPHERD, R. 1988. 'Sensory Influences on Food Acceptance: The Neglected Approach to Nutrition Promotion'. *British Nutrition Foundation Nutrition Bulletin* 13: 39–54.

BOURDIEU, P. 1984. *Distinction: a Social Critique of the Judgement of Taste*. London: Routledge & Kegan Paul. (First published in French as *La Distinction: Critique sociale du jugement* 1979.)

BOWLBY, S. R. 1988. 'From Corner Shop to Hypermarket: Women and Food Retailing', in J. Little, L. Peake and P. Richardson (eds), *Women in Cities: Gender and the Environment*. London: Macmillan, pp. 61–83.

BOWLBY, S. R. and FOORD, J. 1995. 'Relational Contracting between UK Retailers and Manufacturers'. *International Review of Retail, Distribution and Consumer Research* 5:333–61.

BOWLBY, S. R., FOORD, J. and TILLSLEY, C. 1992. 'Changing Consumption Patterns: Impacts on Retailers and their Suppliers'. *International Review of Retail, Distribution and Consumer Research* 2:133–50.

BOYD-ORR, J. 1936. *Food, Health and Income*. London: Macmillan.

BRADBY, H. 1996. 'Cultural Strategies of Young Women of South Asian Origin in Glasgow, with Special Reference to Health'. Unpublished PhD thesis, University of Glasgow.

BRADBY, H. 1997. 'The Salience of Health in Glaswegian Punjabi Women's Thinking about Everyday Food', in P. Caplan (ed.) 1997.

BRADDON, F. E., RODGERS, B., WADSWORTH, M. E. and DAVIES, J. 1986. 'Onset of Obesity in a 36-Year Birth Cohort Study'. *British Medical Journal* 293: 299–303.

BRAH, A. 1993. ' "Race" and "Culture" in the Gendering of Labour Markets: South Asian Young Muslim Women and the Labour Market'. *New Community* 19(3): 441–58.

BRINBERG, D. and DURAND, J. 1983. 'Eating at Fast-food Restaurants: an Analysis Using Two Behavioral Intention Models'. *Journal of Applied Social Psychology* 13: 459–72.

BRINDLEY, D. N., MCCANN, B. S., NIAURA, R., STONEY, C. M. and SUAREZ, E. C. 1993. 'Stress and Lipoprotein Metabolism: Modulators and Mechanisms'. *Metabolism: Clinical & Experimental* 42: 3–15.

BRITISH MEDICAL ASSOCIATION 1950. *Report of the Committee on Nutrition*. London: British Medical Association.

BRODY, G. B. and STONEMAN, Z. (1981) 'Selective Imitation of Same-Age, Older and Younger Peer Models', *Child Development* 52(7) 17–20

BROMLEY, D. W. 1991. *Environment and Economy: Property Rights and Public Policy*. Oxford: Basil Blackwell.

BROWN, C. 1984. *Black and White Britain: the Third PSI Survey*. Aldershot: Gower.

BROWN, P. J. and KONNER, M. 1987. 'An Anthropological Perspective on Obesity'. *Annals of the New York Academy of Sciences* 499: 29–46.

BRUCH, H. 1961. 'Transformation of Oral Impulses in Eating Disorders: a Conceptual Approach'. *Psychiatric Quarterly* 35: 458–81.

BURGESS, R. G. 1983. *Experiencing Comprehensive Education*. London: Methuen.

BURGESS, R. G. 1984. *In the Field*. London: Allen & Unwin.

BURGESS, R. G. and MORRISON, M. 1995. 'Teaching and Learning about Food and Nutrition in Schools'. *Report to ESRC on Grant No. L209252006*. Swindon: ESRC.

BURGESS, R. G., POLE, C., EVANS, K. and PRESTLEY, C. 1994. 'One Study from Four or Four Studies from One?', in A. Bryman and R. G. Burgess (eds), *Analysing Qualitative Data*. London: Routledge.

BURNETT, J. 1968. *Plenty and Want*. Harmondsworth: Penguin Books.

BURT, S. 1992. 'Retail Brands in British Grocery Retailing: a Review'. WP-9204, Institute for Retail Studies, University of Stirling.

BURT, S. and SPARKS, L. 1994. 'Structural Change in Grocery Retailing in Great Britain: a Discount Reorientation'. *International Review of Retail, Distribution and Consumer Research* 4: 195–217.

BURTON, M. P. 1989. 'The Demand for Food in the UK, 1974–84'. *Department of Agricultural Economics Working Paper*. Manchester: University of Manchester.

BURTON, M. P and YOUNG, T. 1992a. 'The Structure of Changing Tastes for Meat and Fish in Great Britain'. *European Review of Agricultural Economics* 19: 165–80.

BURTON, M. P. and YOUNG, T. 1992b. 'Análisis Sobre Cambios Difereciados de Gustos Según Niveles de Renta: Consumo de Carne y Pescado en Gran Bretaña'. *Investigacion Agraria: Economia* 7(2): 231–47.

BURTON, M., DORSETT, R. and YOUNG, T. 1996a. 'Changing Preferences for Meat: Evidence from UK Household Data, 1973–93'. *European Review of Agricultural Economics* 23: 359–72.

BURTON, M., DORSETT, R. and YOUNG, T. 1996b. 'The Decision Not to Eat Meat – an Analysis of Changing Preferences' Mimeo. poster paper prepared for VII EAAE Conference, Edinburgh, September.

BUSH, H. M. and WILLIAMS, R. G. A. forthcoming. 'Opportunities for and Barriers to Good Nutritional Health among Ethnic Minorities'. London: Department of Health.

BUSH, H. M., WILLIAMS, R. G. A., ANDERSON, A. S., LEAN, M.E. and BRADBY, H. 1996. 'Symbolic Meals of Asian and Italian Women in Glasgow'. *Scandinavian Journal of Nutrition* 40: S91–S92.

BUSH, H. M., WILLIAMS, R. G. A., BRADBY, H., LEAN, M. E. J., ANDERSON, A. S. and HAN, T. forthcoming. 'Weight Consciousness and Body Image among South Asian, Italian and General Population Women in Britain' (abstract). *Journal of Epidemiology and Community Health*.

BUTTEL, F., LARSON, O. and G. GILLESPIE 1990. *The Sociology of Agriculture*. New York: Greenwood Press.

CALNAN, M. 1994. 'Lifestyle and its Social Meaning'. *Advances In Medical Sociology* 4: 69–87.

CALNAN, M. and CANT, S. 1990. 'The Social Organisation of Food Consumption: A Comparison of Middle Class and Working Class Households'. *International Journal of Sociology and Social Policy* 10(2): 53–79.

CANNON, G. 1983. 'Censored: A Diet for Life and Death'. *The Sunday Times* 3 July: 1.

CANNON, G. 1987. *The Politics of Food*. London: Century.

CAPLAN, P. 1994. *Feasts, Fasts and Famine: Food for Thought*. Oxford: Berg Occasional Papers in Anthropology No. 2.

CAPLAN, P. 1996. 'Good for Eating, Good for Thinking: Approaches to Food and Diet from a Social Science Perspective'. *Clinical Child Psychology and Psychiatry* 1(2): 213–27.

CAPLAN, P. (ed.) 1997. *Food, Health and Identity*. London: Routledge.

CASTONGUAY, T. W. 1991. 'Glucocorticoids as Modulators in the Control of Feeding'. *Brain Research Bulletin* 27: 423–8.

CATHCART, E. P. and MURRAY, A. M. T. 1931. A Study in Nutrition: 154 St Andrews families'. *Medical Research Council Special Report Series* 151.

CATHCART, E. P., PATON, D. N. and GREENWOOD, M. 1924. 'A Study of Miners' Dietaries'. *Medical Research Council Special Report Series* 87.

CENTRAL STATISTICAL OFFICE 1996. *Annual Abstract of Statistics 1996*. London: HMSO.

CHANG, H. S. and GREEN, R. 1989. 'The Effect of Advertising on Food Demand Elasticities'. *Canadian Journal of Agricultural Economics* 37(3): 481–94.

CHANG, H. S. and KINNUCAN, H. 1991. 'Advertising, Information and Product Quality: the Case of Butter'. *American Journal of Agricultural Economics* 73: 1195–203.

CHAPMAN, G. and MAÇCLEAN, H. 1993. 'Junk Food and Healthy Food: Meanings of Food in Adolescent Women's Culture'. *Journal of Nutrition Eduction* 25(3): 108–13.

CHARLES, N. and KERR, M. 1986a. 'Issues of Responsibility and Control in the Feeding of Families' in S. Rodmell and A. Watts, (eds) 1986.

CHARLES, N. and KERR, M. 1986b. 'Food for Feminist Thought'. *Sociological Review* 34(3): 537–72.

CHARLES, N. and KERR, M. 1988. *Women, Food and Families*. Manchester: Manchester University Press.

CHARSLEY, S. R. 1991. *Rites of Marrying: The Wedding Industry in Scotland*. Manchester: Manchester University Press.

CHARSLEY, S. R. 1992. *Wedding Cakes and Cultural History*. London: Routledge.

CHAVAS, J.-P. 1983. 'Structural Change in the Demand for Meat'. *American Journal of Agricultural Economics* 65: 148–53.

CHESHER, A. 1991. 'Household Composition and Household Food Purchases', in MAFF 1991.

CHISNALL, P.M. 1992. *Marketing Research*. London: McGraw Hill.

CHRISTENSEN, L. 1996. *Diet-Behavior Relationships*. Washington, DC: American Psychological Association.

CIALDINI, R. B., RENO, R. R., and KALLGREN, C. A. 1990. 'A Focus Theory of Normative Conduct: Recycling the Concept of Norms to Reduce Littering in Public Places'. *Journal of Personality and Social Psychology* 58: 1015–26.

CLARK, C, PEACH, C and VERTOVEC, S. (eds.) 1990. *South Asians Overseas: Migration and Ethnicity*. Cambridge: Cambridge University Press.

CLARK, D. 1991. 'Constituting the Marital World. A Qualitative Perspective', in D. Clark (ed.) *Marriage, Domestic Life and Social Change*. London: Routledge, pp. 139–66.

CLARK, F. LE GROS 1943a. *The School Child and the School Canteen*. Hertfordshire County Council.

CLARK, F. LE GROS 1943b. *The School Child's Taste in Vegetables*. Hertfordshire County Council.

CLARK, F. LE GROS 1945. 'Food Advice in a Post-War World'. *Health Education Journal* 3: 75–8.

CLARK, F. LE GROS 1947. 'The Elements of Food Education'. *Health Education Journal*. 5: 134–7.

CLARK, F. LE GROS and BRINTON, L. N. 1936. *Men, Medicine and Food in the USSR*. London: Lawrence & Wishart.

CLARK, F. LE GROS and DUNN, A. C. 1955. *Ageing in Industry*. London: Nuffield Foundation.

CLARK, J. and LOWE, P. 1992. 'Cleaning up Agriculture: Environment, Technology and Social Science'. *Sociologia Ruralis* XXII (1): 11–29.

CLUNIES-ROSS, T. and HILDYARD, N. 1992. *The Politics of Industrial Agriculture*. London: Earthscan.

CMD 278 *DTI – the Department for Enterprise*. London: HMSO.

COHEN, S., KAMARCK, T. and MERMELSTEIN, R. 1983. ' A Global Measure of Perceived Stress'. *Journal of Health and Social Behavior* 24: 386–96.

COLLINS, R. 1985. ' "Horses for Courses": Ideology and the Division of Domestic Labour', in P. Close and R. Collins (eds) *Family and Economy in Modern Society*. London: Macmillan, pp. 63–82.

COLPI, T 1991. *The Italian Factor: The Italian Community in Great Britain*. Edinburgh: Mainstream.

COMMONS AGRICULTURE COMMITTEE 1989. *Salmonella in Eggs, First Report, Minutes of Evidence and Appendices*. London: HMSO.

CONNER, M. T. 1993a. 'Understanding Determinants of Food Choice through Attitude Research'. *British Food Journal* 95(9): 33–7.

CONNER, M. T. 1993b. 'Individualised Measurement of Attitudes Toward Food'. *Appetite*. 20: 235–8.

CONNER, M., and NORMAN, P. 1996. 'The Role of Social Cognition in Health Behaviours', in M. Conner and P. Norman (eds), *Predicting Health Behaviour*. Buckingham: Open University Press, pp. 1–22.

CONNER, M., and SPARKS, P. 1996. 'The Theory of Planned Behaviour and Health Behaviours', in M. Conner and P. Norman (eds) 1996.

COOK, I. 1994. 'New Fruits and Vanity: Symbolic Production in the Global Food Economy', in A. Bonanno *et al.* (eds), *From Columbus to Conagra: the Globalization of Agriculture and Food*. Lawrence, Kansas: University of Kansas Press, pp. 232–48.

COOMBES, G. 1989. 'The Ideology of Health Education in Schools'. *British Journal of the Sociology of Education*. 10(1): 67–80.

CORWIN, R. G. 1983. *Entrepreneurial Bureaucracy*. London: JAI Press.

COTTRELL, R. 1987. *The Sacred Cow*. London: Grafton Books.

COTTERILL, R. W. 1997. 'The Food Distribution System of the Future: Convergence towards the US or UK Model?' *Agribusiness* 13:123–35.

COURNEYA, K. S., NIGG, C. R. and ESTABROOKS, P. A. forthcoming. 'Relationships Among the Theory of Planned Behavior, Stages of Change, and Exercise Behavior in Older Persons over a Three-Year Period'. *Psychology & Health*.

COVELLO, V. 1983. 'The Perception of Technological Risks: A Literature Review'. *Technological Forecasting and Social Change* 23: 285–97.

COX, G., LOWE, P. and WINTER, M. 1986. 'From State Direction to Self-regulation: the Historical Development of Corporatism in British Agriculture'. *Policy and Politics* 14: 475–90.

COX, T. L and WOHLGENANT, M. K. 1986. 'Prices and Quality Effects in Cross-sectional Demand Analysis'. *American Journal of Agricultural Economics* 68: 908–19.

CRAIG, P. L. and TRUSWELL, A. S. 1988. 'Changes in Food Habits when People get Married: Analysis of Food Frequencies', in A. S. Truswell and M. L. Wahlqvist (eds), *Food Habits in Australia*. North Balwyn, Victoria René Gordon.

CRANG, P. and COOK, I. 1996. 'The World on a Plate: Culinary Culture, Displacement and Geographical Knowledge'. *Journal of Material Culture* 1: 131–53.

CREWE, L. and DAVENPORT, E. 1992. 'The Puppet Show: Changing Buyer-supplier Relationships within Clothing Retailers'. *Transactions of the Institute of British Geographers* NS17: 183–97.

CROOK, C. K. 1978. 'Taste Perception in the Newborn Infant', *Infant Behavior and Development*, 1: 52–69.

CRUMB-JOHNSON, R., SMITH-BANES, M., HATCHER, L. and HAGAN, D. W. 1993. 'Assessment of Differences Between Compliers and Non-compliers in Outpatient Research Diet Studies'. *Journal of the American Dietetic Association* 93(9): 1041–2.

CURRY, S. J., KRISTAL, A. R. and BOWEN, D. J. 1992. 'An Application of the Stage Model of Behavior Change to Dietary Fat Reduction'. *Health Education Research: Theory and Practice*. 7(1) 96–105

DALE, A., ARBER, S. and PROCTOR, M. 1988. *Doing Secondary Analysis*. London: Unwin Hyman.

DAVIDOFF, L. 1976. 'The Rationalization of Housework', in D. L. Barker and S. Allen (eds), *Dependence and Exploitation in Work and Marriage*. New York: Longman.

DAVIES, G. 1990. *Tastes of Wales: the Book of the TV Series*. London: BBC Publications.

DAVIES, K. 1990. *Women, Time and the Weaving of the Strands of Everyday Life*. Aldershot: Gower.

DAVIES, K., GILLIGAN, C. and SUTTON, C. 1985. 'Structural Changes in Grocery Retailing: the Implications for Competition'. *International Journal of Physical Distribution and Materials Management* 15: 3–48.

DAVIS, H. L. and RIGAUX, B. P. 1974. 'Perception of Marital Roles in Decision Processes'. *Journal of Consumer Research* 1, June: 5–14.

DAVIS, R. G. 1978. 'Increased Bitter Taste Detection Thresholds in Yucatan Inhabitants Related to Coffee as a Dietary Source of Niacin', *Chemical Senses and Flavour*, 3: 423–9.

DAVISON, C. 1989. 'Eggs and the Sceptical Eater'. *New Scientist* 1655, 11 March: 45–49.

DAVISON, C., FRANKEL, S. and DAVEY-SMITH, G. 1989. 'Inheriting Heart Trouble; the Relevance of Common Sense Ideas to Preventive Measures'. *Health Education Journal Theory and Practice* 4: 329–40.

DAVISON, C., FRANKEL, S. and DAVEY-SMITH, G. 1992. 'The Limits of Lifestyle: Reassessing "Fatalism" in the Popular Culture of Illness Prevention'. *Social Science and Medicine* 34(6): 675–85.

DAWSON, J. 1995. 'Food Retailing and the Food Consumer', in D. Marshall (ed.) 1995.

DAWSON, J. A. and SHAW, S. A. 1989. The Move to Administered Vertical Marketing Systems by British Retailers'. *European Journal of Marketing* 23(7):42–51.

DEACON, J. R. and KONARSKI, E. A. J. 1987. 'Correspondence Training: an Example of Rule–Governed Behavior?', *Journal of Applied Behavior Analysis*, 20: 391–400.

DEATON, A. and MUELLBAUER, J. 1980. *Economics and Consumer Behavior*. Cambridge: Cambridge University Press.

DECI, E. 1971. 'Effects of Externally Mediated Rewards on Intrinsic Motivation', *Journal of Personality and Social Psychology*, 1: 105–15.

DECI, E. L. 1975. *Intrinsic Motivation*. New York: Plenum Press.

DECI, E. L. and RYAN, R. M. 1985. *Intrinsic Motivation and Self Determination in Human Behavior*. New York: Plenum Press.

de CHERNATONY, L. 1989 'Branding in an Era of Retailer Dominance'. *International Journal of Advertising* 8: 245–60.

DEGUCHI, H. 1984. 'Observational Learning from a Radical–Behavioristic Viewpoint', *The Behavior Analyst*, 7: 83–95.

DELPHY, C. 1979. 'Sharing the Same Table: Consumption and the Family', in C. Harris (ed.), *The Sociology of the Family: New Directions for Britain*. Sociological Review Monograph 28, Keele: University of Keele.

DENTON, D. 1982. *The Hunger for Salt*. New York: Springer Verlag.

DEPARTMENT OF THE ENVIRONMENT 1993. *Planning Policy Guidance (PPG6): Town Centres and Retail Developments.* Department of the Environment, London: HMSO.

DEPARTMENT OF THE ENVIRONMENT 1994. *Planning Policy Guidance (PPG13): Transport.* Department of the Environment, London: HMSO.

DEPARTMENT OF THE ENVIRONMENT 1996. *Planning Policiy Guidance (PPG6): Town Centres and Retail Developments.* Department of the Environment, London: HMSO.

DEPARMENT FOR EDUCATION (DFE) 1994. *News Circular* 271/94.

DEPARTMENT OF EDUCATION AND SCIENCE (DES) 1977. *Education in Schools: a Consultative Document.* London: HMSO.

DEPARTMENT OF EDUCATION AND SCIENCE (DES) 1981. *West Indian Children in Our Schools: The Rampton Report.* London: HMSO.

DEPARTMENT OF HEALTH 1992. *The Health of the Nation: a Strategy for Health in England* (White Paper). London: HMSO.

DEPARTMENT OF HEALTH 1994. *Nutritional Aspects of Cardiovascular Disease.* London: Department of Health.

DEPTFORD CITY CHALLENGE 1993. *Year One Process Report,* Deptford City Challenge Evaluation Project. London: Goldsmiths College.

DEPTFORD CITY CHALLENGE 1994a. *Baseline Update Report, 1994,* Deptford City Challenge Evaluation Project. London: Goldsmiths College.

DEPTFORD CITY CHALLENGE 1994b. *Year Two Process Report,* Deptford City Challenge Evaluation Project. London: Goldsmiths College.

DESOR, J. A., MALLER, O. and TURNER, R. E. 1973. 'Taste in Acceptance of Sugars by Human Infants', *Journal of Comparative and Physiological Psychology,* 84: 496–501.

DEVAULT, M. L. 1991. *Feeding the Family: the Social Organisation of Caring as Gendered Work.* Chicago: Chicago University Press.

DICKINSON, A. M. 1989. 'The Detrimental Effects of Extrinsic Reinforcement on "Intrinsic Motivation"', *The Behavior Analyst,* 12: 1–15.

DOWEY, A. J. 1996. *Psychological Determinants of Children's Food Preferences.* Unpublished Doctoral Dissertation, University of Wales, Bangor.

DUNCKER, K. 1938. 'Experimental Modification of Children's Food Preferences Through Social Suggestion', *Journal of Abnormal and Social Psychology,* 33: 489–507.

DOBSON, B., BEARDSWORTH, A., KEIL, T. and WALKER, R. 1994. *Diet, Choice and Poverty: Social, Cultural and Nutritional Aspects of Food Consumption among Low Income Families.* London: Family Policy Studies Centre.

DOEL, C. 1995. 'Market Development, Organizational Change and the Food Industry'. Unpublished PhD thesis, Unversity of Cambridge.

DOEL, C. 1996. 'Market Development and Organizational Change: the Case of the Food Industry', in N. Wrigley and M. S. Lowe (eds), *Retailing, Consumption and Capital: Towards the New Retail Geography.* Harlow: Longman, pp. 48–67.

DOEL, C. 1998. 'Towards a Supply Chain Community? Insights from

Governance Processes in the Food Industry'. *Environment and Planning A* 30.

DONO, G. and THOMPSON, G. 1994. 'Explaining Changes in Italian Consumption of Meat: Parametric and Non-parametric Analysis'. *European Review of Agricultural Economics* 21–2: 175–98.

DOUGLAS, M. 1966. 'The Abominations of Leviticus', in *Purity and Danger*. London: Routledge & Kegan Paul.

DOUGLAS, M. and NICOD, M. 1974. 'Taking the Biscuit: The Structure of British Meals'. *New Society* 30 (637): 744–7.

DOUGLAS, M. 1975. 'Deciphering a Meal', in M. Douglas, *Implicit Meanings*. London: Routledge & Kegan Paul.

DOUGLAS, M. (ed.) 1984. *Food and the Social Order*. New York: Russell Sage Foundation.

DOWEY, A. J. 1996. 'Psychological Determinants of Children's Food Preferences'. Unpublished doctoral dissertation, University of Wales, Bangor.

DOWLER, E. and RUSHTON, C. 1994. *Diet and Poverty in the UK: Contemporary Research Methods and Current Experience: a Review*, Department of Public Health and Policy Publication 11. London: London School of Hygiene and Tropical Medicine.

DUKE, R. 1996 'Buyer-supplier Relationships in UK Grocery Retailing'. Paper presented at 3rd International Conference on Recent Advances in Retailing and Services', Telfs/Buchen, Austria, 22–25 June 1996).

DUNCKER, K. 1938. 'Experimental Modification of Children's Food Preferences through Social Suggestion'. *Journal of Abnormal and Social Psychology* 33: 489–507.

DURKHEIM, E. 1952. (original edition 1895). *Suicide: a Study in Sociology*, London: Routledge & Kegan Paul.

EAGLY, A. H. and CHAIKEN, S. 1993. *The Psychology of Attitudes*. Fort Worth: Harcourt Brace Jovanovich.

EALES, J. S. and UNNEVEHR, L. J. 1988. 'Demand for Beef and Chicken Products: Separability and Structural Change'. *American Journal of Agricultural Economics* 70: 522–32.

ELDRIDGE, J., KITZINGER, J. and WILLIAMS, K. 1996. *Mass Media Power in Modern Britain*. Oxford: Oxford University Press.

ELLIS, R. 1983. 'The Way to a Man's Heart: Food in the Violent Home', in A. Murcott (ed.) 1983b.

ERICSON, R., BARANEK, P. and CHAN, J. 1989. *Negotiating Control: a Study of News Sources*. Milton Keynes: Open University Press.

EVETTS, J. 1966. *Gender and Career in Science and Engineering*. London: Taylor & Francis.

FALLON A 1990. 'Culture in the Mirror: Sociocultural Determinants of Body Image', in T. F. Cash, T. Prizinsky (eds), *Body Images: Development, Deviance and Change*. New York: Guilford.

FARB, P. and ARMELAGOS, G. 1980. *Consuming Passions: The Anthropology of Eating*. Boston: Houghton Mifflin.

FEHILY, A. M., VAUGHN-WILLIAMS, E. and SHIELS, K. *et al.* 1989. 'The Effect of Dietary Advice on Nutrient Intakes: Evidence from the Diet and Re-infarction Trial (DART)'. *Journal of Human Nutrition and Dietetics* 2(4): 225–36.

FERNIE, J. 1992. 'Distribution Strategies of European Retailers'. *European Journal of Marketing* 26 (8/9): 35–47.

FERNIE, J. 1994. 'Quick Response: an International Perspective' *International Journal of Physical Distribution and Logistics Management* 24(6): 38–46.

FIDANZA, A. A. 1990. 'Mediterranean Meal Patterns', in J. C. Somogyi and E. H. Koskinen (eds), *Nutritional Adaptation to New Lifestyles.* Basel: Karger.

FIDDES, N. 1991. *Meat: a Natural Symbol.* London and New York: Routledge.

FIDDES, N. 1995. 'The Omnivore's Paradox', in D. Marshall (ed.) 1995, pp. 131–51.

FINE, B. 1993a. 'Modernity, Urbanism, and Modern Consumption – a Comment'. *Environment and Planning D, Society and Space* 11: 599–601.

FINE, B. 1993b. 'Resolving the Diet Paradox'. *Social Science Information* 32(4) Dec. 669–87.

FINE, B. 1994a. 'Towards a Political Economy of Food'. *Review of International Political Economy* 1(3): 519–45.

FINE, B. 1994b. 'Towards a Political Economy of Food: a Response to my Critics'. *Review of International Political Economy* 1(3): 579–86.

FINE, B. 1995. 'From Political Economy to Consumption', in D. Miller (ed.) 1995.

FINE, B. 1995a. 'Towards a Political Economy of Anorexia'. *Appetite* 24: 231–42.

FINE, B. 1995b. 'Towards a Political Economy of Consumption', in D. Miller (ed.) 1995.

FINE, B. and HEASMAN M. 1997. *Consumption in the Age of Affluence: Diet, Health, Information and Policy.* London: Routledge.

FINE, B. and LEOPOLD, E. 1993. *The World of Consumption.* London: Routledge.

FINE, B. and SIMISTER J. 1995. 'Consumption Durables: Exploring the Order of Acquisition'. *Applied Economics* 27: 1049–57.

FINE, B. and WRIGHT 1991. 'Digesting the Food and Information Systems'. *Birkbeck Discussion Paper* 7(91) Dec.

FINE, B., HEASMAN, M. and J. WRIGHT 1996. *Consumption in the Age of Affluence: the World of Food.* London: Routledge.

FINKELSTEIN, J. 1989. *Dining Out: a Sociology of Modern Manners.* Cambridge: Polity Press.

FISCHLER, C. 1988. 'Cuisines and Food Selection' in D. H. Thomson (ed.), *Food Acceptability.* London: Elsevier, pp. 193–206.

FISCHER, R., GRIFFIN, F., ENGLAND, S. and GARN, S. M. 1961. 'Taste Thresholds and Food Dislike', *Nature,*

FISKE, S. T., and TAYLOR, S. E. 1991. *Social Cognition.* (2nd edn). New York: McGraw-Hill.

FITCHEN, J. M. 1988. 'Hunger, Malnutrition and Poverty in the Contemporary US: some Observations on their Social and Cultural Context'. *Food and Foodways* 2: 309– 33.

FLETCHER, T., WHEELER, G. and WRIGHT, M.E. 1990. 'The use of Database Marketing'. *Quarterly Review of Marketing* 34: 14–26.

FLORA, S. R. 1990. 'Undermining Intrinsic Interest from the Standpoint of a Behaviorist', *The Psychological Record*, 40: 323–46.

FLYNN, A. and MARSDEN, T. 1992. 'Food Regulation in a Period of Agricultural Retreat: the British Experience'. *Geoforum* 23: 85–93.

FLYNN, A., MARSDEN, T. and WARD, N. 1991. 'Managing Food? A Critical Perspective on the British Experience'. *Changement technique et restructuration de l'industrie agro-alimentaire en Europe*. INRA Actes et Communications 7: 159–81.

FOREMAN, S. 1989. *Loaves and Fishes.* London: HMSO.

FOORD, J., BOWLBY, S. R. and TILLSLEY, C. 1992. 'Changing Relations in the Retail-supply Chain: Geographical and Employment Implications'. *International Journal of Retail and Distribution Management* 20: 23–30.

FRANK, R. H. 1989. *Microeconomics and Behaviour* (2nd edn). New York: McGraw-Hill.

FREDRICKS, A. J. and DOSSETT, D. L. 1983. 'Attitude-behavior Relations: a Comparison of the Fishbein–Ajzen and Bentler–Speckart Models'. *Journal of Personality and Social Psychology* 45: 501–12.

FREEDMAN, R. 1986. *Beauty Bound.* Massachusetts: Lexington Books.

FREEMAN, B. 1996 (1980). *First Catch Your Peacock: Her Classic Guide to Welsh Food.* Talybont, Ceredigion: Y Lolfa.

FRIEDMAN, M. 1962. *Price Theory: A Provisional Text.* London: Cass.

GARDNER, C. and SHEPHERD, J. 1989. *Consuming Passion: The Rise of Retail Culture.* London: Unwin Hyman.

GARN, S. M. and CLARK, D. C. 1976. 'Trends in Fatness and the Origins of Obesity'. *Pediatrics* 57(4): 443–56.

GATES, R. and MCDANIEL, C. 1992. *Contemporary Marketing Research.* St Paul, Minneapolis, MD: West Publishing.

GEER, B. 1964. 'First Days in the Field', in P. Hammond (ed.) *Sociologists at Work.* New York: Basic Books.

GELDARD, F. A. 1972. *The Human Senses.* New York: John Wiley and Sons.

GEORGES, E., MUELLER W. H. and WEAR, M. L. 1991. 'Body Fat Distribution: Associations with Socioeconomic Status in the Hispanic Health and Nutrition Examination Survey'. *American Journal of Human Biology* 3: 489–501.

GEWIRTZ, J. L. and STINGLE, K. G. 1968. 'Learning of Generalized Imitation as the Basis for Identification', *Psychological Review*, 75: 374–97.

GILLESPIE, A. H. and ACHTERBERG, C. L. 1989. 'Comparison of Family Interaction Patterns Related to Food and Nutrition'. *Journal of the American Dietetic Association, Aoruk* 89(4): 509–12.

GILLIE, O. 1985. 'Guide to Healthy Eating Blocked'. *Sunday Times* 4 August: 3a.

GILLMAN, M. W. 1996. 'Enjoy Your Fruits and Vegetables: Eating Fruit and Vegetables Protects Against the Common Chronic Diseases of Adulthood', *British Medical Journal*, 313, 765–6.

GINTIS, H. 1974. 'Welfare Criteria with Endogenous Preferences: the Economics of Education'. *International Economic Review* 15(2): 415–30.

GLANVILLE, E. V. and KAPLAN, A. R. 1965. 'Food Preference and Sensitivity of Taste for Bitter Compounds', *Nature, 205,* 851–3.

GLENNIE, P. and THRIFT, N. 1992. 'Modernity, Urbanism, and Modern Consumption'. *Environment and Planning D: Society and Space* 10(4): 423–43.

GLENNIE, P. and THRIFT, N. 1993. 'Modern Consumption: Theorising Commodities and Consumers'. *Environment and Planning D: Society and Space* 11: 603–6.

GODIN, G. and KOK, G. 1996. 'The Theory of Planned Behavior: A Review of its Applications to Health-related Behaviors'. *American Journal of Health Promotion* 11: 87–98.

GODIN, G., DESHARNAIS, R., VALOIS, P. and BADET, R. 1995. 'Combining Behavioral and Motivational Dimensions to Identify and Characterise the Stages in the Process of Adherence to Exercise'. *Psychology and Health* 10: 333–44.

GOFTON, L. R. 1983. 'Real Men, Real Ale'. *New Society* 86: 271–3.

GOFTON, L. R. 1986. 'Social Change, Market Change'. *Food and Foodways* 1(3): 253–77.

GOFTON, L.R. 1990. 'On the Town; Drink and the New Lawlessness'. *Youth and Policy* 29: 33–9.

GOFTON, L. and MARSHALL, D. 1992. *Fish: a Marketing Problem.* Horton, Yorkshire: Horton Publishing.

GOLDBERG, J. P., GORN, G. J. and GIBSON, W. 1978. 'TV Messages for Snack and Breakfast Foods: Do They Influence Children's Preferences?', *Journal of Consumer Research,* 5: 73–81.

GOLDBLATT, P. B., MOORE, M. E. and STUNKARD, A. J. 1965. 'Social Factors in Obesity'. *Journal of the American Medical Association* 192(12): 97–102.

GOLDING, P. and MURDOCK, G. 1996. 'Culture, Communications and Political Ecoanomy', in J. Curran and M. Gurevitch (eds), *Mass Media and Society.* London: Edward Arnold.

GOLLWITZER, P. M. 1996. 'The Volitional Benefits of Planning', in P. Gollwitzer and J. A. Bargh (eds), *Psychology of Action.* New York: Guilford, pp. 287–312.

GOODENOUGH, S. 1977. *Jam and Jerusalem.* Glasgow and London, Collins.

GOODMAN, D. and WATTS, M. 1994. 'Reconfiguring the Rural or Fording the Divide? Capitalist Restructuring and the Global Agro-Food System'. *Journal of Peasant Studies* 22(7): 1–49.

GOODY, J. 1982. *Cooking, Cuisine and Class.* Cambridge: Cambridge University Press.

GORN, G. J. and GOLDBERG, M. E. 1982. 'Behavioural Evidence of the Effects of Televised Food Messages on Children', *Journal of Consumer Research,* 9: 200–5.

GORN, G. J. and GOLDBERG, M. E. 1987. 'Television and Children's Food Habits: A Big Brother/Sister Approach' in M.E. Manley–Casimir and C.Luke eds, *Children and Television: a Challenge for Education.* New York: Praeger Publishers, pp. 34–48.

GOULD, B. W. 1992. 'At-home Consumption of Cheese: a Purchase-infrequency Model'. *American Journal of Agricultural Economics* 74(2): 453–9.

GOVE, W. R. , Hughes, M. and Style, C. B.. 1983. 'Does Marriage have Positive Effects on the Psychological Well-being of the Individual?' *Journal of Health and Social Behaviour* 24: 122–31.

GRAHAM, H. 1984. *Women, Health and the Family.* Sussex: Harvester Wheatsheaf.

GRAHAM, H. 1987. 'Being Poor: Perceptions and Coping Strategies of Lone Mothers', in J. Brannen and G. Wilson (eds), *Give and Take in Families: Studies in Resource Distribution.* London: Allen & Unwin.

GRANOVETTER, M. 1985. 'Economic Action and Social Structure: the Problem of "embeddedness" '. *American Journal of Sociology* 91: 491–510.

GRANT, R. 1987. 'Manufacturerer–retailer Relations: the Shifting Balance of Power', in G. Johnson (ed.), *Business Strategy and Retailing.* London: Wiley, pp. 43–58.

GRANT, W. 1983. 'The National Farmers' Union: the Classic Case of Incorporation', in D. Marsh (ed.)*Pressure Politics.* London: Junction Books.

GREENE, G. W., ROSSI, S. R., RICHARDS REED, G., WILLEY, C. and PROCHASKA, J. O. 1994. 'Stages of Change for Reducing Dietary Fat to 30% of Energy or Less'. *Journal of the American Dietetic Association* 94: 1105–10.

GREENO, C. G. and WING, R. R. 1994. 'Stress-induced Eating. *Psychological Bulletin* 115: 444–64.

GREER, R. D., DOROW, L., WILLIAMS, G., McCORKLE, N. and ASNES, R. 1991. 'Peer–Mediated Procedures to Induce Swallowing and Food Acceptance in Young Children'. *Journal of Applied Behavior Analysis,* 24, 783–90.

GREGORY, J., FOSTER, K., TYLER, H. and WISEMAN, M. 1990. *The Dietary and Nutritionary Survey of British Adults.* London: HMSO.

GREGSON, N. and LOWE, M. 1993. 'Renegotiating the Domestic Division of Labour? A Study of Dual Career Households in North East and South East England. *Sociological Review* 41(3): 475–505.

GUBA, E. G. and LINCOLN, Y. S. 1982. 'Epistemological and Methodological Bases of Naturalistic Enquiry', *Educational Communication and Technology Journal* 30: 233–52.

GUY, C. M. 1988. 'Retail Planning Policy and Large Grocery Store Development'. *Land Development Studies* 5:31–45.

GUY, C. M. 1994. *The Retail Development Process.* London: Routledge.

GUY, C. M. 1996. 'Corporate Strategies in Food Retailing and their Local Impacts: a Case Study of Cardiff'. *Environment and Planning A* 28:1575–1602.

GUY, C. M. 1997. 'Fixed Assets or Sunk Costs? An Examination of Retailers' Land and Property Investment in the UK'. *Environment and Planning A* 29.

HALL, M. J., BARTOSHUK, L. M., CAIN, W. S. and STEVENS, J. C. 1975. 'PTC Taste Blindness and the taste of Caffeine', *Nature* 253, 442–3.

HALL, P., LAND, H., PARKER, R. and WEBB, A. 1975. *Change, Choice and Conflict in Social Policy.* London: Heinemann.

346

HAMMERSLEY, M. and ATKINSON, P. 1983. *Ethnography: Principles and Practice.* London: Tavistock.

HANDEN, B. L., MANDELL, F. and RUSSO, D. C. 1986. 'Feeding Induction of Children Who Refuse to Eat', *American Journal of Diseases of Children.* 140: 52–4.

HARGREAVES HEAP, S., HOLLIS, M., LYONS, B., SUGDEN, R. and WEALE, A. 1992. *The Theory of Choice: A Critical Guide.* Oxford: Blackwell.

HARPER, L. and SANDERS, K. 1975. 'The Effect of Adults' Eating on Young Children's Acceptance of Unfamiliar Foods', *Journal of Experimental Child Psychology,* 20: 200–14.

HARRIS, B. J. 1995. *The Health of the Schoolchild.* Oxford: Oxford University Press.

HARRISON, M., FLYNN, A. and MARSDEN, T. forthcoming. 'Contested Regulatory Practice and the Implementation of Food Policy: Exploring the Local and National Interface'. *Transactions of the Institute of British Geographers.*

HARRISS, B. 1990. 'The Intra-family Distribution of Hunger in South Asia', in J. Dreze and A. Sen. (eds), *The Political Economy of Hunger,* vol. 2. Oxford: Clarendon Press.

HATCHER, R. P. 1979. 'Treatment of Food Refusal in a Two Year–old Child'. *Journal of Behavior Therapy and Experimental Psychology,* 10: 363–7.

HEALTH EDUCATION AUTHORITY (HEA) 1989. *Diet, Nutrition and 'Healthy Eating' in Low Income Groups.* London: Health Education Authority.

HEARD, P., HEARD, J. and CORDER, R. 1994. *Dining with Angels.* Tregynon, Gwaun Valley, Pembrokeshire: Bluestone Books.

HEASMAN, M. 1990. 'Nutrition and Technology: The Development of the Market for "Lite" Products'. *British Food Journal* 92(2): 5–13.

HECHTER, M. 1978. 'Group Formation and the Cultural Division of Labour'. *American Journal of Sociology* 84: 293–318.

HECKHAUSEN, H. 1991. *Motivation and Action.* Berlin: Springer-Verlag.

HENDERSON CROSTHWAITE 1992. 'Three Plus One'. Food Retail Report No. 10, Henderson Crosthwaite Institutional Brokers Ltd, 32 St Mary-at-Hill, London, EC3P 3AJ.

HENSON, S. 1992. 'From High Street to Hypermarket. Food retailing in the 1990s', in National Consumer Council (ed.), *Your Food: Whose Choice?* London: HMSO.

HENSON, S., GREGORY, S., HAMILTON, M. and WALKER, A. 1995. 'The Effect on the Family of One Member's Change in Diet', in E. Feichtinger and B. Köhler (eds), *Current Research into Eating Practices: Contributions of Social Sciences* (Proceedings of the European Interdisciplinary Meeting) Frankfurt am Main: AGEV Publication Series, Vol. 10.

HIRSCHON, R. 1989. *Heirs of the Greek Catastrophe.* Oxford: Clarendon Press.

HOBSBAWM, E. and RANGER, T. 1983. *The Invention of Tradition.* Cambridge: Cambridge University Press.

HOGARTH-SCOTT, S. and PARKINSON, S. T. 1993. 'Retailer-supplier

Relationships in the Food Channel: a Supplier Perspective'. *International Journal of Retail and Distribution Management* 21: 11–18.

HORNE, P. J. and LOWE, C. F. 1993. 'Determinants of Human Performance on Concurrent Schedules.' *Journal of Experimental Analysis of Behavior*, 59: 29–60.

HORNE, P. J., LOWE, C. F., FLEMING, P. F. J. and DOWEY, A. J. 1995. 'An Effective Procedure for Changing Food Preferences in 5–7 Year–old Children.' *Proceedings of the Nutrition Society*, 54: 441–52.

HORNE, P. J. and LOWE, C. F. 1996. 'On the Origins of Naming and Other Symbolic Behavior.' *Journal of the Experimental Analysis of Behavior*, 65: 185–241.

HOMANS, H. 1983. 'A Question of Balance: Asian and British Women's Perceptions of Food in Pregnancy', in A. Murcott (ed.) 1983b, pp. 73–83.

HORTON, T. and BERTHOUD, R. 1990. *The Attendance Allowance and the Costs of Caring*. London, Policy Studies Institute.

HOUTHAKKER, H. S. 1957. 'An International Comparison of Household Expenditure Patterns, Commemorating the Century of Engel's Law'. *Econometrica* 25.

HOUTHAKKER, H. S. and TAYLOR, L. D. 1966. *Consumer Demand in the United States: Analysis and Projections*. Cambridge, USA: Harvard University Press.

HUGHES, A. L. 1996a 'Changing Food Retailer-manufacturer Power Relations within National Economies: a UK–USA Comparison.' Unpublished PhD thesis, Unversity of Southampton.

HUGHES, A. L. 1996b. 'Retail Restructuring and the Strategic Significance of Food Retailers' Own Labels: a UK–USA Comparison'. *Environment and Planning A* 28:2201–26.

HUGHES, A. L. 1996c. 'Forging New Cultures of Food Retailer-manufacturer Relations?' in N. Wrigley and M. S. Lowe (eds), *Retailing, Consumption and Captial: Towards the New Retail Geography*. Harlow: Longman, pp. 90–115.

HUGHES, A. L. 1997. 'The Changing Organization of New Product Development for Retailers' Private Labels: a UK–US Comparison'. *Agribusiness* 13:169–84.

HUGHES, A. L. 1998. 'Constructing Competitive Spaces: on the Corporate Practice of British Retailer-supplier Relationships'. *Environment and Planning A*, 30.

HUGHES, D. 1994. *Breaking with Tradition*. London: Wye College Press.

HURREN, C. A. and BLACK, A. E. 1991. *The Food Network: Achieving a Healthy Diet by the Year 2000*. London: Smith Gordon.

HURST, R. 1990. 'Care Maintenance'. *Search*, Winter.

HYDE, S., BALLOCH, S. and AINLEY, P. 1989. *A Social Atlas of Poverty in Lewisham*. London: Centre for Inner City Studies, Goldsmiths College.

IRWIN, A. and WYNNE, B. 1996. *Misunderstanding Science? The Public Reconstruction of Science and Technology*. Cambridge: Cambridge University Press.

IRWIN, S. 1996. 'Rites of Passage'. PhD thesis: Edinburgh University.

JAMES, A. 1997. 'How British is British Food? A View from Anthropology', in A. P. Caplan (ed.) 1997.

JEFFERSON, S. C. and ERDMAN, A. M. 1970. 'Taste Sensitivity and Food Aversions of Teenagers,' *Journal of Home Economics*, 62: 605–8.

JEFFREY, D. B., McLELLARN, R. W. and FOX, D. T. 1982. 'The Development of Children's Eating Habits: the Role of Television Commercials,' *Health Educational Quarterly*, 9: 174–89.

JEFFERY, P. 1976. *Migrants and Refugees: Muslim and Christian Pakistani Families in Bristol.* Cambridge: Cambridge University Press.

JEFFERY, P., JEFFERY, R. and LYON, A. 1989, *Labour Pains and Labour Power: women and childbearing in India.* London: Zed Books.

JOHNSON, M. L. with DI GREGARIO, S. and HARRISON, B. 1981. *Ageing, Needs and Nutrition: A Study of Voluntary and Statutory Collaboration in Community Care for Elderly People.* London: Policy Studies Institute.

JONES, A. M. 1989. 'A Double-hurdle Model of Cigarette Consumption'. *Journal of Applied Econometrics* 4: 23–39.

JONES, T. 1993. *Britain's Ethnic Minorities.* London: Policy Studies Institute.

JORDANOVA, L. J. 1981. 'The History of the Family', in *The Cambridge Woman's Studies Group. Women in Society.* London: Virago, pp. 41–54.

JOURNAL OF THE ROYAL COLLEGE OF PHYSICANS OF LONDON 1983. 'The health consequences of overweight and obesity'. Vol. 17: 6–65.

J. P. MORGAN SECURITIES INC 1995. 'Private Brands and Food Retail Consolidation'. New York: J. P. Morgan Securities Inc.

KAGEL, J. H., BATTALIO, R. C., RACHLIN, H. and GREEN, L. 1981. 'Demand Curves for Animal Consumers'. *Quarterly Journal of Economics* XCVI (1): 1–15.

KAPLAN, K. J. 1972. 'On the Ambivalence-indifference Problem in Attitude Theory and Measurement: a Suggested Modification of the Semantic Differential Technique'. *Psychological Bulletin* 77: 361–72.

KAZDIN, A. E. 1982. *Single–case Research Design.* New York: Oxford University Press.

KEANE A. 1997. 'Too Hard to Swallow? the Palatability of Healthy Eating Advice', in P. Caplan (ed), *Food, Health and Identity.* London: Routledge.

KEANE, A. and WILLETTS, A. 1993. 'A Bellyful of Words'. *Guardian* 7 August.

KEANE, A. and WILLETTS, A. 1994. 'Factors that Affect Food Choice'. *Nutrition and Food Science* 4. July–Aug.:15–17.

KEANE, A. and WILLETTS, A. 1996. *Concepts of Healthy Eating: an Anthropological Investigation in South-East London.* London: Goldsmiths College Occasional Paper.

KEITH, M. and CROSS, M. 1993. 'Racism and the postmodern city', in M. Cross and M. Keith (eds), *Racism, the City and the State.* London: Routledge.

KELLEHER, D. 1996. 'A Defence of the Use of the Terms "ethnicity" and "culture" ', in D. Kelleher and S. Hillier (eds), *Researching cultural differences in health*. London: Routledge.

KEMMER, D., ANDERSON, A. S. and MARSHALL, D. M. forthcoming. 'Living together and eating together: changes in food choice and eating habits during the transition from single to married or cohabiting. *Sociological Review*.

KESTELOOT, H. and JOOSSENS, J. V. 1992. 'Nutrition and International Patterns of Disease', in M. Marmot and P. Elliott (eds), *Coronary Heart Disease Epidemiology*. Oxford: Oxford University Press, pp. 152–65.

KEY, T. J. A., THOROGOOD, M., APPLEBY, P. N. and BURR, M. L. 1996. 'Dietary Habits and Mortality in 11,000 Vegetarians and Health Conscious People: Results of a 17-year Follow Up.' *British Medical Journal, 313*, 775–9.

KHAN, M. A. 1981. 'Evaluation of Food Selection Patterns and Preferences'. *Critical Reviews in Food Science and Nutrition* 15:129–53.

KIRMAN, A. P. 1992. 'Whom or What Does the Representative Individual Represent?' *Journal of Economic Perspectives* 6(2):117–36.

KITZINGER, J. and REILLY, J. forthcoming. 'The Rise and Fall of Risk Reporting'. *European Journal of Communication* 12(3).

KNETSCH, J. L. 1992. 'Preferences and Nonreversibility of Indifference Curves'. *Journal of Economic Behaviour and Organization* 17:131–9.

KNOX, S. D. and WHITE, H. F. M. 1991. 'Retail Buyers and their Fresh Produce Suppliers: a Power or Dependency Scenario in the UK', *European Journal of Marketing* 25(1):40–52.

KOIVISTO, U., FELLENIUS, J. and SJODEN, P. 1994. 'Relations Between Parental Mealtime Practices and Children's Food Intake'. *Appetite*, 22: 245–58.

KUHL, J. 1985. 'Volitional Mediators of Cognition-behavior Consistency: Self-regulatory Processes and Action Versus State Orientation', in J. Kuhl and J. Beckman (eds), *Action control: From Cognition to Behavior*. New York: Springer, pp. 101–28.

LAMBERT, H. and ROSE, H. 1996. 'Disembodied Knowledge? Making Sense of Medical Science', in A. Irwin and B. Wynne (eds) 1996, pp. 65–83.

LANGSTON, P., CLARKE, G. P. and CLARKE, D. B. 1997. 'Retail Saturation, Retail Location and Retail Competition: an Analysis of British Grocery Retailing'. *Environment and Planning A* 29:77–104.

LAVIN, M. 1993. 'Husband-Dominant, Wife-Dominant, Joint: A Shopping Typology for Baby Boom Couples'. *Journal of Consumer Marketing* 10:33–42.

LAZARUS, R. S. and FOLKMAN, S. 1989. *Manual for the Hassles and Uplifts Scales*. Palo Alto: Consulting Psychologists Press.

LEAHY, T. 1987. 'Branding–the Retailer's Viewpoint', in J. M. Murphy (ed.), *Branding: a Key Marketing Tool*. London: Macmillan, pp. 116–24.

LEAT, D. 1990. *For Love and Money: the Role of Payment in Encouraging the Provision of Care*. York: Joseph Rowntree Foundation.

LEAT, D. 1993. *Managing Across Sectors*. London: City University Business School.

LEAT, D. and GAY, P. 1987. *Paying for Care: An Exploratory Study of the Issues Raised by Paid Care Schemes.* London: Policy Studies Institute.

LEATHER, S. 1992. 'Less Money, Less Choice: Poverty and Diet in the UK Today', in The National Consumer Council (ed.), *Your Food, Whose Choice?* London: HMSO.

LEATHER, S. 1994. 'What Changes in National Policy could Improve Children's Eating Patterns?', in *Food for Children: Influencing Choice and Investing in Health.* London: The National Forum for Coronary Heart Disease Prevention.

LEIGH, D. 1980. *The Frontiers of Secrecy.* London: Junction Books.

LENGUA, L. *et al.* 1992. 'Using Focus Groups to Guide the Development of a Parenting Programme for Difficult-to-research, High Risk Families'. *Family Relations* 41: 163–8.

LEONARD, D. 1980. *Sex and Generation: A Study of Courtship and Weddings.* London: Tavistock.

LEPPER, M. R. and GREENE, D. 1978. 'Overjustification Research and Beyond: Towards a Means–end Analysis of Intrinsic and Extrinsic Motivation' in M. R. Lepper and D. Greene eds, *The Hidden Costs of Reward: New Perspectives on the Psychology of Human Motivation.* Hillsdale: Lawrence Erlbaum, pp.109–43.

LEPPER, M., SAGOTSKY, G., DAFOE, J. and GREENE, D. 1982. 'Consequences of Superfluous Social Constraints: Effects on Young Children's Social Inferences and Subsequent Intrinsic Interest', *Journal of Personality and Social Psychology,* 42: 51–65.

LÉVI-STRAUSS, C. 1968 (1958). *Structural Anthropology* vol 1. Harmondsworth: Penguin Books.

LÉVI-STRAUSS, C. 1965. 'The Culinary Triangle'. *Partisan Review* 33:586–9.

LÉVI-STRAUSS, C. 1992 (1964). *The Raw and the Cooked: Introduction to the Science of Mythology* 1. Harmondsworth: Penguin Books.

LEWBEL, A. 1989. 'Exact Aggregation and a Representative Consumer'. *Quarterly Journal of Economics* 104:622–33.

LIN, C.-T. and MILON, J. W. 1993. 'Attribute and Safety Perceptions in a Double Hurdle Model of Shellfish Consumption'. *American Journal of Agricultural Economics* 75:724–9.

LLOYD, H. M., PAISLEY, C. M. and MELA, D. J. 1993. 'Changing to a Low Fat Diet: Attitudes and Beliefs of UK Consumers'. *European Journal of Clinical Nutrition* 47:361–73.

LOBSTEIN, T. 1988. *Fast Food Facts: A Compendium of the Hidden Secrets of Fast Food Catering.* London: Camden Press.

LOBSTEIN, T. 1991. *The Nutrition of Women on Low Incomes* mimeo. London: The Food Commission.

LOEWENSTEIN, G. 1996. 'Out of Control: Visceral Influences on Behavior'. *Organizational Behavior and Human Decision Processes* 65:272–92.

LOGUE, A. W. 1991. *The Psychology of Eating and Drinking: an Introduction* (2nd edn). New York: W. H Freeman.

LONDON COUNCIL OF SOCIAL SERVICE 1944. *The Communal Restaurant:*

A Study of the Place of Civic Restaurants in the Life of the Community. London.

LONDON COUNCIL OF SOCIAL SERVICE 1948. *Young Workers at Meal Time*. London.

LONG, B. C. and KAHN, S. E. (eds) 1993. *Women, Work, and Coping*. Montreal: McGill-Queen's University Press.

LOWE, C. F. 1979. 'Determinants of Human Operant Behaviour' in M. D. Zeiler and P. Harzem eds, *Advances in Analysis of Behaviour* Vol. 1. Chichester, England: Wiley, pp. 159–92.

LOWE, C. F. 1983. 'Radical Behaviourism and Human Psychology' in G. C. L. Davey (ed.) *Animal Models of Human Behaviour*. Chichester, England: Wiley.

LOWE, C. F., HORNE, P. J. and HIGSON, P. J. 1987. 'Operant Conditioning: the Hiatus Between Theory and Practice in Clinical Psychology' in H. J. Eysenck and I. Martin (eds). *Theoretical Foundations of Behavior Therapy*. New York: Plenum Press, pp. 153–65.

LOWE, C. F. and HORNE, P. J. 1996. 'Reflections on Naming and Other Symbolic Behavior.' *Journal of the Experimental Analysis of Behavior*, 65, 315–40.

LURIA, A. R. 1961. *The Role of Speech in the Regulation of Normal and Abnormal Behaviors*. New York: Liveright.

MAAN, B. 1992. *The New Scots*. Edinburgh: John Donald.

MACDIARMID, J. I. and HETHERINGTON, M. 1995. 'Mood Modulation by Food: an Exploration of Affect and Cravings in "Chocolate Addicts" '. *British Journal of Clinical Psychology* 34:129–38.

MACINTYRE, S. 1995. 'The Public Understanding of Science or the Scientific Understanding of the Public? A Review of the Social Context of the New Genetics. *Public Understanding of Science* 4:223–32.

MADIGAN, R., JOHNSON, S. and LINTON, P. 1995. 'The Language of Psychology'. *American Psychologist* 50(6):428–36.

MANSFIELD, P. and COLLARD, J. 1988. *The Beginning of the Rest of Your Life*. London: Macmillan.

MANSTEAD, A. S. R., PLEVIN, C. E. and SMART, J. L. 1983. 'Predicting and Understanding Mothers' Infant-feeding Intentions and Behavior'. *Journal of Personality and Social Psychology* 44:657–71.

MARCUS, B. H., EATON, C. A., ROSSI, J. S. and HARLOW, L. L. 1994. 'Self-efficacy, Decision-making, and Stages of Change – An Integrative Model of Physical Exercise'. *Journal of Applied Social Psychology* 24:489–508.

MARET, E. and FINLAY, B. 1984. 'The Distribution of Household Labor Among Women in Dual Earner Families'. *Journal of Marriage and the Family* 46, May:357–64.

MARINHO, H. 1942. 'Social Influence in the Formation of Enduring Preferences', *Journal of Abnormal and Social Psychology*, 37: 448–68.

MARSDEN, D. and DUFF, E. 1975. *Workless*. Harmondsworth: Penguin Books.

MARSDEN, T. and WRIGLEY, N. 1995. 'Regulation, Retailing and Consumption'. *Environment and Planning A* 27(12): 1180–92.

MARSDEN, T., HARRISON, M. and FLYNN, A. 1998. 'Creating Competitive

Space: Exploring the Social and Political Maintenance of Retail Power'. *Environment and Planning A* (forthcoming).

MARSHALL, D. 1993. 'Appropriate Meal Occasions: Understanding Conventions and Exploring Situational Influences on Food Choice'. *International Review of Retail, Distribution and Consumer Resarch* 3(3):279–301.

MARSHALL, D. (ed.) 1995. 'Eating at Home: Meals and Food Choice' in *Food Choice and the Consumer*. London: Blackie Academic.

MARSHALL, D., KEMMER, D. and ANDERSON, A. S. 1996. 'Negotiation in the Shopping Aisle: Pre-marital Food Shopping Experiences'. Working paper presented at Joint Annual Meetings of the Association for the Study of Food and Society, Agriculture, Food, and Human Values Society, and the International Food Choice Conference. Missouri: St Louis University.

MARTENS, L. and WARDE, A. 1995. 'The Future of Eating Out'. Paper to ESRC/Flora Nation's Diet Conference, London, November.

MARTIN, W. and PORTER, D. 1985. 'Testing for Changes in the Structure of the Demand for Meat in Australia'. *Australian Journal of Agricultural Economics* 16:16–31.

MCCANN, B., WARNICK, G. and KNOPP, R. 1990. 'Changes in Plasma Lipids and Dietary Intake Accompanying Shifts in Perceived Workload and Stress'. *Psychosomatic Medicine* 52:97–108.

MCCORRISTON, S. and SHELDON, I. M. 1997. 'Vertical Restraints and Competition Policy in the US and UK Food Marketing Systems'. *Agribusiness* 13:237–52.

MCINTOSH, W. A. 1996. *Sociologies of Food and Nutrition.* London: Plenum Press.

MCINTOSH, W. A. and ZEY, M. 1989. 'Women as Gatekeepers of Food Consumption: A Sociological Critique'. *Food and Foodways* 34(4): 317–32.

MCKEE, F. 1997. 'The Popularisation of Milk as a Beverage During the 1930s', in D. F. Smith 1997b, pp. 123–42.

MCKEIGUE, P. M. and CHATURVEDI, N. 1996. 'Epidemiology and Control of Cardiovascular Disease in South Asians and Afro-Caribbeans', in W. Ahmad, T. Sheldon and O. Stuart (eds), *Ethnicity and Health: Reviews of Literature and Guidance for Purchasers in the Areas of Cardiovascular Disease, Mental Health and Haemoglobinopathies.* CRD Report No. 5. York: University of York, NHS Centre for Reviews and Dissemination.

MCKENZIE, J. C. and YUDKIN, J. 1963. 'The Food we Fancy'. *New Scientist* 17:280–1.

MCKIE, L. J., WOOD, R. C. and GREGORY, S. 1993. 'Women Defining Health: Food, Diet and Body Image'. *Health Education Research* 8(1):35–41.

MCKINNON, A. C. 1989. *Physical Distribution Systems.* London: Routledge.

MCNAIR, D. M., LORR, N. and DROPPLEMAN, L. F. 1981. *Manual for the Profile of Mood States.* San Diego: Education and Industrial Testing Service.

MCRAE, S. 1987. 'The Allocation of Money in Cross-class Families'. *Sociological Review* 35(1):9–122.

MEAD, G. H. 1934. *Mind, Self and Society*. Chicago: University of Chicago Press.

MENNELL, S. 1985. *All Manners of Food: Eating and Taste in England and France from the Middle Ages to the Present*. Oxford: Blackwell.

MENNELL, S., MURCOTT, A. and VAN OTTERLOO, A. 1992. *The Sociology of Food: Eating, Diet and Culture*. London: Sage.

MERTON, R.K. 1987. 'The Focused Interview and Focus Groups: Continuities and Discontinuities'. *Public Opinion Quarterly* 51: 550–6.

MERTON, R.K. and KENDALL, P. L. 1946. 'The Focused Interview'. *American Journal of Sociology* 51; 541–57.

MESSER, E. (1984) 'Anthropological Perspectives on Diet'. *Annual Review of Anthropology* 13:205–49.

M'GONIGLE, G. C. M. and KIRBY, J. 1936. *Poverty and Public Health*. London: Gollancz.

MICHAUD, C., KAHN, J. P., MUSSE, N., BURLET, C., NICOLES, J. P. *et al.* 1990. 'Relationships Between a Critical Life Event and Eating Behaviour in High-school Students'. *Stress Medicine* 6:57–64.

MIKULA, G. 1989. 'Influencing Food Preferences of Children by "If–then" Type Instruction', *European Journal of Social Psychology*, 19: 225–41.

MILES, R. 1982. *Racism and Migrant Labour*. London: Routledge & Kegan Paul.

MILLER, D. (ed.) 1995. *Acknowledging Consumption*. London: Routledge.

MILLER, D. and REILLY, J. 1995. *Food Scares in the Media*. Glasgow: Glasgow University Media Group.

MINISTRY OF AGRICULTURE, FISHERIES AND FOOD (MAFF) 1991. *Household Food Consumption and Expenditure 1990*. London: HMSO.

MINISTRY OF AGRICULTURE, FISHERIES AND FOOD (MAFF) 1995. *National Food Survey 1994*. London: HMSO.

MINISTRY OF HEALTH 1932. *Certain Recommendations of the Advisory Committee on Nutrition*. London: HMSO.

MINTEL 1990. *Eggs. Market Intelligence*. London: Mintel.

MINTZ, S. 1985. *Sweetness and Power: the Place of Sugar in Modern History*. New York: Viking.

MINTZ, S. 1992. 'A taste of history'. *The Times Higher Education Supplement* 8 May.

MMC 1981. *Discounts to Retailers*. Monopolies and Mergers Commission, HC311, London: HMSO.

MORGAN, D. 1991. 'Ideologies of Marriage and Family Life', in D. Clark (ed.) 1991.

MOIR, C. 1990. 'Competition in the UK Grocery Trades', in C. Moir and J. A. Dawson (eds), *Competition and Markets: Essays in Honour of Margaret Hall*. London: Macmillan, pp. 91–1181.

MOROKVASIC, M. 1993. ' "In and Out" of the Labour Market: Immigrant and Minority Women in Europe'. *New Community* 19(3):459–83.

MORRIS, L. 1990. *The Workings of the Household*. Oxford: Polity Press.

MORRISON, M. 1996a. 'A Curriculum for Food: Places Left at the School Table'. *The Curriculum Journal* 7(1):51–73.

MORRISON, M. 1996b. 'Cross-cultural Perspectives on Eating: a Hidden Curriculum for Food', in R. Chawla-Duggan and C. Pole (eds), *Reshaping Education in the 1990s: Perspectives on Primary Schooling*. Lewes: Falmer Press.

MOSCHINI, G. and MEILKE, K. D. 1989. 'Modeling the Pattern of Structural Change in US Meat Demand'. *American Journal of Agricultural Economics* 71:255–61.

MURCOTT, A. 1982. 'On the Social Significance of the Cooked Dinner in South Wales'. *Social Science Information* 21(4/5):677–96.

MURCOTT, A. 1983a. 'Its a Pleasure to Cook for Him: Food, Meal Times and Gender in South Wales Households', in E. Gamarnikow, D. Morgan, J. Purvis and D. Taylorson (eds), *The Public and the Private*. London: Heinemann.

MURCOTT, A. 1983b. 'Cooking and the Cooked: a Note on the Domestic Preparation of Meals', in A. Murcott (ed.), *The Sociology of Food and Eating*. Aldershot: Gower.

MURCOTT, A. 1986. 'Opening the "Black Box"; Food, Eating and Household Relationships'. *Sosioaaliliaaketieteellinen Aikakauslehti* 23 (Vuosikerta 2):85–92.

MURCOTT, A. 1988. 'Sociological and Social Anthropological Approaches to Food and Eating'. *World Review of Nutrition and Dietetics* 55:1–40.

MURCOTT, A. 1995. 'Social Science, Food and Eating: Opportunities for Multi-Disciplinary Research', in E. Feichtinger and B. Köhler (eds), *Current Research into Eating Practices: Contributions of Social Sciences* (Proceedings of the European Interdisciplinary Meeting). Frankfurt am Main: AGEV Publication Series, Vol. 10.

MURCOTT, A. 1996. 'Food as an Expression of National Identity', in S. Gustavsson and L. Lewin (eds), *The Future of the Nation State: Essays on Cultural Pluralism and Political Integration*. Stockholm: Nerenius & Santérus.

MURCOTT, A. 1997. 'Family Meals in Britain: a Thing of the Past?', in A. P. Caplan (ed.) 1997.

MURCOTT, A. forthcoming. ' "The Nation's Diet" and the Policy Contexts', in J. Germov and L. Wiliams. (eds), *The Social Appetite*. Sydney: Oxford University Press.

NASSER, M. 1988. 'Culture and Weight Consciousness', *The Journal of Psychosomatic Research* 32(6):573–7.

NATIONAL CHILDREN'S HOME 1991 *Poverty and Nutritional Survey*. London: National Children's Home.

NATIONAL CONSUMER COUNCIL 1988. *Consumers and the Common Agricultural Policy*. London: HMSO.

NATIONAL CURRICULUM COUNCIL 1990b. *Curriculum Guidance 5, Health Education*. York: NCC.

NEWMAN, G. 1924. *Public Education in Health*. London: HMSO.

NEWMAN, G 1931. *On the State of Public Health 1930*. London: HMSO.

NEWMAN, J. and TAYLOR, A. 1992. 'Effect of a Means–end Contingency on Young Children's Food Preferences', *Journal of Experimental Child Psychology*, 64: 200–16.

NIAURA, R., HERBERT, P. N., SARITELLI, A. L., GOLDSTEIN, M. G., FLYNN, M. *et al.* 1991. 'Lipid and Lipoprotein responses to Episodic Occupational and Academic Stress'. *Archives of Internal Medicine* 151:2172–9.

NICOLAAS, G. 1995. *Cooking Attitudes and Behaviour*. London: HMSO.

NISBETT, R. E. and WILSON, T. D. 1977. 'Telling More than we can Know: Verbal Reports on Mental Processes', *Psychological Review*, 8: 231–59.

NORMAN, P. and CONNER, M. 1996. 'The Role of Social Cognition Models in Predicting Health Behaviours', in M. Conner and P. Norman (eds) 1996.

NUTRITION BULLETIN 1947a. 1(1).

NUTRITION BULLETIN 1947b. 1(4).

O'DONNELL, L. *et al.* 1987. 'Plasma Catecholamines and Lipoproteins in Chronic Psychological Stress'. *Journal of the Royal Society of Medicine* 80:339–42.

OFFICE OF POPULATION CENSUSES AND SURVEYS (OPCS) 1991. 'Social Class Based on Occupation: Definitions in Terms of Standard Occupational Classification (SOC) Unit Groups and Employment Status', in *1991 Census User Guide*, 44. London: Office of Population Censuses and Surveys.

OFFICE OF POPULATION CENSUSES AND SURVEYS (OPCS) 1995. *General Household Survey April 1993–March 1994*. London: HMSO.

OFT 1985. *Competition and Retailing*. Office of Fair Trading, Field House, Bream Buildings, London EC4 1PR.

OLSON, J. M. and ZANNA, M. P. 1993. Attitudes and Attitude Change'. *Annual Review of Psychology* 44:117–54.

OMAR, O. E. 1995. 'Retail Influence on Food Technology and Innovation'. *International Journal of Retail and Distribution Management* 23(3):11–16.

PAHL, J. 1983. 'The Allocation of Money and the Structuring of Inequality within Marriage'. *Sociological Review* 31(2):237–62.

PAHL, J. 1990. 'Household Spending, Personal Spending and the Control of Money in Marriage'. *Sociology* 24(1):119–38.

PAHL, R. 1984. *Division of Labour*. Oxford: Blackwell.

PAISLEY, C. M. and SPARKS, P. forthcoming. 'Expectations of Reducing Fat Intake: the Role of Perceived Need with the Theory of Planned Behaviour'. *Psychology and Health*.

PAPANEK, H. 1990. 'To Each Less Than She Needs; From Each More Than She Can Do: Allocations, Entitlements and Value', in I. Tinker (ed.), *Persistent Inequalities*. Oxford: Oxford University Press.

PARKER, N. (ed.) 1988. *Charities and Broadcasting*. London, Directory of Social Change.

PARKER, D., MANSTEAD, A. S. R. and STRADLING, S. G. 1995. 'Extending the Theory of Planned Behaviour: the Role of Personal Norm. *British Journal of Social Psychology* 34:127–37.

PEAK, H. 1955. 'Attitude and Motivation', in M. R. Jones (ed.), *Nebraska*

Symposium on Motivation Vol. 3. Lincoln: University of Nebraska Press.

PETERSON, P. E., JEFFREY, D. B., BRIDGEWATER, C. A. and DAWSON, B. 1984. 'How Pronutrition Television Programming Affects Children's Dietary Habits', *Developmental Psychology*, 2: 55–63.

PETTY, C. 1987. 'The Impact of the Newer Knowledge of Nutrition: Nutrition Science and Nutrition Policy, 1900–1939.' Unpublished PhD thesis, London University.

PETTY, C. 1989. 'Primary Research and Public Health: the Prioritisation of Nutrition Research in Inter-war Britain', in J. Austoker and L. Bryder, *Historical Perspectives on the Role of the MRC*. Oxford: Oxford University Press.

PETTY, R. E. and KROSNICK, J. A. (eds) 1995. *Attitude Strength: Antecedents and Consequences*. Hillsdale, NJ: Erlbaum.

PICKARD, D. and CORI, R. 1964. 'The Role of the Sociologist in Changes in Food Choice', in J. Yudkin and J. C. McKenzie 1964.

PILL, R. 1983. 'An Apple a Day. Some Reflections on Working-class Mothers' Views on Food and Health', in A. Murcott (ed.) 1983b.

PILL, R. and PARRY, O. 1989. 'Making Changes – Women, Food and Families'. *Health Education Journal* 44(3):51–4.

PILLOW, D. R., ZAUTRA, A. J. and SANDLER, I. 1996. 'Major Life Events and Minor Stressors: Identifying Mediational Links in the Stress Process'. *Journal of Personality and Social Psychology* 70:381–94.

PITT-RIVERS, J. 1977. 'The Law of Hospitality', in J. Pitt-Rivers (ed) *The Fate of Shechem*. Cambridge: Cambridge University Press.

PLINER, P. 1982. 'The Effects of Mere Exposure on Liking for Edible Substances'. *Appetite*. 3: 283–90.

PLINER, P. and HOBDEN, K. 1992. 'Development of a Scale to Measure the Trait of Food Neophobia in Humans.' *Appetite* 19:105–20.

POLEGATO, R and ZAICHKOWSKY, J. L. 1994. 'Family Food Shopping: Strategies Used by Husbands and Wives'. *The Journal of Consumer Affairs* 28(2):278–99.

POLIVY, J., HERMAN, C. P. and MCFARLANE, T. 1994. 'Effects of Anxiety on Eating: Does Palatability Moderate Distress-induced Over-eating in Dieters?' *Journal of Abnormal Psychology* 103:505–10.

POLLAK, R. A. 1978. 'Endogenous Tastes in Demand and Welfare Analysis'. *Papers and Proceedings of the American Economics Association* 68:374–9.

POLLARD, T., STEPTOE, A., CANAAN, L., DAVIES, G. J. and WARDLE, J. 1995. 'The Effects of Academic Examination Stress on Eating Behavior and Blood Lipid Levels'. *International Journal of Behavioral Medicine* 2:299–320.

PRÄTTÄLÄ, R., EKSTRÖM, M., HOLM, L. and KJAEARNES, U. (eds) 1991. *Palatable Worlds: Sociocultural Food Studies*. Oslo: Solum.

PROCHASKA, J. O. and DICLEMENTE, C. C. 1984. *The Transtheoretical Approach: Crossing Traditional Boundaries of Therapy*. Homewood, IL: Dow Jones Irwin.

PROCHASKA, J. O., DICLEMENTE C. C. and NORCROSS, J. C. 1992. 'In search of how people change: applications to addictive behaviours'. *American Psychologist* 47, 1102–1114

PURVIS, J. 1985. 'Domestic Subjects since 1870', in I. Goodson (ed.), *Social Histories of the Secondary Curriculum*. Lewes: Falmer Press.

QUEEN ELIZABETH COLLEGE 1960. *Annual Report 1959–60*. London: QEC.

RAUDENBUSH, B., VAN DEN KLAAUW, N. J. and FRANK, R. A. 1995. 'The Contribution of Psychological and Sensory Factors to Food Preference Patterns as Measured by the Food Attitudes Survey (FAS)'. *Appetite* 25:1–15.

REYNOLDS, J. 1997. 'Retailing in Computer-mediated Environments: Electronic Commerse across Europe'. *International Journal of Retail and Distribution Management* 25(1):29–37.

RICHARDS, J. and MACNEARY, A. 1991. 'A City View of Retailing: Challenge and Opportunity in the Nineties', in A. Treadgold (ed.), *The City View of Retailing*. Harlow: Longman.

RICHARD, R., VAN DER PLIGT, J. and DE VRIES, N. 1995. 'Anticipated Affective Reactions and Prevention of AIDS'. *British Journal of Social Psychology* 34:9–21.

RICHARD, R., VAN DER PLIGT, J. and DE VRIES, N. 1996. 'Anticipated Affect and Behavioral Choice'. *Basic and Applied Social Psychology* 18:111–29.

RIMM, I. J. and RIMM, A. A. 1974. 'Association Between Socioeconomic Status and Obesity in 59,556 Women'. *Preventive Medicine* 3:543–72.

RIORDAN, M., IWATA, B. A., FINNEY, J. W., WOHL, M. K. and STANLEY, A. E. 1984. 'Behavioral Assessment of and Treatment of Chronic Food Refusal in Handicapped Children.' *Journal of Applied Behavior Analysis*, 1: 327–41.

RITSON, C. and HUTCHINS, R. 1995. 'Supply and Food Availability', in D. Marshall (ed.), *Food Choice and the Consumer*. Glasgow: Chapman & Hall.

RIZVI, N. 1991. 'Socio-economic and Cultural Factors Affecting Inter-household and Intra-household Food Distribution in Rural and Urban Bangladesh', in A. Sharman, J. Theophano, K. Curtis and E. Messer (eds), *Diet and Domestic Life in Society*. Philadelphia: Temple University Press.

RODMELL, S. and WATTS, A. (eds) 1986. *The Politics of Health Education: Raising the Issues*. London: Routledge & Kegan Paul.

ROGERS, P. J. and BLUNDELL, J. E. 1990. 'Psychological Bases of Food Choice' in D. Ashwell (ed.), *Why We Eat What We Eat*, Proceedings of the Twelfth British Nutrition Foundation Annual Conference, London: The British Nutrition Foundation, pp. 31–40.

ROSCH, P. 1995. 'The Stress-food-mood Connection: Are There Stress-reducing Foods and Diets?'. *Stress Medicine* 11:1–6.

ROTHA, P. 1973. *Documentary Diary: an Informal History of the British Documentary Film, 1928–1939*. London: Secker & Warburg.

ROYAL SOCIETY OF LONDON 1985. *The Public Understanding of Science*. London: Royal Society.

ROYAL TOWN PLANNING INSTITUTE 1988. *Planning for Shopping in the 21st Century: a Report of the Retail Planning Working Party*. London: RTPI.

ROZIN, P. 1982. 'Human Food Selection: the Interaction of Biology, Culture and Individual Experience' in L. M. Barker (ed.) *The Psychobiology of Human Food Selection*. Chichester: Wiley, Ch. 13.

ROZIN, P. 1990. 'Acquisition of Stable Food Preferences,' *Nutrition Reviews*, 4: 106–13.

ROZIN, P. 1990. 'The Importance of Social Factors in Understanding the Acquisition of Food Habits', in E. D. Capaldi and T. L. Powley (eds), *Taste, experience and feeding*. Washington: American Psychological Association.

ROZIN, P and VOLLMECKE, T. 1986. 'Food Likes and Dislikes'. *Annual Review of Nutrition* 6:433–56.

SAIFULLAH-KHAN, V. 1976. 'Purdah in the British Situation', in D. L. Barker and S. Allen (eds), *Dependence and Exploitation in Work and Marriage*. London: Longman.

SAYER, A. and WALKER, R. 1992. *The New Social Economy: Reworking the Division of Labour*. Oxford: Blackwell.

SCHELLING, T. C. 1992. 'Self-command: A New Discipline', in G. Lowenstein and J. Elster (eds), *Choice Over Time*. New York: Russell Sage Foundation.

SCHLUNDT, D. G., VIRTS, K. I., SBROCCO, T. and POPE-CORDLE, J. 1993. 'A Sequential Behavioral Analysis of Craving Sweets in Obese Women'. *Addictive Behaviors* 18:67–80.

SCHNEIDER, D. J. 1991. 'Social Cognition'. *Annual Review of Psychology* 42:527–61.

SCHUMAN, H and JOHNSON, M. P. 1976. 'Attitudes and Behavior'. *Annual Review of Sociology* 2:161–207.

SCHUTZ, A. 1970. *On Phenomenology and Social Relations: Selected Writings*, H. R. Wagner (ed.). Chicago: University of Chicago Press.

SCHUTZ, A. 1973. 'Choosing Among Projects of Action', in *Collected Papers*, vol. 1, M. Natanson (ed.). The Hague: Martinus Nijhoff.

SCOTTISH OFFICE 1994. *The Scottish Diet: Report of a Working Party to the Chief Medical Officer for Scotland*. Edinburgh: The Scottish Office Home and Health Department, revised edn.

SELF, P and STORING, H. 1962. *The State and the Farmer*. London: Allen & Unwin.

SEN, A. K. 1990. 'Gender and Cooperative Conflicts', in I. Tinker (ed.), *Persistent Inequalities*. Oxford: Oxford University Press.

SENKER, J. 1986. 'Technological Cooperation between Manufacturers and Retailers to meet Market Demand'. *Food Marketing* 2(3):88–100.

SHARMAN, A., THEOPHANO, J., CURTIS, K. and MESSER, E. (eds) 1991. *Diet and Domestic Life in Society*. Philadelphia: Temple University Press.

SHAW, S. A., DAWSON, J. A. and BLAIR, L. M. A. 1992. 'The Sourcing of Retailer Brand Food Products by a UK Retailer'. *Journal of Marketing Management* 8:127–46.

SHAW, S. A., NISBET, D. J. and DAWSON, J. A. 1989. 'Economies of Scale in UK Supermarkets: Some Preliminary Findings'. *International Journal of Retailing* 4(5):12–26.

359

SHEPHERD, R. 1989. 'Factors Influencing Food Preferences and Choice', in R. Shepherd (ed.), *Handbook of the Psychophysiology of Human Eating.* Chichester: Wiley.

SHEPHERD, R. and STOCKLEY, L. 1985. 'Nutrition Knowledge, Attitudes and Fat Consumption'. *Journal of the American Dietetic Association* 87:615–19.

SHEPPARD, B. H., HARTWICK, J. and WARSHAW, P. R. 1988. 'The Theory of Reasoned Action: a Meta-analysis of Past Research with Recommendations for Modifications and Future Research'. *Journal of Consumer Research* 15:325–39.

SIDMAN, M. 1960. *Tactics of Scientific Research.* New York: Basic Books.

SIEGAL, L. J. 1982. 'Classical and Operant Procedures in the Treatment of a Case of Food Aversion in a Young Child.' *Journal of Clinical Child Psychology*, 1: 167–72.

SIMOONS, F. J. 1969. 'Primary Adult Lactose Intolerance and the Milking Habit: a Problem in Biological and Cultural Interrelations I: Review of the Medical Research.' *American Journal of Digestive Disorders*, 1: 819–36.

SIMOONS, F. J. 1970. 'Primary Adult Lactose Intolerence and the Milking Habit: a Problem in Biological and Cultural Interrelations II: A Cultural–Historical Hypothesis.' *The American Journal of Digestive Diseases*, 1: 695–710.

SINCLAIR, I., PARKER, R., LEAT, D. and WILLIAMS, J. 1990. *The Kaleidoscope of Care: a Review of Research on Welfare Provision for Elderly People.* London: HMSO.

SKINNER, B. F. 1969. *Contingencies of Reinforcement.* Englewood Cliffs, NJ: Prentice–Hall, Inc.

SMITH, A. 1904. *An Inquiry into the Nature and Causes of the Wealth of Nations.* London: Methuen.

SMITH, D. F. 1987. 'Nutrition in Britain in the Twentieth Century'. Unpublished PhD thesis, Edinburgh University.

SMITH, D. F. 1992a. 'Nutrition Science and Nutrition Politics during the Second World War'. Typescript of paper prepared for Historians and Nutritionists Seminar, King's College, London, 8 July 1992.

SMITH, D. F. 1992b. 'The Food Leaders Scheme, 1942–52', in E. M. Prisk (ed.), *The Urban Context.* Liverpool: John Moores University.

SMITH, D. F. 1995. 'The Social Construction of Dietary Standards: The British Medical Association – Ministry of Health Advisory Committee on Nutrition Report of 1934', in D. Maurer and J. Sobal (eds), *Eating Agendas.* New York: Aldine de Gruyter, pp. 279–304.

SMITH, D. F. (ed.) 1997a. *Nutrition in Britain, Science, Scientists and Politics in the Twentieth Century.* London: Routledge.

SMITH, D. F. 1997b. 'Nutrition Science and the Two World Wars', in D. F. Smith (ed.), *Nutrition in Britain, Science, Scientists and Politics in the Twentieth Century.* London: Routledge.

SMITH, D. F. and NICOLSON, M. 1989. 'The "Glasgow School" of Paton, Findlay and Cathcart: Conservative Thought in Chemical Physiology, Nutrition and Public Health'. *Social Studies in Science* 19:195–238.

SMITH, D. L. G. and SPARKS, L. 1993. 'The Transformation of Physical Distribution in Retailing: the Example of Tesco plc'. *International Review of Retail, Distribution and Consumer Research* 3:35–64.

SMITH, M. J. 1990. *The Politics of Agricultural Support in Britain.* Aldershot: Dartmouth.

SMITH, P. 1991. 'Ethnic Minorities in Scotland'. Scottish Office Central Research Unit Papers. Edinburgh: The Scottish Office.

SMITH, V. H. and GOODWIN, B. K. 1992. 'Consumer Demand for Speciality Beef Products'. *Review of Agricultural Economics* 14:289–97.

SOBAL, J. and STUNKARD, A. J. 1989. 'Socioeconomic Status and Obesity: a Review of the Literature'. *Psychological Bulletin* 105(2):260–75.

SOOMAN, A., MACINTYRE, S. and ANDERSON, A. 1993. 'Scotland's Health: a More Difficult Challenge for Some? The Price and Availability of Health Foods in Socially Contrasting Localities in the West of Scotland'. *Health Bulletin* 51:276–84.

SOUTHON, V. 1986. *Children in Care: Paying Their New Families.* London: DHSS.

SPARKS, L. 1994. 'Delivering Quality: the Role of Logistics in the Post-war Transformation of British Food Retailing', in G. Jones and N. J. Morgan (eds), *Adding Value: Brands and Marketing in Food and Drink.* London: Routledge, pp. 310–35.

SPARKS, L. 1996a. 'Challenge and Change: Shoprite and the Restructuring of Grocery Retailing in Scotland'. *Environment and Planning A,* 28: 261–84.

SPARKS, L. 1996b. 'Space Wars: Wm Low and the "auld enemy" '. *Environment and Planning A* 28:1465–84.

SPARKS, L. 1997. 'From Coca-colonization to Copy-cotting: the Cott Corporation and Retailer Brand Soft Drinks in the UK and the US'. *Agribusiness* 13:153–67.

SPARKS, P. 1994. 'Food Choice and Health: Applying, Assessing, and Extending the Theory of Planned Behaviour', in D. R. Rutter and L. Quine (eds), *Social Psychology and Health: European Perspectives.* Aldershot: Avebury.

SPARKS, P. and SHEPHERD, R. 1992. 'Self-identity and the Theory of Planned Behaviour: Assessing the Role of Identification with "Green Consumerism" '. *Social Psychology Quarterly* 55:388–99.

SPARKS, P., HEDDERLY, P. and SHEPHERD, R. 1992. 'An Investigation into the Relationship Between Perceived Control, Attitude Variability and the Consumption of Two Common Foods'. *European Journal of Social Psychology* 22:55–71.

SPENCER, C. 1990. 'All the Food Fit to Eat'. *Guardian* 4 August: 10.

SPRADLEY, J. P. 1979. *The Ethnographic Interview.* New York: Holt Rinehart & Winston.

STANWAY, P. and STANWAY, A. 1978. *Breast is Best: a Commonsense Approach to Breast Feeding.* London: Pan.

STARK, L., COLLINS, F., OSNES, P. and STOKES, T. 1986. 'Using Reinforcement and Cueing to Increase Healthy Snack Food Choices in Preschoolers.' *Journal of Applied Behavior Analysis,* 1: 367–79.

STEINER, J. E. 1977. 'Facial Expressions of the Neonate Infant Indicating the Hedonics of Food Related Chemical Stimuli' in J. M. Weiffenbach (ed.) *Taste and Development*, Bethesda, MD: US Department of Health, Education and Welfare.

STEPTOE, A. 1991. 'The Links Between Stress and Illness'. *Journal of Psychosomatic Research* 35:633–44.

STEPTOE, A. forthcoming. 'Psychophysiological Bases of Disease', in M. Johnston and D. Johnston (eds), *Comprehensive Clinical Psychology, Vol. 8: Health Psychology*. New York: Elsevier.

STEPTOE, A. and WARDLE, J. (eds) 1994. *Psychosocial Processes and Health: A Reader*. Cambridge: Cambridge University Press.

STEPTOE, A., POLLARD, T. M. and WARDLE, J. 1995. 'The Development of a Measure of the Motives Underlying the Selection of Food: the Food Choice Questionnaire'. *Appetite* 25:267–84.

STEPTOE, A., WARDLE, J., POLLARD, T. M., CANAAN, L. and DAVIES, G. J. 1996. 'Stress, Social Support and Health-related Behavior: a Study of Smoking, Alcohol Consumption and Physical Exercise'. *Journal of Psychosomatic Resarch* 41:171–80.

STEWART, D. and SHAMDASANI, P. 1990. *Focus Groups; Theory and Practice*. Newbury Park, CA: Sage.

STIGLER, G. J. 1954. 'The Early History of Empirical Studies of Consumer Behavior'. *Journal of Political Economy* LXII(2):95–113.

STIGLER, G. and BECKER, G. 1977. 'De Gustibus non est Disputandum'. *American Economic Review* 67:76–90.

STITT, S. 1995. 'Schooling for Capitalism: Cooking and the National Curriculum'. Paper presented at the 4th International Multidisciplinary Conference on Food Choice, University of Birmingham, 24–26 April.

STITT, S. 1996. 'When Health Promotion Doesn't Work: Food Poverty in the UK'. Paper for the International Conference on Health Promotion and Nutrition, Wageningen, January.

STONE, A. A. and BROWNELL, K. D. 1994. 'The Stress-eating Paradox: Multiple Daily Measurements in Adult Males and Females'. *Psychology and Health* 9:435–6.

STONEMAN, Z. and BRODY, G. H. 1981. 'Peers as Mediators of Television Food Advertisements Aimed at Children.' *Developmental Psychology*, 1: 853–8.

STRAUGHAN, R. 1992. 'Freedom of Choice. Principles and Practice', in National Consumer Council (ed.), *Your Food: Whose Choice?* London: HMSO.

STUNKARD, A. J. 1988. 'Some Perspectives on Human Obesity: its Causes'. *Bulletin of the New York Academy of Medicine* 64:902–23.

STUNKARD, A. J., HARRIS, J. R., PEDERSEN, N. L. and McCLEARN, G. E. 1990. 'The Body Mass Index of Twins who Have Been Reared Apart'. *The New England Journal of Medicine* 322(21): 1483–7.

SUTTON, S. 1996. 'Can "Stages of Change" Provide Guidance in the Treatment of Addictions? A Critical Examination of Prochaska and DiClemente's model', in G. Edwards and C. Dare (eds), *Psychotherapy: Psychological Treatments and the Addictions*. Cambridge: Cambridge University Press.

TANSEY, G. and WORSLEY, T. 1995. *The Food System: a Guide.* London: Earthscan.

TEUTEBERG, H. J. (ed.) 1992. *European Food History: A Research Review.* Leicester: Leicester University Press.

The Times 1942. Special Article: Food and Food Values. From the Scientist to the Administrator. Nutrition as an Aid to Health'. *The Times* 28 August.

THOMAS, C. J. and BROMLEY, R. D. F. 1993. 'The Impact of Out-of-centre Retailing', in R. D. F. Bromley and D. J. Thomas (eds), *Retail Change: Contemporary Issues.* London: UCL Press, pp. 126–52.

THOMAS, R. L. 1987. *Applied Demand Analysis.* Harlow: Longman.

THOMAS, W. J. (ed.) 1972. *The Demand for Food. An Exercise in Household Budget Analysis.* Manchester: Manchester University Press.

THOMPSON, M. M., ZANNA, M. P. and GRIFFIN, D. W. 1995. 'Let's not be Indifferent about (Attitudinal) Ambivalence', in R. E. Petty and J. A. Krosnick (eds), *Attitude Strength: Antecedents and Consequences.* Hillsdale, NJ: Erlbaum.

THURMAN, W. N. 1987. 'The Poultry Sector: Demand Stability and Industry Structure'. *American Journal of Agricultural Economics* 69:30–7.

TIBBOTT, S. M. 1976. *Welsh Fare: a Selection of Traditional Recipes.* Cardiff: National Museum of Wales, Welsh Folk Museum.

TOMATIS, L. 1990. *Cancer: Causes, Occurrence and Control.* Oxford: Oxford University Press.

TOWLER, G. and SHEPHERD, R. 1991. 'Modification of Fishbein and Ajzen's Theory of Reasoned Action to Predict Chip Consumption'. *Food Quality and Preference* 3:37–45.

TOWNSEND, P. 1979. *Poverty.* Harmondsworth: Penguin Books.

TRAVERS, C. J. and COOPER, C. L. 1996. *Teachers Under Pressure.* London: Routledge.

TROVATO, F. and LAURIS, G. 1989. 'Marital Status and Mortality in Canada 1951–1981'. *Journal of Marriage and the Family* 51, Nov: 907—22.

TROWELL, H. 1975. 'Obesity in the Western World'. *Plant Foods for Man* 1:157–65.

TROYNA, B. 1983. 'Multicultural Education: Just Another Brick in the Wall'. *New Community* 10:424–8.

TROYNA, B. 1989. 'Beyond Multiculturalism', in B. Moon, P. Murphy and J. Raynor (eds), *Policies for the Curriculum.* London: Hodder & Stoughton.

TROYNA, B. and WILLIAMS, J. 1986. *Racism, Education and the State: the Racialisation of Education Policy.* Beckenham: Croom Helm.

TULL, G. and HAWKINS, T. 1992. *Marketing Research: Measurement and Method.* New York: Macmillan.

TUORILA, H. 1987. 'Selection of Milks with Varying Fat Contents and Related Overall Liking, Attitudes, Norms and Intentions'. *Appetite* 8:1–14.

TURNER, F. M. 1980. 'Public Science in Britain, 1880–1918'. *ISIS* 71: 589–608.

363

TYLER, P. and CUSHWAY, D. 1992. 'Stress, Coping and Mental Well-being in Hospital Nurses'. *Stress Medicine* 8:91–8.

VYGOTSKY, L. S. 1987. 'Thinking and Speech' in R. W. Rieber and A. S. Carlton (eds.), *The Collected Works of L. S. Vygotsky* Vol. 1, New York: Plenum, pp. 39–285. (Originally published in Russian 1934).

WALKER, C. and CANNON, G. 1984. *The Food Scandal.* London: Century Publishing.

WARD SCHOFIELD, J. 1993. 'Increasing the Generalisability of Qualitative Research', in M. Hammersley (ed.), *Social Research, Philosophy, Politics, and Practice.* London: Sage.

WARDE, A. 1996a. 'The Pleasures of Consumption: a Conceptual and Empirical Analysis'. Paper to European Sociological Association Symposium. 'The Sociology of Consumption', Tallinn, August.

WARDE, A. 1996b. 'Eating Out and Eating In: Households and Food Choice'. *Report to ESRC on Grant No. L209252044.* Swindon: ESRC.

WARDE, A. 1997. *Consumption, Food and Taste: Culinary Antinomies and Commodity Culture.* London: Sage.

WARDE, A., MARTENS, L. and OLSEN, W. 1997. 'The Pursuit of Variety: Status Competition and Dining Out'. Paper to European Sociological Association Conferences, Essex University, August.

WARDLE, J. 1987. 'Eating Style: a Validation Study of the Dutch Eating Behaviour Questionnaire in Normal Subjects and Women with Eating Disorders'. *Journal of Psychosomatic Research* 31:161–9.

WARDLE, J. and BEALES, S. 1988. 'Control and Loss of Control Over Eating: an Experimental Investigation'. *Journal of Abnormal Psychology* 97:35–40.

WARTIME NUTRITION BULLETIN 1941. 'Composition and Function of a Local CNC', No. 12.

WARTIME NUTRITION BULLETIN 1943. 'Editorial Note', No. 26.

WARTIME NUTRITION BULLETIN 1944. 'The Problem of "Food Advice" in Post-war Reconstruction', No. 32.

WARTIME NUTRITION BULLETIN 1945. What is Meant by "Social Nutrition"?', No. 34.

WEBER, M. 1947. *Theory of Social and Economic Organisation.* London: Collier-Macmillan.

WEBER, M. 1948. 'Class, Status and Party', in H. H. Gerth and C. W. Mills (eds), *From Max Weber: Essays in Sociology.* London: Routledge & Kegan Paul.

WEBSTER, C. 1982. 'Healthy or Hungry Thirties?' *History Workshop* 13:110–29.

WEIDNER, G., KOHLMANN, C.-W., DOTZAUER, E. and BURNS, L. R. forthcoming. 'The Effects of Academic Stress on Health Behaviors in Young Adults'. *Anxiety, Stress and Coping.*

WEINSTEIN, N. D. 1988. 'The Precaution Adoption Proceess'. *Health Psychology* 7:355–86.

WERBNER, P. 1990. *The Migration Process.* Oxford: Berg.

WESTLAKE, T. 1993. 'The Disadvantaged Consumer: Problems and Policies', in R. D. F. Bromley and C. J. Thomas (eds), *Retail Change: Contemporary Issues.* London: UCL Press, pp. 172–91.

WESTON, P. B., BARRETT, E. and JAMIESON, J. 1992. *Quest for Coherence: The Whole Curriculum*. Slough: NFER.

WHIT, W. C. 1995. *Food and Society: a Sociological Approach*. Dix Hills, NY: General Hall.

WHITE, A., FREETH, S. and O'BRIEN, M. 1992. *Infant Feeding 1990*. London: HMSO.

WILLETTS, A. 1997. 'Meat Eating and Vegetarianism in South-east London', in A. P. Caplan (ed.) 1997.

WILLETTS, A. and KEANE, A. 1995. 'You Eat What You Are'. *Guardian* 15 April:42–3.

WILLIAMS, J. 1996. 'Globalization in Rural Wales: Some Dietary Changes and Continuities on Welsh Farms'. London: Goldsmiths College Occasional Paper.

WILLIAMS, J. 1997. ' "We Never Eat Like This at Home": Food on Holiday in South-west Wales', in A. P. Caplan (ed.) 1997.

WILLIAMS, Lord 1965. *Digging for Britain*. London: Hutchinson.

WILLIAMS, R., BHOPAL, R. and HUNT, K. 1994. 'Coronary Risk in a British Punjabi Population: Comparative Profile of Non-biochemical Risk Factors'. *International Journal of Epidemiology* 23:28–37.

WILLIAMS, R. G. A., BUSH, H. M., ANDERSON, A. S., LEAN, M. E. J. and BRADBY, H. 1996. 'Dietary Change in South Asian and Italian Women in the West of Scotland'. *Report to ESRC on Grant No. X2092252023*. Swindon: ESRC.

WILSON, G. 1977. *Special Interests and Policy-Making: Agricultural Policy and Politics in Britain and the USA 1956–70*. Chichester: Wiley.

WILSON, G. 1989. 'Family Food Systems, Preventive Health and Dietary Change: A Policy to Increase the Health Divide'. *Journal of Social Policy* 18(2):167–85.

WOOD, R. 1994. 'Dining Out on Sociological Neglect'. *British Food Journal* 96(10):10–14.

WORLD HEALTH ORGANIZATION 1990. *Diet, Nutrition and the Prevention of Chronic Diseases*. Geneva: WHO.

WORSLEY, A. 1988. 'Co-habitation-gender Effects on Food Consumption'. *International Journal of Biosocial Research* 10(2):107–22.

WRIGLEY, N. 1991. 'Is the "Golden Age" of British Grocery Retailing at a Watershed?' *Environment and Planning A* 23: 1537–44.

WRIGLEY, N. 1992. 'Antitrust Regulation and the Restructuring of Grocery Retailing in Britain and the USA'. *Environment and Planning A* 24: 727–49.

WRIGLEY, N. 1993. 'Abuses of Market Power? Further Reflections on UK Food Retailing and the Regulatory State'. *Environmeot and Planning A* 25:1545–57.

WRIGLEY, N. 1994. 'After the Store Wars? Towards a New Era of Retail Competition?' *Journal of Retail and Consumer Services* 1:5–20.

WRIGLEY, N. 1996. 'Sunk Costs and Corporate Restructuring: British Food Retailing and the Property Crisis', in N. Wrigley and M. S. Lowe (eds), *Retailing, Consumption and Capital: Towards the New Retail Geography*. Harlow: Longman, pp. 116–36.

WRIGLEY, N. 1997a. 'Exporting the British Model of Food Retailing to the US: Implications for the EU–US Food Systems Convergence Debate'. *Agribusiness* 13:137–52.

WRIGLEY, N. 1997b. 'British Food Retail Capital in the USA – Part 1: Sainsbury and the Shaw's experience'. *International Journal of Retail and Distribution Management* 25(1):7–21.

WRIGLEY, N. 1997c. 'British Food Retail Capital in the USA – Part 2; Giant Prospects?'. *International Journal of Retail and Distribution Management* 25 (2):48–58.

WRIGLEY, N. 1998a. 'Understanding Store Development Programmes in Post-property-crisis UK Food Retailing'. *Environment and Planning A* 30.

WYKE, S. and FORD, G. 1992. 'Competing Explanations for Associations Between Marital Status and Health', *Social Science and Medicine* 34(5):523–32.

WYNNE, B. 1996. 'Misunderstood Misunderstandings: Social Identities and Public Uptake of Science', in A. Irwin and B. Wynne (eds), *Misunderstanding Science? The Public Reconstruction of Science and Technology.* Cambridge: Cambridge University Press.

YANAGISAKO, S. J. 1979. 'Family and Household: the Analyses of Domestic Groups'. *Annual Review of Anthropology* 8:161–205

YOUNG, D. 1996. 'Changing Tastes and Endogenous Preferences: Some Issues in Modelling the Demand for Agricultural Products'. *European Review of Agricultural Economics* 23:281–300.

YOUNG, I. 1994. 'The Health Promoting School' in *Food for Children: Influencing Choice and Investing in Health.* London: The National Forum for Coronary Heart Disease Prevention.

YUDKIN, J. 1944a. 'The Nutritional Status of Cambridge Schoolchildren' *British Medical Journal* II:201–5.

YUDKIN, J. 1944b. 'Nutrition and Family Size'. *The Lancet* II:384–7.

YUDKIN, J. 1952. 'Nutrition', in T. Horder (ed.), *The British Encyclopaedia of Medical Practice: Medical Progress.* London: Butterworth.

YUDKIN, J. 1953a. 'Fighting Food Faddism'. *Nutrition, Dietetics, Catering* 7:186–90.

YUDKIN, J. 1953b. 'The Teaching of Nutrition'. *Proceedings of the Nutrition Society* 12:198–9.

YUDKIN, J. 1956. 'Man's Choice of Food'. *Lancet* i:645–9.

YUDKIN, J. 1958. *This Slimming Business.* London: MacGibbon & Kee.

YUDKIN, J. 1959. 'Aetiology of Cardiac Infarction'. *American Medical Association Archives of Internal Medicine* 104:681–3.

YUDKIN, J. 1964. 'Beware the Malnutrition of Affluence'. *New Scientist* 21: 273.

YUDKIN, J. and McKENZIE, J. C. 1964. 'Conspectus', in J. Yudkin and J. C. McKenzie (eds), *Changing Food Habits.* London: MacGibbon & Kee.

ZANNA, M. P. and REMPEL, J. K. 1988. 'Attitudes: a New Look at an Old Concept', in D. Bar-Tal and A. W. Kruglanski (eds), *The Social Psychology of Knowledge.* New York: Cambridge University Press.

ZWEININGER-BARGIELOWSKA, I. 1993. 'Bread rationing in Britain, July 1946–July 1948'. *Twentieth Century British History* 4:57–85.

Index of Authors

Index of Principal Topics

Learning and Information Services
University of Wales Institute, Cardiff
Colchester Avenue
Cardiff
CF3 7XR